Contemporary Understanding and Management of Renal Cortical Tumors

Guest Editor

PAUL RUSSO, MD, FACS

UROLOGIC CLINICS OF NORTH AMERICA

www.urologic.theclinics.com

November 2008 • Volume 35 • Number 4

SAUNDERS an imprint of ELSEVIER, Inc.

W.B. SAUNDERS COMPANY
A Division of Elsevier Inc.

1600 John F. Kennedy Blvd. ● Suite 1800 ● Philadelphia, PA 19103-2899

http://www.theclinics.com

UROLOGIC CLINICS OF NORTH AMERICA Volume 35, Number 4
November 2008 ISSN 0094-0143, ISBN-13: 978-1-4160-6367-4, ISBN-10: 1-4160-6367-6

Editor: Kerry Holland
Developmental Editor: Donald Mumford

Urologic Clinics of North America (ISSN 0094-0143) is published quarterly by Elsevier Inc., 360 Park Avenue South, New York, NY 10010-1710. Months of issue are February, May, August, and November. Business and Editorial Offices: 1600 John F. Kennedy Blvd., Suite 1800, Philadelphia, PA 19103-2899. Customer Service Office: 6277 Sea Harbor Drive, Orlando, FL 32887-4800. Periodicals postage paid at New York, NY and additional mailing offices. Subscription prices are $269.00 per year (US individuals), $429.00 per year (US institutions), $308.00 per year (Canadian individuals), $526.00 per year (Canadian institutions), $383.00 per year (foreign individuals), and $526.00 per year (foreign institutions). Foreign air speed delivery is included in all *Clinics* subscription prices. All prices are subject to change without notice. **POSTMASTER:** Send address changes to *Urologic Clinics of North America*, Elsevier Periodicals Customer Service, 11830 Westline Industrial Drive, St. Louis, MO 63146. Customer Service: 1-800-654-2452 (US). From outside the United States, call 1-314-453-7041. Fax: 1-314-453-5170. E-mail: JournalsCustomerServiceusa@elsevier.com (for print support) and JournalsOnlineSupport-usa@elsevier.com (for online support).

Reprints. For copies of 100 or more, of articles in this publication, please contact the Commercial Reprints Department, Elsevier Inc., 360 Park Avenue South, New York, New York 10010-1710. Tel.: 212-633-3813; Fax: 212-462-1935; E-mail: reprints@elsevier.com.

Urologic Clinics of North America is covered in MEDLINE/PubMed (*Index Medicus*), *Excerpta Medica, Current Contents/ Clinical Medicine, Science Citation Index,* and *ISI/BIOMED*.

Printed in the United States of America.

Contributors

GUEST EDITOR

PAUL RUSSO, MD, FACS
Attending Surgeon and Professor, Department
of Surgery, Urology Service, Weill Cornell
College of Medicine, Memorial Sloan Kettering
Cancer Center, New York, New York

AUTHORS

ARIADNE M. BACH, MD
Associate Professor, Department of Radiology,
Memorial Sloan Kettering Cancer Center,
Weill Medical College of Cornell University,
New York, New York

MICHAEL L. BLUTE, MD
Professor of Urology, Mayo Clinic, Rochester,
Minnesota

STEVEN C. CAMPBELL, MD, PhD
Professor of Surgery, Section of Urological
Oncology, Glickman Urological and Kidney
Institute, Cleveland Clinic Foundation,
Cleveland, Ohio

JONATHAN A. COLEMAN, MD
Assistant Professor, Department of Surgery/
Urology Division, Weill Cornell Medical
College, Memorial Sloan Kettering Cancer
Center, New York, New York

G. JOEL DeCASTRO, MD, MPH
Resident, Department of Urology, Columbia
University/New York Presbyterian Hospital,
New York, New York

CHAITANYA DIVGI, MD
Professor of Radiology, Division of Nuclear
Medicine and Clinical Molecular Imaging,
Department of Radiology, University of
Pennsylvania, Philadelphia, Pennsylvania

ANURADHA GOPALAN, MD
Instructor, Department of Pathology, Memorial
Sloan-Kettering Cancer Center, New York,
New York

HARRY W. HERR, MD
Department of Urology, Memorial
Sloan-Kettering Cancer Center, Weill Cornell
Medical College, New York, New York

WILLIAM HUANG, MD
Assistant Professor, Department of Urology,
New York University School of Medicine,
New York, New York

MICHAEL A. S. JEWETT, MD
Professor, Division of Urology, Department
of Surgical Oncology, Princess Margaret
Hospital and the University Health Network,
University of Toronto, Toronto, Ontario,
Canada

MICHAEL W. KATTAN, PhD
Chairman, Department of Quantitative Health
Sciences, Cleveland Clinic, Cleveland, Ohio

TOBIAS KLATTE, MD
Research Fellow in Urologic Oncology,
Department of Urology, David Geffen School
of Medicine, University of California–Los
Angeles, Los Angeles, California

GLENN S. KROOG, MD
Assistant Member, Genitourinary Oncology Service, Division of Solid Tumor Oncology, Department of Medicine, Memorial Sloan-Kettering Cancer Center, New York, New York

BRIAN R. LANE, MD, PhD
American Urologic Association Foundation Research Scholar, Glickman Urological and Kidney Institute, Cleveland Clinic, Cleveland, Ohio

BRADLEY C. LEIBOVICH, MD
Associate Professor of Urology, Mayo Clinic, Rochester, Minnesota

JOHN A. LIBERTINO, MD
Chairman, Department of Urology, Lahey Clinic, Burlington, Massachusetts

JAMES M. McKIERNAN, MD
Associate Professor, Department of Urology, Columbia University/New York Presbyterian Hospital, New York, New York

ROBERT J. MOTZER, MD
Member, Genitourinary Oncology Service, Division of Solid Tumor Oncology, Department of Medicine, Memorial Sloan-Kettering Cancer Center, New York, New York

CARVELL T. NGUYEN, MD, PhD
Resident, Glickman Urological & Kidney Institute, Cleveland Clinic Foundation, Cleveland, Ohio

ANDREW C. NOVICK, MD
Chairman, Glickman Urological & Kidney Institute, Cleveland Clinic Foundation, Cleveland, Ohio

MATTHEW FRANCIS O'BRIEN, MD
Fellow, Urological Oncology, Memorial Sloan Kettering Cancer Center, New York, New York

ALLAN J. PANTUCK, MD
Associate Professor of Urology, Department of Urology, David Geffen School of Medicine, University of California–Los Angeles, Los Angeles, California

RODOLFO PERINI, MD
Chief Resident, Division of Nuclear Medicine and Clinical Molecular Imaging, Department of Radiology, University of Pennsylvania, Philadelphia, Pennsylvania

DANIEL PRYMA, MD
Assistant Professor of Radiology, Division of Nuclear Medicine and Clinical Molecular Imaging, Department of Radiology, University of Pennsylvania, Philadelphia, Pennsylvania

PAUL RUSSO, MD, FACS
Attending Surgeon and Professor, Department of Surgery, Urology Service, Weill Cornell College of Medicine, Memorial Sloan Kettering Cancer Center, New York, New York

SATISH K. TICKOO, MD
Associate Attending Pathologist, Department of Pathology, Memorial Sloan-Kettering Cancer Center, New York, New York

CHAD WOTKOWICZ, MD
Urology Resident, Department of Urology, Lahey Clinic, Burlington, Massachusetts

MATTHEW F. WSZOLEK, MD
Urology Resident, Department of Urology, Lahey Clinic, Burlington, Massachusetts

JINGBO ZHANG, MD
Assistant Professor, Department of Radiology, Memorial Sloan Kettering Cancer Center, New York, New York

ALVARO ZUNIGA, MD
Fellow, UroOncology Fellowship Program, University of Toronto, Toronto, Ontario, Canada

Contents

> The modern era of renal surgery began on August 2, 1869 when the first planned nephrectomy on a living human being was performed. Eighteen years later in 1887, the first partial nephrectomy to remove a renal tumor was performed. Both total and partial nephrectomy have become the hallmark surgical procedures used today to treat renal tumors, and their conception and evolution represent two of the most important advances in medicine and surgery. Surgery for kidney cancer continues to evolve. This article traces the history of surgical management for renal tumors.

> Our better understanding of the morphologic spectrum of renal cortical tumors has resulted in a clinically more relevant classification of these tumor types. We now recognize that "granular cell" and "sarcomatoid" renal cell carcinoma are only nonspecific descriptors, and that such features are seen in a variety of types of renal tumors. The authors believe that the recently gained knowledge about molecular-driven antigen expression will play an important role in the characterization, development, and evaluation of targeted therapies in kidney cancer in the coming years.

> Hereditary and familial forms of kidney cancer are encountered routinely in urologic practice. Discoveries in the genetic and molecular biology of these diseases have had a critical impact on the understanding of kidney cancer pathogenesis in nearly all subtypes of renal cortical neoplasms and their clinical features. Developing knowledge in the field has helped formulate new diagnostic and molecular therapeutic strategies for patients who have kidney cancer. This article aims to familiarize the reader with the current understanding of identified syndromes, their biology, and approaches to treatment.

The last 10 years have witnessed a dramatic evolution in our understanding of renal cell carcinoma (RCC) biology, which has led to the development of novel medical therapies and revolutionized the approach to their clinical management. This review considers the genetic basis of RCC and the molecular mechanisms of the hypoxia-induced pathway, the mammalian target of rapamycin pathway, the extracellular signal-regulated kinase pathway, and the ubiquitin-proteasome pathway. All these molecular pathways are involved in RCC biology, tumorigenesis, and progression, and serve as the source of new rational treatment strategies based on the design of small molecule inhibitors directed against their targets.

The increasing incidence of renal cell carcinoma over the past 2 decades can be partly explained by the expanding use of abdominal imaging. As a result, the most incident renal cancers today are small, localized, and asymptomatic. However, the well-documented rise in *all* stages of RCC calls into question the nature of these asymptomatic lesions. The expected "screening effect" of detecting RCC when it is small and localized, with subsequent decreases in disease-specific mortality, has not been observed. Disease-specific mortality is actually rising, especially in African American patients. Effective interventions aimed at reducing obesity, hypertension, and smoking may help in reducing the incidence of RCC in the future.

Contemporary radiologic imaging has resulted in an increasing number of smaller renal cortical tumors being identified. The ability of imaging to classify these tumors is limited, although certain features may help classify the renal cortical neoplasm. The important role of radiologic imaging in tumor detection, characterization, staging, and follow-up of patients who have renal cortical tumors is reviewed in this article.

The recent identification of agents that have significantly influenced the therapy of clear cell renal carcinoma and the decreasing size of renal masses, usually detected serendipitously, have led to a resurgence in imaging for this condition. Although structural methods continue to be used routinely for identification of renal masses, functional and molecular techniques are showing considerable promise in their ability to characterize unique features of the renal cancer phenotype. This article discusses the evolving role of molecular imaging in the evaluation of renal cancer, including current and future applications.

Prognostic Models and Algorithms in Renal Cell Carcinoma   613

Brian R. Lane and Michael W. Kattan

Although surgical treatment is curative for localized renal cell carcinoma (RCC), 25% of patients present with locally advanced or disseminated disease, and disease will recur systemically in another 20% to 30% of those who have localized disease at presentation. Many clinical, histologic, and molecular factors have been identified that place patients who have localized RCC at greater risk for recurrence and those who have metastatic disease at risk for progression or death. This article reviews the major prognostic factors for RCC and the most commonly used algorithms developed for use before or after nephrectomy and before initiation of systemic therapy. These RCC nomograms allow more accurate counseling of patients regarding their likely clinical course and facilitate treatment planning.

Renal Tumor Natural History: the Rationale and Role for Active Surveillance   627

Michael A.S. Jewett and Alvaro Zuniga

Renal cell carcinoma (RCC) is the most common malignancy of the kidney. Despite widespread treatment at diagnosis, overall mortality rates associated with RCC have not decreased. Partly because of the more frequent use of abdominal imaging, diagnosis as an incidental finding has increased. The largest increase in incidence is in tumors smaller than 4 cm, termed small renal masses (SRMs). SRMs that are RCC may frequently be growth slowly and have a low risk of early progression. Initial active surveillance with delayed treatment for progression for selected patients should be considered. This should result in an overall decrease in treatment burden and cost saving.

The Medical and Oncological Rationale for Partial Nephrectomy for the Treatment of T1 Renal Cortical Tumors   635

Paul Russo and William Huang

This article presents the oncological and medical rationale for partial nephrectomy as the treatment of choice whenever possible for T1 renal tumors. The value of partial nephrectomy in the management of small renal cortical tumors is gaining wider recognition thanks to (1) enhanced understanding of the biology of renal cortical tumors; (2) better knowledge about tumor size and stage migration to small tumors at the time of presentation; (3) studies indicating the oncologic efficacy of kidney-sparing surgery, and (4) increasing awareness of the wide prevalence of chronic kidney disease. The overzealous use of radical nephrectomy for small renal tumors must now be considered detrimental to the long-term health and safety of the patient with a small renal cortical tumor.

Choice of Operation for Clinically Localized Renal Tumor   645

Carvell T. Nguyen, Steven C. Campbell, and Andrew C. Novick

The cornerstone of treatment for localized renal tumors is surgical excision, which until recently was accomplished primarily through radical nephrectomy. The last 2 decades have seen a rapid evolution in the surgical management of renal cell carcinoma, marked by the increased use of nephron-sparing surgery and the application of minimally invasive techniques. A plethora of surgical options now are available. This article discusses the optimal surgical approach to renal tumors in various clinical scenarios. In all these discussions we assume that a proactive approach to treatment is indicated and desired, recognizing that active surveillance is always an additional option to consider in certain subpopulations such as the elderly or infirm.

Surgical resection of renal cell carcinoma remains the mainstay for the management of patients who suffer from this disease. Five percent to 10% of renal cell carcinomas develop a tumor thrombus that propagates into the renal vein or the inferior vena cava. Radical nephrectomy and inferior vena cava thrombectomy can provide longstanding survival rates comparable to those for tumors confined to the renal parenchyma. In general the surgical approach is dictated by the cephalad extension of tumor thrombus. This article reviews the authors' experience with 243 patients who suffered from renal cell carcinoma with extension into the venous system with specific reference to the surgical techniques and the long-term outcomes.

Radical nephrectomy and regional lymphadenectomy have been the cornerstone of therapy for renal cell carcinoma for several decades; however, debate regarding the potential advantages of lymph node dissection for renal cell carcinoma continues. Currently, there are no definitive data indicating a survival advantage to lymphadenectomy, and systematic complete lymph node dissection adds time to the procedure and requires manipulation of the great vessels, which some surgeons may find challenging. This article examines the rationale for lymphadenectomy in the management of renal cell carcinoma and reviews the limited literature on the subject.

For patients with metastatic renal cancer, prognostic factors defined in systemic therapy clinical trials stratify patients into good, intermediate, and poor risk groups with median survival varying from 4 to 13 months. These same factors also stratify patients whose renal cancers were initially resected completely and who then developed subsequent metastatic disease. Metastasectomy performed in low-risk patients was significantly associated with enhanced survival when compared with low-risk patients not undergoing metastasectomy. Two randomized, prospective clinical trials demonstrated a modest survival advantage of approximately 6 months for patients undergoing cytoreductive nephrectomy followed by interferon alfa-2b. Once effective systemic agents are developed, both metastasectomy and cytoreductive nephrectomy will play greater roles in consolidating clinical responses.

Systemic Therapy for Metastatic Renal Cell Carcinoma   687

Glenn S. Kroog and Robert J. Motzer

Renal cell cancer (RCC) is the most common form of cancer of the kidney and accounts for approximately 44,000 cases per year in the United States. Historically, only immunotherapy showed activity in metastatic RCC. The improved survival and quality of life for patients with metastatic RCC over the last several years are direct results of advances made in understanding the development of RCC. Three targeted therapies—sunitinib, sorafenib, and temsirolimus—have been approved for use in the United States recently. Current research is aimed at developing new drugs and combining available drugs to improve upon the responses and survival seen with approved single agents.

GOAL STATEMENT

The goal of *Urologic Clinics of North America* is to keep practicing urologists and urology residents up to date with current clinical practice in urology by providing timely articles reviewing the state of the art in patient care.

ACCREDITATION

The *Urology Clinics of North America* is planned and implemented in accordance with the Essential Areas and Policies of the Accreditation Council for Continuing Medical Education (ACCME) through the joint sponsorship of the University of Virginia School of Medicine and Elsevier. The University of Virginia School of Medicine is accredited by the ACCME to provide continuing medical education for physicians.

The University of Virginia School of Medicine designates this educational activity for a maximum of *15 AMA PRA Category 1 Credits™*. Physicians should only claim credit commensurate with the extent of their participation in the activity.

The American Medical Association has determined that physicians not licensed in the US who participate in this CME activity are eligible for *15 AMA PRA Category 1 Credits™*.

Credit can be earned by reading the text material, taking the CME examination online at: http://www.theclinics.com/home/cme, and completing the evaluation. After taking the test, you will be required to review any and all incorrect answers. Following completion of the test and evaluation, your credit will be awarded and you may print your certificate.

FACULTY DISCLOSURE/CONFLICT OF INTEREST

The University of Virginia School of Medicine, as an ACCME accredited provider, endorses and strives to comply with the Accreditation Council for Continuing Medical Education (ACCME) Standards of Commercial Support, Commonwealth of Virginia statutes, University of Virginia policies and procedures, and associated federal and private regulations and guidelines on the need for disclosure and monitoring of proprietary and financial interests that may affect the scientific integrity and balance of content delivered in continuing medical education activities under our auspices.

The University of Virginia School of Medicine requires that all CME activities accredited through this institution be developed independently and be scientifically rigorous, balanced and objective in the presentation/discussion of its content, theories and practices.

All authors/editors participating in an accredited CME activity are expected to disclose to the readers relevant financial relationships with commercial entities occurring within the past 12 months (such as grants or research support, employee, consultant, stock holder, member of speakers bureau, etc.). The University of Virginia School of Medicine will employ appropriate mechanisms to resolve potential conflicts of interest to maintain the standards of fair and balanced education to the reader. Questions about specific strategies can be directed to the Office of Continuing Medical Education, University of Virginia School of Medicine, Charlottesville, Virginia.

The faculty and staff of the University of Virginia Office of Continuing Medical Education have no financial affiliations to disclose.

The authors/editors listed below have identified no professional/financial affiliations for themselves or their spouse/partner:
Ariadne M. Bach, MD; Michael L. Blute, MD; Jonathan Andrew Coleman, MD; Guarionex Joel DeCastro, MD, MPH; Chaitanya R. Divgi, MD; Anuradha Gopalan, MD; Harry W. Herr, MD; Kerry K. Holland (Acquisitions Editor); William C. Huang, MD; Michael A.S. Jewett, MD; Michael W. Kattan, PhD; Tobias Klatte, MD; Brian R. Lane, MD, PhD; Bradley C. Leibovich, MD; John A. Libertino, MD; Carvell T. Nguyen, MD, PhD; Andrew C. Novick, MD; Matthew Francis O'Brien, MD; Allan J. Pantuck, MD; Rodolfo Fleury Perini, MD; Daniel A. Pryma, MD; William Steers, MD (Test Author); Satish K. Tickoo, MD; Chad Wotkowicz, MD; Matthew F. Wszolek, MD; Jingbo Zhang, MD; and Alvaro Zuniga, MD.

The authors/editors listed below have identified the following professional or financial affiliations for themselves or their spouse/partner:
Steven C. Campbell, MD, PhD is an industry funded research/investigator for Pfizer and Novartis, serves on the Advisory Committee for Pfizer and Sanofi Aventis, and serves on the Speakers Bureau for Sanofi Aventis.
Glenn S. Kroog, MD serves on the Advisory Committee for Merck and Novartis, and owns stock in Merck and Pfizer.
James M. McKiernan, MD is a consultant for Sanofi Aventis.
Robert J. Motzer, MD is an industry funded research/investigator for Pfizer, Inc., Wyeth, Novartis, and Bayer/Onyx and serves on the Speakers Bureau for Bayer/Onyx.
Paul Russo, MD, FACS (Guest Editor) is a consultant for Wilex Ag.

Disclosure of Discussion of non-FDA approved uses for pharmaceutical products and/or medical devices:
The University of Virginia School of Medicine, as an ACCME provider, requires that all faculty presenters identify and disclose any "off label" uses for pharmaceutical and medical device products. The University of Virginia School of Medicine recommends that each physician fully review all the available data on new products or procedures prior to instituting them with patients.

TO ENROLL

To enroll in the *Urologic Clinics of North America* Continuing Medical Education program, call customer service at 1-800-654-2452 or visit us online at: http://www.theclinics.com/home/cme. The CME program is available to subscribers for an additional fee of $195.00.

Urologic Clinics of North America

RELATED INTEREST

Radiologic Clinics of North America, January 2008 (Vol. 46, No. 1)
Genitourinary Tract Imaging
Michael A. Blake, MRCPI, FFR(RCSI), FRCR and Mannudeep K. Kalra, MD
Guest Editors

THE CLINICS ARE NOW AVAILABLE ONLINE!

Access your subscription at:
www.theclinics.com

Preface

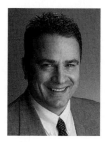

Paul Russo, MD, FACS
Guest Editor

In 2008 there will be an estimated 54,390 new cases of renal tumors and 13,010 deaths attributable to renal cancer in the United States. Compared with 1971, this represents a fivefold increase in the incidence and twofold increase in the mortality of renal cancer. Associated risk factors include hypertension, obesity, and African American race. Despite the abdominal imaging–related tumor size and stage migration observed over the past decade and increased surgical treatment for all renal tumors, particularly the smaller ones, epidemiologic evidence suggests an increase in all stages of renal cancer, including the advanced and metastatic cases. Approximately 30% to 40% of renal tumor patients either present with or later develop metastatic disease. This "treatment disconnect" may be a result of unaccounted-for etiologic factors increasing the incidence of all renal cortical tumors. The increased treatment and cure of small, incidentally discovered renal tumors, greater than 90% of which must be considered nonlethal in nature, does not seem to offset the increased mortality caused by the more advanced and metastatic tumors.

Over the last decade several factors working in parallel have changed our approach to the management of both clinically localized and advanced renal cortical tumors. The oncologic effectiveness of partial nephrectomy for tumors of 7 cm or less coupled with the medical benefits of renal functional preservation, which delays or prevents the onset of chronic kidney disease (CKD), has been clearly elucidated. For advanced disease, the enhanced understanding of the molecular mechanisms responsible for the development of malignant renal tumors has led to the development of systemic agents that have been highly effective in causing remission of metastatic disease and regression of primary tumors with prolonged survival achieved in patients formerly facing a grave prognosis. In this issue of the *Urologic Clinics of North America* numerous experts in this field present a contemporary understanding of the epidemiology, pathology, molecular biology, radiology, and clinical management of renal cortical tumors with an encouraging eye toward the future.

A historical view of kidney surgery reveals the dangers and high mortality rates associated with total nephrectomy in the latter years of the nineteenth century (>40%) and the beginning of the twentieth century (>20%) until the time of the urologist Edwin Beer in 1920 (<4%). In the first half of the twentieth century, patients were only diagnosed with large, symptomatic (palpable masses with hematuria and pain), and usually locally advanced renal tumors, which provided a surgical challenge to the urologists. At that time, incidentally detected renal tumors represented less than 5% of the total. Charles Robson's published experience with transthoracic radical nephrectomy (including ipsilateral adrenal, all perinephric soft tissues, and regional retroperitoneal lymph nodes) in 1963 provided the mainstay surgical approach to all renal tumors during the pre-CT era until the mid 1980s when elective kidney-sparing operations were first described. A perioperative mortality rate of 3% was further improved on as post–World War II methods of anesthesia, blood banking, and perioperative care were integrated into the surgical management of renal tumors.

The discovery and widespread use of the modern abdominal imaging techniques (CT, MRI, and abdominal ultrasound) over the last 2 decades changed the profile of the renal tumor patient

Urol Clin N Am 35 (2008) xiii–xvii
doi:10.1016/j.ucl.2008.07.016

urologic.theclinics.com

from one who had a massive, symptomatic tumor at presentation to the current patient who has a small, asymptomatic renal mass (<4 cm) incidentally discovered in 70% of the cases after evaluation of nonspecific abdominal and musculoskeletal pain or during unrelated cancer diagnosis and follow-up care. At the same time as this clinical size and stage migration was occurring, an enhanced understanding of the pathology of renal tumors was underway. Until the 1980s, renal cortical tumors were classified only by descriptive terms, such as clear, granular, papillary, sarcomatoid, and renal oncocytoma. The realization that the renal cortical tumors were, in fact, members of a complex family with unique pathologic appearances, cytogenetic and molecular defects, familial and hereditary syndromes, and variable metastatic potentials lead to the development of the current Heidelberg Classification of renal tumors in 1997. We now know that granular and sarcomatoid tumors are not specific histologic subtypes, whereas chromophobe, papillary, conventional clear cell, medullary, collecting duct, metanephric adenoma, and oncocytoma are. Approximately 90% of the renal tumors that are metastatic have the conventional clear cell histology.

Focused research into hereditary and familial tumor syndromes, which account for less than 5% of all renal cortical tumors, also provided molecular insight into the sporadic cases within each of the histologic subtypes. Investigators from the National Cancer Institute discovered that the tumor suppressor gene *VHL*, located at chromosome 3p25, could be inactivated by various mutations, loss of heterozygosity, hypermethylations, or alterations in VHL modifier genes, and was responsible for the von Hippel-Lindau syndrome. This autosomal dominant syndrome is characterized by retinal hemangiomas, conventional clear cell renal cell carcinoma, renal cysts, cerebellar and spinal hemangioblastomas, pheochromocytomas, endocrine pancreatic tumors, and epididymal cysts. The dysfunction of the VHL protein increases hypoxia-induced factor (HIF) 1 alpha resulting in a marked overexpression of vascular and endothelial growth factors and the hypervascular state observed in the VHL syndrome of tumors in general and its associated conventional clear cell carcinomas of the kidney. Loss of *VHL* gene function also occurs in at least 50% of sporadic conventional clear cell carcinomas. Similar intensive research into other hereditary renal tumor syndromes, including hereditary papillary RCC (cMet mutation at chromosome 7q34), hereditary leiomyomatosis syndrome and renal cell carcinoma (HLRCC, mutation in fumarate hydratase gene),

and Birt Hogge Dube syndrome of fibrofolliculomas, chromophobe and oncocytic predominant renal tumors, pneumothorax, and bronchiectasis (recently mapped to 17q12) has provided tremendous insight into the molecular mechanisms by which these tumors operate. Similar cytogenetic and molecular defects were observed in the histologic subtypes of the sporadic forms of renal cancer. The research and development of new systemic agents, tyrosine kinase and mTOR inhibitors, which specifically target pathways that stimulate renal tumor regulation and growth, allowed for clinical trials in metastatic renal cell carcinoma with marked improvement in response rates compared with traditional chemotherapy and cytokines. In addition, tumor-specific immunohistochemical stains and molecular probes can now precisely diagnose and subclassify renal tumors far better than traditional pathologic assessment.

Modern imaging with ultrasound, MRI, and contrast-enhanced CT provides clarity and precision for the diagnosis and extent of disease evaluation of patients who have renal masses. Ultrasound can be a highly useful adjunct in assessing cystic lesions and allowing for a preoperative correlate to intraoperative ultrasound, which is particularly useful when a partial nephrectomy for an endophytic tumor is planned. MRI is the method of choice for assessing the extent of renal vein and inferior vena cava extension, which is essential for assembling the proper surgical team and equipment for such major operations. Unfortunately, none of these modalities can distinguish with certainty a benign from malignant renal mass or define the histologic subtype. A new molecular imaging strategy, termed "immunoPET" scanning, is under active investigation and uses the cG250, whose target, CA9, is abundant in the malignant conventional clear cell carcinoma. cG250 is linked to iodine-124, which has a 4-day half-life and 23% positron emission, permitting adequate PET imaging. In a pilot study of 25 patients who had renal masses imaged before resection, the G250 scan accurately predicted the clear cell histology in 13 of 14 cases with only one false negative. This imaging approach is currently being evaluated in a large, multi-institutional national trial of 158 patients. If these initial results are confirmed, the implications for the use of this clear cell–specific immunoPET scan are broad and could include a rational approach to active surveillance, molecular determination of extent of disease, extension of kidney-sparing operations, and a molecular means of following the impact of novel local treatments (renal tumor ablations) and systemic agents (multitargeted kinases).

Surgeons managing renal cortical tumors confront two distinct patient groups. The first group, approximately 30% of the total, is the large, usually symptomatic, and locally advanced tumors often with regional adenopathy, adrenal invasion, and extension into the renal vein or inferior venacava. Most of these tumors have the conventional clear cell histology (90%) and differ little from the symptomatic tumors treated surgically by Robson after World War II. Approximately 4% to 10% of patients have renal cancers that involve the renal vein and inferior vena cava. In 1% of patients, the thrombus can extend into the right atrium of the heart. Surgical resection of these tumors can require complex cardiovascular techniques, with and without bypass, and can lead to safe resection with perioperative mortality rates of less than 10% depending on the extent of the thrombus. In the absence of nodal or distant metastases, 5-year survival rates of greater than 50% are possible. The incidence of occult positive lymph nodes in 3% to 5% of patients has lead many surgeons to recommend thorough retroperitoneal node dissections, especially for large T3 and T4 tumors, which may provide a therapeutic benefit in otherwise well patients who have limited metastatic disease and provide enhanced pathologic staging that can facilitate entry into adjuvant clinical trials.

Despite radical resection of these massive tumors, whether by open or laparoscopic surgical techniques, in conjunction with regional lymphadenectomy and adrenalectomy, progression to distant metastasis and death from disease occurs in approximately 30% of these patients. For patients presenting with or developing isolated metastatic disease with good performance status, metastasectomy has been associated with long-term survival. For patients who have diffuse metastatic disease and good performance status, cytoreductive nephrectomy may add several additional months of survival as opposed to cytokine therapy alone. The integration of surgical therapy for locally advanced and metastatic renal cancer in the new era of effective systemic multitargeted kinase inhibitors is currently under active investigation in neoadjuvant and adjuvant clinical trials.

The second group, approximately 70% of the total, is those who have small renal tumors (median tumor size <4cm, T1a), usually incidentally discovered in asymptomatic patients during ultrasound, CT, or MRI obtained for other reasons. A survival rate of 90% or greater, depending on the tumor histology, is expected whether partial or radical nephrectomy is performed. Approximately 20% of patients are found to have a benign lesion, such as angiomyolipoma, oncocytoma, metanephric adenoma, or hemorrhagic cyst. Although CT-guided percutaneous renal biopsy can easily be performed, the differentiation between a benign and malignant tumor and the determination of tumor histologic subtypes by current radiologic and biopsy techniques alone can be difficult (70% accurate) although the development of immunohistochemical and cytogenetic techniques may substantially improve this accuracy to 90%. Various prognostic models, nomograms, and algorithms have been constructed based on clinical and pathologic factors, such as tumor size, histologic subtype, stage, grade, performance status, and serum laboratory values to assist clinicians in counseling patients regarding their prognosis, designing appropriate follow-up exams and imaging, predicting renal functional outcomes, and assisting in clinical trial design.

Trends in surgical oncology toward organ preservation (ie, breast cancer, soft tissue sarcoma), wherein the oncologic efficacy of more limited operations was confirmed, lead to similar approaches for the management of renal tumors. Well-done studies first showed that for tumors of 4 cm or less, and later for tumors of 7 cm or less, elective partial nephrectomy (PN) was equally effective as radical nephrectomy (RN) in local tumor control and metastases-free survival. Reports comparing renal functional outcomes between patients undergoing PN or RN for small renal tumors revealed that closely matched patients undergoing RN were more likely to have proteinuria and an elevated serum creatinine (>2.0 mg/dL). Recent studies, using the calculation of estimated glomerular filtration rate (eGFR) obtained from the MDRD formula, confirmed the deleterious impact of RN on renal function. In one large study, the 3-year probability of freedom from new onset of GFR less than 60 mL/min/1.73 m^2 was 80% after PN but only 35% after RN. Corresponding values for the 3-year probability of freedom from GFR less than 45 mL/min/1.73 m^2, a more severe level of CKD, was 95% for PN but only 64% for RN. Multivariable analysis indicated that RN was an independent risk factor for the development of new-onset CKD.

In addition, before kidney tumor resection in apparently healthy patients who had a normal contralateral kidney, it was reported that 26% of patients had pre-existing CKD as defined by an eGFR of less than 60 mL/min/1.73 m^2. The pathologic basis of this pre-existing CKD in renal tumor patients was recently elucidated when the non–tumor-bearing portion of kidneys was examined and only 10% was found to be normal.

The remaining patients had vascular sclerotic changes and other intrinsic renal abnormalities, including diabetic nephropathy, glomerular hypertrophy, mesangial expansion, and diffuse glomerulosclerosis.

Before the morbid traditional endpoint of end-stage renal failure and dialysis (eGFR <15 mL/min/1.73 m^2), CKD (eGFR 15–60 mL/min/1.73 m^2) is associated with increasing risk for cardiovascular events, hospitalization, and death, the likelihood of which increases as the eGFR decreases. It is now estimated that there are 19 million adults in the United States who have CKD. Unlike the carefully selected and much younger kidney donors, renal tumor patients have a median age of older than 60 years and often have common medical conditions, such as diabetes, hypertension, and peripheral vascular disease, that can affect baseline kidney function. Careful, prospective renal tumor tracking studies in patients initially not treated surgically coupled with meta-analysis of the published literature suggests that small renal tumors have a slow yearly growth rate (approximately 0.3 cm/y). A substantial percentage of small renal masses have benign or indolent histology (45%), and even if the patient has a conventional clear cell carcinoma, the likelihood of metastatic disease for tumors of 4 cm or less is believed to be 5% to 7%. The clinical logic of offering active surveillance to select patients who have small renal masses with or without a confirmatory biopsy, particularly those who are elderly or comorbidly ill, is gaining increasing acceptance particularly in light of concerns that overly aggressive application of radical nephrectomy can worsen or cause CKD. Despite this robust literature in favor of kidney preservation strategies, evidence from large cross-sectional national databases indicates that RN is overused in the United States and abroad and still accounts for 90% of kidney operations for small renal (T1) tumors. Overuse of RN is a quality-of-care issue that needs to be carefully addressed through educational programs and increased training in open and laparoscopic kidney-sparing operations. New approaches to the small renal mass, including laparoscopic and robotic partial nephrectomy, and thermal ablative approaches (radiofrequency ablation, cryoablation) have been actively pursued by committed clinician investigators in the United States and abroad. Careful case selection and increased experience with the laparoscopic approach to partial nephrectomy has rendered this a reasonable alternative in skilled hands; however, concerns relating to the impact of warm ischemia on long-term renal function and greater perioperative urologic and non-urologic complications compared with open partial nephrectomy may limit its widespread application beyond certain centers of excellence committed to minimally invasive surgery. For the ablative procedures, concerns regarding the pathologic completeness of the ablation, the best method to follow the ablated kidney lesion and to determine if it is still viable, and difficulties in achieving surgical salvage without completion nephrectomy in cases of documented recurrence remain to be completely addressed before the widespread acceptance of these approaches.

The observation that an intense immune response can be elicited by renal cell cancers, sufficient enough on rare occasions to lead to spontaneous regression and even complete remission of metastatic disease sites, lead to numerous clinical trials with cytokines, such as interferon alpha 2a and interleukin 2. Although these agents could induce durable remissions in rare cases, patient selection factors seemed to be important in predicting responses and toxicities were substantial. Partial responses (<20%), and occasional complete remissions (<4%) were documented with median survival times usually less than 12 months. Numerous attempts to treat metastatic renal cancer with systemic chemotherapies were also unsuccessful and were marked by limited responses and substantial drug toxicities. Based on research described above into the molecular pathways involved in the pathogenesis of the conventional clear cell carcinoma, two new multi-tyrosine kinase inhibitors (sunitinib, sorafenib) and one mammalian target of rapamycin (mTOR) inhibitor (temsirolimus) have been recently approved by the US Food and Drug Administration (FDA) after showing superior responses in placebo-controlled randomized trials involving both treatment-naïve and previously treated patients, compared with interferon alpha 2a with improvement in progression-free survival from 5 to 11 months. Temsirolimus is effective in improving overall and progression-free survival in patients who have poor-risk renal cell cancer. Interesting and substantial responses in the primary tumor have opened the door to neoadjuvant clinical trials with these agents for patients who may be unresectable at presentation. Unfortunately, significant toxicities (fatigue, rash, hand-foot syndromes) and the lack of durable, complete responses have stimulated the oncology community to seek new agents and actively study drug combinations (ie, TKI inhibitors and bevacizumab). Another hurdle to confront is metastatic non–clear cell tumor (chromophobe, papillary, medullary, collecting duct) that seem not to use the above-described pathways to the same degree as the clear cell tumors and are therefore less responsive to the newly FDA-approved agents.

The authors of this issue of the *Urologic Clinics of North America* provide a comprehensive review of the great progress made, on numerous fronts, in the understanding and management of renal cortical tumors. Their work illuminates a clear and hopeful path to our future goal of further decreasing the morbidity and mortality of renal cancer.

Paul Russo, MD, FACS
Attending Surgeon and Professor
Weill College of Medicine, Cornell University
Memorial Sloan Kettering Cancer Center
New York, New York, USA

E-mail address:
russop@MSKCC.org (P. Russo)

Dedication

I dedicate this issue of the *Urologic Clinics of North America* to my father, Dr. Carmine Paul Russo of Ithaca, New York. Dr. Russo was born in New York City in 1914 and was a 1938 graduate of the College of Physicians and Surgeons of Columbia University. He did residency training in Urology at Queens General Hospital and the Long Island College Hospital. He was a Major in the United States Army and served 4 years at a military hospital in Coventry, England during World War II, as a result of which he received the Bronze Star. On his return to the United States and under the advice of Dr. Victor Marshall, Dr. Russo established the first urology practice in Ithaca, New York, in 1947. At that time, most major urologic operations were done by general surgeons. Dr. Russo brought innovative techniques and procedures to upstate New York, including intravenous pyelograms, transurethral resections, transaortic renal angiograms, perineal radical prostatectomies, and partial nephrectomy. He retired from clinical practice in 2004, a difficult year in which he lost his wife, my mother Rose Russo, to cancer after 62 years of marriage. Today, Dr. Russo remains active in the Ithaca community and recently had a showing of nearly 40 years of his paintings and artwork, which was very well received.

As a youngster, I knew that my father was a busy and respected physician. When I was older and worked alongside him as a hospital orderly and premedical student, I understood for the first time the full dimensions and responsibilities of his profession. Keeping current with his specialty was extremely important to my father, and he was an avid and committed reader of the literature in his and other medical specialties. I was always amazed at how knowledgeable and thoughtful he was about the contemporary problems in urology and urologic oncology. When I interviewed for residency positions I found that many academic urologists knew my father, who had referred patients to them when their expertise represented the best care.

His career spanned most of the twentieth century, from the discovery of antibiotics to the cloning of the human genome. Most importantly, C. Paul Russo was a loving and dedicated parent to my sisters and me, and a devoted spouse to my mother. For this, especially, I will always be grateful.

Paul Russo, MD, FACS

Urol Clin N Am 35 (2008) xix
doi:10.1016/j.ucl.2008.07.017

urologic.theclinics.com

Surgical Management of Renal Tumors: A Historical Perspective

Harry W. Herr, MD

KEYWORDS

• Renal tumors • Surgery • History

FOUNDATIONS

The modern era of renal surgery began on August 2, 1869, just 139 years ago, when Gustav Simon (1824–1876), then Professor of Surgery at Heidelberg, performed the first planned nephrectomy on a living human being.[1] His patient was a 46-year-old woman named Margaretha Kleb, who suffered from a pervious urinary fistula caused by an injury to the ureter sustained during a prior laparotomy to remove an ovarian cyst. She survived removal of her kidney and was permanently cured of her fistula. Eighteen years later in 1887, Vincenz Czerny (1842–1915), Simon's successor at Heidelberg, performed the first partial nephrectomy to remove a renal tumor.[2] Both total and partial nephrectomy have become the hallmark surgical procedures used today to treat renal tumors, and their conception and evolution represent two of the most important advances in medicine and surgery.

Simon (**Fig. 1**) arrived at his decision to remove a healthy, functioning kidney, plagued with many questions for which he had no sure answers. Would the remaining kidney supply the needs of the body? Could the ligated renal artery withstand the blood pressure of the aorta following absorption of the ligature? Could the initial hemorrhage be controlled? Could wounds and infection of the peritoneum be avoided? Still, there was historical precedent for the operation.

For many years, physiologists had established the fact that animals could survive after removal of one kidney. In 1670, Zambecarri, along with Rounhuysen, extirpated sound kidneys without causing death; he was also the first to contemplate the operation of nephrectomy in man.[3] Between 1690 and 1841, Blancard, Blundell, Claude Bernard and others repeated similar experiments, concluding that any adverse effects following nephrectomy were more a result of the operation itself than to the absence of one kidney. During the nineteenth century, abdominal surgery flourished, particularly to remove large ovarian cysts or tumors. In a few cases this had resulted in unintentional nephrectomies, as in those by Wolcott (1861), Spiegelberg (1867), and Peaslee (1868). Although the patients died eventually from infections, in each case the remaining kidney worked well. Many autopsies also showed that for an indefinite time before death, only one kidney had been functioning.[4]

The animal experiments and surgical misadventures of the ovariotomists impressed Simon, but he was still not ready to remove a healthy kidney without witnessing the consequences himself. He nephrectomized 30 dogs and observed they lived in perfect health after ablation of one kidney. He noted compensatory hypertrophy and convinced himself that the physiologic function of the kidneys could be maintained by one kidney. He dissected cadavers to work out the anatomic details, steps of the operation, and the best access to the retroperitoneum. Only then was he ready to proceed with his landmark nephrectomy. In 1869, before a live audience, he removed Kleb's left kidney through a lumbar incision. Simon completed the operation in 40 minutes and lost just 50 mL of blood. Renal surgery was born.

Department of Urology, Memorial Sloan-Kettering Cancer Center, Weill Cornell Medical College, 1275 York Avenue, New York, NY 10021, USA
E-mail address: herrh@mskcc.org

Urol Clin N Am 35 (2008) 543–549
doi:10.1016/j.ucl.2008.07.010
0094-0143/08/$ – see front matter © 2008 Elsevier Inc. All rights reserved.

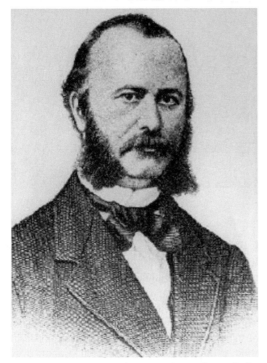

Fig. 1. Gustav Simon, (1824–1876), performed first planned nephrectomy in 1869.

EARLY RENAL SURGERY

Simon had no imitators for nearly a year. In April 1870, Parker removed a kidney from a 12-year-old girl, for hydronephrosis, but the patient died from shock the following day. In December 1870, Gilmore,[5] an American surgeon, removed a painful floating kidney in a woman, aged 39 years, who recovered without mishap. In 1875, Langenbuch[6] performed the first nephrectomy for a malignant tumor, followed by Jessop[7] in 1877, who removed a Wilms tumor. Both patients survived the operation. The first decade after Simon (1870–1879) saw 28 nephrectomies, but the mortality rate was a frightful 64%. With the wide acceptance of antisepsis in 1876, and later adopting Lister's methods of asepsis in 1880, the next 5 years (from 1880 to 1884) saw the mortality rate fall to 24% after 219 nephrectomies.[8] Most surgeons used the lumbar approach, believing that it was safer; however, in 1876 Kocher was forced to use the transperitoneal route to remove a bulky tumor and concluded that it afforded a fairly easy approach to the kidney.[9] Some surgeons adopted this approach because they could ascertain the condition of the opposite kidney by palpation. However, the invention of the cystoscope by Nitze in 1877, and the practical applications of ureteral catheterization, soon gave adequate information on the opposite kidney; transperitoneal operations fell into disfavor, except for removal of large tumors.

Every decade up the dawn of the twentieth century, survival rates after nephrectomy improved. In 1901, von Schmieden reported on 1,118 nephrectomies, collecting the operations of the first three decades following the first deliberate nephrectomy by Simon. He showed that nephrectomy by the lumbar route was followed by a mortality of 44% in the first, by 27% in the second, and by 17% in the third decade. The abdominal method had a mortality of 55% in the first, 48% in the second, and 19% in the last decade.[10] In 1902, Kuster[11] collected the statistics of 1,521 nephrectomies performed by different surgeons around the world, giving mortality for all cases of 34% for the transperitoneal and 12% for the extraperitoneal removal of kidneys. By 1900 though, techniques of abdominal surgery had improved markedly so that both approaches were comparable. During the early twentieth century, mortality reported by specialists or skilled urologists was markedly less than nephrectomy done by general surgeons. In 1912, Gerster[12] in New York reported mortality in 21% of 112 nephrectomies done by general surgeons in the last 16 years. During the same time, renal cases segregated, studied, and operated upon by urologists under the direction of Edwin Beer[13] had a mortality rate of only 3.8% among 207 nephrectomies.

The usual indications for nephrectomy were stones, movable kidney, hydronephrosis, renal abscess, urinary fistulae, and tumors. Many of these diseases affected only a part of the kidney, and partial or heminephrectomy developed rapidly owing to the successes of total nephrectomy. In November 1887, Czerny (**Fig. 2**) performed the first deliberate partial resection when he removed an angiosarcoma from the kidney of a 30-year-old gardener. The patient recovered. Fears of uncontrollable hemorrhage were dispelled by the work of Tuffier[14], who in 1889 showed that gentle pressure could control bleeding from the kidney, and animal experiments by Thiriar in 1888[15] and Bardenheuer[16] in 1891 proved that incisions made into the kidney often healed primarily without fistula formation. They investigated renal repair mechanisms, compensatory hypertrophy, renal function, changes in body functions, and the amount of renal tissue necessary for life after partial resection.

Surgeons then began to perform partial nephrectomy in various types of cases, but the operation soon lost favor and it was more or less abandoned because of an unwarranted fear of

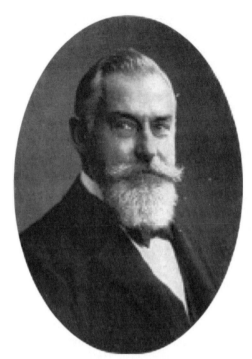

Fig. 2. Vinsenz Czerny, (1842–1915), performed first partial nephrectomy for renal tumor.

extensive hemorrhage at operation, delayed bleeding following surgery, frequent and persistent urinary fistula, and poor results owing to the injudicious use of partial resection to treat tuberculosis and neoplasms of the kidney. Kummell (1890), Bardenheuer (1891), and Block (1895) attempted partial nephrectomy for tumors but their patients died of atrophy of the kidney, shock, and uremia. During this early period, lumbar nephrectomy became established as the only effective operation for malignant diseases of the kidney.

In spite of better surgical methods, nephrectomy for kidney tumors was followed by a high mortality, varying from 50% (Squier, 1909) to 11% (Braasch, 1913). As late as 1920, Hyman[15] reported a mortality of 23% to 37%. The reasons for the unusually high mortality in nephrectomy for tumor were attributed to shock resulting from toxins released during the manipulation necessary to remove large tumors, and hemorrhage. Another frequent cause was fatal tumor emboli, owing to dislodged cancer cells entering the circulation during surgery. Block[16] noted an extension of cancer cells into the renal vein in 13 of 86 cases studied. Enthusiasm for conservative surgery for renal tumors was especially discouraged by autopsy and nephrectomy specimens showing frequent tumor spread into fat around the kidney and involvement of renal veins, as well as that almost all patients during this time had palpable and symptomatic renal cancers.

In 1903, Gregoire[17] reported removing kidney tumors en bloc with the fatty capsule, adrenal gland, and adjacent lymph nodes. This was the first description of the modern radical (perifascial) nephrectomy popularized later in the twentieth century. Its advantages were articulated by Chute[18], who in 1926 advocated anterior abdominal removal of kidney cancers because the pedicle is more easily reached and can be ligated immediately, minimizing the danger of forcing metastases into the renal veins, causing less trauma and affording palpation of the retroperitoneal glands. In large tumors, control of the renal pedicle posed problems. In 1902, Pasteau[19] recommended ligating the renal artery and vein separately, whereas Legueu (1921) and others advised tying off the pedicle en masse. Early surgeons emphasized that dividing the upper ureter facilitated greater mobility of the kidney and easier ligation of the pedicle, and they did not hesitate to resect a rib to secure better exposure. Most surgeons continued to perform a lumbar or flank nephrectomy, however; and although they believed that total nephrectomy was the only effective treatment of malignant kidney tumors, despite such aggressive surgery for the times, 33% of patients died of disease within 1 year and 65% died in less than 5 years.

In 1921, Rosenstein[20] performed a partial nephrectomy to palliate a kidney cancer and urged that this operation should be done in similar cases in which the contralateral kidney was incapable of satisfactory function following nephrectomy. In 1937 Goldstein and Abeshouse collected 296 cases of partial resection (1901–1935), of which 34 (11%) were done for renal tumors. They noted one death among 21 malignant tumors and no deaths for 13 benign tumors, and there were no cases of secondary hemorrhage or urinary fistula. They concluded that "small tumors and tumors of moderate size situated at one of the poles of the kidney, may be removed by partial resection out of necessity, but was contraindicated if the opposite kidney was healthy."[21] From 1937 to 1950 another 25 cases were added with similar results, although suspected renal tumors were primarily treated by total nephrectomy and only a few patients with poor renal function underwent local excision. Most surgeons regarded partial nephrectomy as technically more demanding than nephrectomy, associated with a higher complication rate, and simply unnecessary in most patients.

In 1950, Vermooten laid the foundation for modern nephron sparing surgery for renal neoplasms. "There are certain instances, when, for the patient's well being, it is unwise to do a nephrectomy, even in the presence of a malignant growth involving the kidney. The question is, whether such a procedure is ever justifiable when the opposite kidney is normal. I am inclined to think that in certain circumstances it may be."[22] In 1948 he removed a 10-cm carcinoma from the left kidney of a 52-year-old woman with a normal right kidney. His decision was based on the pathologic studies by Cahill (1948), showing that clear cell carcinomas arose from the cortex, were localized, surrounded by a capsule, grew by expansile growth, rarely invaded surrounding structures, and generally spread by the bloodstream. He was also aware that the autopsy studies by Bell and others (1938–1944) had revealed few metastases from small renal tumors. Bell[23] reported that only 7% of tumors less than 5 cm had metastasized, compared with 83% of tumors larger than 10 cm. In fact, small tumors rarely broke through the capsule and only one isolated metastasis was noted among 38 tumors 3 cm or smaller in size. Microscopic studies of tissue adjacent to tumors persuaded Vermooten that some tumors could be excised with only a 1-cm margin without fear of local recurrence, and local tumor excision should be attempted, especially in a solitary kidney or when there was markedly impaired function of the opposite kidney.

Few urologists paid much attention to Vermooten or to the observations of Bell except to argue that, because small tumors might metastasize, that warranted total nephrectomy for all renal tumors, especially in cases with two kidneys. During the next 40 years, partial nephrectomy was done mostly for tumors in a solitary kidney, poor renal function, or bilateral renal tumors. From 1950 to 1967, Zinman and Dowd collected only 18 essential cases of partial nephrectomy, adding 3 of their own. At the same time, other progressive surgeons reported individual cases of partial nephrectomy for unilateral renal tumors when the other kidney was considered satisfactory. Still, most urologists believed that partial nephrectomy was unwarranted unless there was a compelling reason to preserve renal function. Textbooks published between 1937 and 1970 do not mention partial nephrectomy.[24]

MODERN RADICAL NEPHRECTOMY

In 1949, Charles Robson in Toronto was searching for a safer method to remove large tumors when he became aware of simultaneous descriptions in 1948 by Chute and colleagues[25] in Boston and Mortensen[26] in New Zealand, where large renal carcinomas were removed through a thoraco-abdominal incision. The kidney mass was removed together with the perinephric fat and overlying peritoneum, but no attempt was made to excise the draining lymphatic field. Robson[27] performed his first thoraco-abdominal radical nephrectomy in 1949, and in 1963 he published his results in a landmark article, reporting survival rates of 56% at 3 years and 48% at 5 years among 62 cases. He updated his experience in 88 patients in 1969, showing similar superior results over historical reports and only a 3% surgical mortality.[28] He also became the first to correlate survival with extent (stage) and grade of kidney cancer. Robson believed the improved survival he saw over lumbar nephrectomy was because of early occlusion of the renal pedicle before manipulation of the tumor, removal of the kidney within its envelope of perinephric fat, and dissection of the regional lymph glands, which were involved in 22% of the cases. Although claims of superior survival over simple nephrectomy favored in the past were never substantiated[29], there is no doubt that Robson's Halstedian approach to kidney cancer was right for the times. Most patients presented then with symptomatic or locally advanced tumors, mandating radical excision of the kidney and involving adjacent tissues and organs. Radical nephrectomy became established as the standard surgical treatment for localized kidney tumors and all solid renal masses were considered to be potentially lethal cancers. These attitudes would prevail for much of the rest of the twentieth century.

MODERN PARTIAL NEPHRECTOMY

Amid a climate of radical surgery, the 1960s also saw significant advances in nephron-sparing surgery. Poutasse (1962) improved the surgical technique of partial nephrectomy by tracing the segmental blood supply to the kidney, and Kerr (1959) and Klotz (1960) introduced renal hypothermia, which prevented ischemic damage, and permitted longer operations and complicated reconstructions of the kidney in a bloodless field. As a result of these surgical advances and the earlier favorable experiences of a few surgeons, partial nephrectomy began to be done more frequently in essential cases.[24] Local recurrence in the partially resected kidney ranged from 4% to 10%, but overall survival was similar to radical nephrectomy. In 1975, Wickham[30] reviewed the world literature (1954–1974) and reported a 5-year survival rate of 72% in 37 patients after partial nephrectomy for tumors in a solitary kidney or bilateral renal tumors, setting the stage to expand the indications for partial nephrectomy to include patients with a healthy opposite kidney.

In the 1970s, Puigvert (1976), Herr (1976), Novick (1977), and later Marberger (1981) began to seriously question the wisdom of removing a mostly healthy kidney containing a unilateral, localized renal tumor, even in patients with a normal opposite kidney. This was hardly an original idea, as Vermooten (1950), Ljunggren (1960), and Semb (1965) had come to similar conclusions more than a decade earlier. During the 1980s, although a few urologists advocated routine elective partial nephrectomy for small renal tumors, the majority still showed little interest in pursuing conservative surgery over radical nephrectomy for renal cancers. However, that was about to change.[24]

The 1980s marked the beginning of the era of elective nephron-sparing surgery for renal tumors. Although the topic was hotly debated among the urological community for the next two decades, all the important pieces were in place to predict successful partial nephrectomy for most renal tumors. These included knowledge of intra-renal vascular anatomy, better surgical methods to 'reconstruct the kidney-reducing complications, renal hypothermia, an increasing number of smaller cortical tumors detected incidentally by later generation high resolution CT and MRI scans, and few local recurrences reported after partial nephrectomy for tumors in solitary kidneys. Many urologists remained skeptical, however, of removing only the tumor and preserving the diseased kidney when the patient had another perfectly good kidney. Their major concern was the possibility of local recurrence because of inadequate excision or multicentric tumors after partial excision. In 1988 that fear was amplified by Mukamel when he reported evidence of occult renal tumors in up to 30% of nephrectomy specimens, which might recur if only the primary tumor was removed. Although this rate would later fall to 5%, there was little evidence at the time that such information dissuaded committed surgeons from pursuing elective nephron-sparing surgery. However, it strengthened the arguments of those who were philosophically opposed to a conservative approach and undoubtedly deterred some from performing partial nephrectomy, even for small tumors.

In 1993, Licht and Novick[31] reported early favorable results in 241 cases collected from the literature (1967–1991) of partial nephrectomy with a normal opposite kidney. Although the average tumor size was less than 3.5 cm and follow-up was short (3 years), only two local recurrences were reported and 95% of patients survived. In addition, improved surgical techniques using the argon beam coagulator, newer hemostatic agents, and intraoperative ultrasound allowed more precise resection, reducing the risk of serious postoperative complications. Subsequently, Herr[32] and Novick[33] provided 10-year follow-up on more

than 100 patients, showing a rare local recurrence and almost 100% survival, especially in patients with unilateral tumors less than 4 cm in size. At the dawn of the twenty-first century, only then did urologists widely accept elective partial nephrectomy as a viable surgical treatment of localized renal tumors.

LAPAROSCOPIC NEPHRECTOMY

Although Kelling was the first to try laparoscopy using Nitze's cystoscope in 1901, laparoscopic surgery evolved slowly and was largely limited to the removal of small pieces of solid tissues (ovary, lymph nodes) or excision of hollow organs (gallbladder). In 1991, Ralph Clayman took a laparoscopic leap forward when he and his team in St. Louis successfully removed the right kidney and a 3-cm tumor from an 85-year-old woman. The operative time was 7 hours and became the first operation where laparoscopic techniques were used to remove a major solid organ from a human being. Clayman knew he was breaking new ground. Like Simon had done more than a century before, Clayman performed successive nephrectomies in pigs to learn the laparoscopic operation and to perfect a sack to contain the kidney in the abdomen. Engineers also devised an effective morcellator/evacuator to remove the specimen.[34] Published as a simple letter[35], Clayman's innovative and bold first laparoscopic nephrectomy touched off urology's enduring courtship with laparoscopic surgery (**Fig. 3**).

Advances then progressed rapidly. The first partial nephrectomy went from bench to bedside in less than a year. Seminal work done by Elspeth McDougall and colleagues[36] in the laboratory was translated into clinical reality in 1993 when Howard Winfield[37], in Iowa, performed the first laparoscopic partial nephrectomy. Still in the development stage today, laparoscopic partial

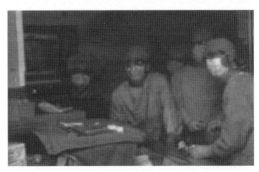

Fig. 3. Laparoscopic nephrectomy team at Washington University in St. Louis (circa 1991). Ralph Clayman is at far right.

nephrectomy for renal tumors is a technically demanding procedure that has yet to recapitulate all of the favorable features marking the successful open operation, and its final place in the armamentarium of the surgical treatment of renal tumors remains to be defined. Improvements are being made regularly, however; and these, and robot assisted surgery now widely available, are likely to extend laparoscopic capabilities beyond imagination.

THE TWENTY-FIRST CENTURY

Surgery for kidney cancer continues to evolve. Today, the majority of nephrectomies for malignant renal tumors are performed laparoscopically. Partial nephrectomy is mostly done by open surgery, although laparascopic approaches are becoming more common, and the current trend is toward nephron-sparing surgery. For example, most renal tumors are now small and serendipitously diagnosed, half are benign or subtypes associated with favorable biology compared with clear cell carcinoma, global renal function is better preserved, onset of chronic kidney disease may be prevented or delayed, and survival improved after local tumor excision compared with nephrectomy.[38] Such considerations have led to expanding the indications of partial nephrectomy to include centrally located and larger tumors.[39]

If we look ahead into the twenty-first century, it is a safe bet we will not treat renal tumors the same way we do now. Surgery will still predominate, but using minimally invasive approaches. Parallel advances in tumor biology, radiologic imaging, and technology already suggest that laparoscopic, robotic, and percutaneous energy-ablation procedures promise to control renal tumors with less morbidity than open surgery. There is every reason to believe that such treatments and aims will prove to be successful. Eventually, a simple needle biopsy or a targeted image will characterize renal tumors at the molecular level, identifying which need or do not need treatment. This will become important in the future to deal with the increasing incidence of renal tumors in an aging population.

In 1950, Abeshouse said it best: "Few procedures provide the urologist with more satisfaction than those that preserve renal function." If we want to gaze into the future, we need only look to the past.

REFERENCES

1. Simon G. Chirugie der Nieren. Stuttgart: Ferdinand Enke, vol. II, p. 314, 1871.
2. Czerny V. Reported by Herczel E: Uber Nierenexsirpation. Beitr. Z. Klinik. Chir. 1890;6:485.
3. Newman D. History of renal surgery. Lancet 1901;6: 884–5.
4. Morris H. On the origin and progress of renal surgery. Philadelphia: P. Blakiston, Son & Co; 1898.
5. Gilmore JT. Case of successful removal of a kidney from a woman. Am J Obst 1871;4:74–5.
6. Langenbuch C. Berlin Klin. Wchnschr 1877;14:337.
7. Jessop TR. Lancet 1877;1:889 [Annotation].
8. Riches E. Annual oration on the development of renal surgery. Trans Med Soc Lond 1970;86:200.
9. Mathe CP. Kidney surgery. In: History of Urology, vol 1. American Urological Association, Williams & Wilkins Co.; 1932. p. 298.
10. von Schmieden V. Die Erfolge der Nierenchirugie. Deutsche Ztschr. f. Chir. 1901;1xii:205.
11. Kuster EGF. Die Chirugirschen Krankheiten der Nieren. Stuttgart (Germany): Deutsche Chirugie; 1896–1902. Lfg. 52b, p. 174.
12. Gerster AG. Nephrectomy. Ann Surg 1912;1vi:1.
13. Beer E, Hyman A. Progress in nephrectomy. JAMA 1920;1xxv:1180.
14. Tuffier T. Etudes experimentales sur la chirugie du rein. Steinheil G, Paris, 1889, vol. 1, p. 166.
15. Hyman A. Tumors of the kidney. Tr Am Urol A 1920; xii:242.
16. Block G. Folia Urol 1910;161.
17. Gregoire W. Les propagations du cancer du rein. Bull Med Soc Anat (Paris) 1903;78:764–9.
18. Chute AL. A study of some cases of hypernephroma. Boston: Medical and Surgical Journal; 1926;cxciv, 471.
19. Pasteau O. Technique de la ligature du pedicule renal dans la nephrectomie. Bull Soc Anat 1902;1xxvii: 89.
20. Rosenstein P. J Urol 1921;15:447.
21. Goldstein AE, Abeshouse BS. Partial resections of the kidney. J Urol 1937;38:15–9.
22. Vermooten V. Indications for conservative surgery in certain renal tumors: a study based on growth pattern of the clear cell carcinoma. J Urol 1950;64: 200.
23. Bell ET. A classification of renal tumors with observations on the frequency of the various types. J Urol 1938;39:238.
24. Herr HW. History of partial nephrectomy. J Urol 2005;173:705–8.
25. Chute R, Soutter L, Kerr WS. Value of thoraco-abdominal incision in removal of kidney tumors. New Engl. J Med 1949;241:951.
26. Mortensen H. Transthoracic nephrectomy. J Urol 1948;60:855.
27. Robson CJ. Radical nephrectomy for renal cell carcinoma. J Urol 1963;89:37.
28. Robson CJ, Churchill BM, Anderson W. The results of radical nephrectomy for renal cell carcinoma. J Urol 1969;101:297–301.

29. Skinner D, Colvin R, Vermillion C, et al. Diagnosis and management of renal cell carcinoma. Cancer 1971; 28:1165–73.
30. Wickham JE. Conservative renal surgery for adenocarcinoma. Br J Urol 1975;47:25.
31. Licht MR, Novick AC. Nephron sparing surgery for renal cell carcinoma. J Urol 1993;149:1–10.
32. Herr HW. Partial nephrectomy for unilateral renal carcinoma and a normal contralateral kidney: 10-year followup. J Urol 1999;161:33–7.
33. Fergany AF, Hafez KS, Novick AC. Long-term results of nephron sparing surgery for localized renal cell carcinoma: 10-year followup. J Urol 2000;163:442–6.
34. Clayman RV, Kavoussi LR, Leng SR, et al. Laparoscopic nephrectomy: initial report of pelviscopic organ ablation in the pig. J Endourol 1990;4:247.
35. Clayman RV, Kavoussi L, Soper NJ, et al. Laparoscopic nephrectomy. N Engl J Med 1991;324: 1370–1.
36. McDougall EM, Clayman RV, Chandhoke PJ, et al. Laparoscopic partial nephrectomy in the pig model. J Urol 1993;149:1633–6.
37. Winfield HN, Donovan JF, Clayman RV. Laparoscopic partial nephrectomy: initial case report for benign disease. J Endourol 1993;7:521–6.
38. Huang WC, Sevey AS, Russo P. Chronic kidney disease after nephrectomy in patients with renal cortical tumors. Lancet Oncol 2006;9: 735–40.
39. Russo P, Goetzl M, Simmons R, et al. Partial nephrectomy: the rationale for expanding indications. Ann Surg Oncol 2002;9:680–7.

Pathologic Features of Renal Cortical Tumors

Satish K. Tickoo, MD*, Anuradha Gopalan, MD

KEYWORDS

- Renal cell carcinoma • Oncocytoma • Pathology
- Morphologic features • Immunohistochemistry

Until the 1980s, renal cortical tumors had been traditionally classified as clear cell, granular cell, papillary and sarcomatoid carcinoma, or renal oncocytoma. In 1985, Thöenes and colleagues[1,2] first described chromophobe renal cell carcinoma (RCC) in human beings, followed soon by its eosinophilic variant. This led to a reassessment of the morphologic classification of renal tumors and laid the framework for the clinicopathologically more valid classification used today (**Box 1**). We know now that "granular cell carcinoma" and "sarcomatoid carcinoma" are not specific entities, and that granular and sarcomatoid features can be seen in a variety of renal tumors with markedly diverse biologic potential. The current histologic classification has also been validated by a number of molecular studies.[3–5] The implications of this now universally accepted classification system are that publications about clinicopathologic aspects of renal tumors from the pre-1985 era may not correspond to the current knowledge about these tumors.

The better understanding of the molecular aspects of renal tumors in the recent past has resulted in the realization that differing molecular pathways are involved in different renal tumors. This has resulted in the development and usage of multiple targeted therapies, particularly for advanced clear cell RCC, with promising initial results.[6] At the same time, this knowledge has provided pathologists with additional tools to investigate molecular pathway markers in different subtypes of kidney tumors, and to potentially use them for their differential diagnostic and prognostic evaluation. Therefore, the challenges to the genitourinary pathologists are to (i) understand the morphologic diversity seen in different tumors to classify them more precisely, (ii) understand the antigenic diversity in these tumors and its application to targeted therapy, and (iii) be able to classify these tumors on minimal material, such as needle biopsies and aspirates.

GRADING AND STAGING OF RENAL TUMORS

Among the several grading schemes proposed for renal tumors over the years, Fuhrman's system is the most widely used. It uses nuclear grades based on nuclear size, irregularity of the nuclear membrane, and nucleolar prominence. For practical purposes, easily identifiable nucleoli at low magnification ($10\times$) examination are characteristic of nuclear grade 3 or 4, with grade 4 nuclei also showing marked pleomorphism and multilobulation. Grade 1 or 2 nuclei generally require examination at high magnification ($40\times$) to identify and evaluate the level of prominence of the nucleoli. While the utility of Fuhrman's grading system in clear cell RCC is well established, its value in papillary and chromophobe RCC remains controversial. Renal oncocytomas are not graded, as they are benign tumors.

The TNM classification of the American Joint Committee on Cancer (AJCC) and Union Internationale Contre le Cancer is the most widely used and clinically relevant staging system for renal tumors. Over the years it has been modified and improved multiple times; the latest modifications

Department of Pathology, Memorial Sloan-Kettering Cancer Center, 1275 York Avenue, New York, New York 10065, USA
* Corresponding author.
E-mail address: tickoos@mskcc.org (S.K. Tickoo).

Urol Clin N Am 35 (2008) 551–561
doi:10.1016/j.ucl.2008.07.001

Box 1
Classification of adult renal cortical tumors

Benign

Renal oncocytoma

Papillary adenoma

Metanephric adenoma

Metanephric adenofibroma

Malignant

Clear Cell (conventional) RCC

Papillary RCC

Chromophobe RCC

Collecting duct carcinoma

Medullary carcinoma

Tubulocystic RCC

Acquired cystic disease of kidney-associated RCC

RCC, unclassified

Mucinous tubular and spindle cell carcinoma

Translocation associated carcinomas

Tumors of indefinite malignant potential

Multilocular cystic RCC

---

were made in 2002. While it cannot claim to be a perfect staging system, at present the usage of TNM classification is recommended in the hope of establishing uniformity in reporting, while future AJCC staging criteria will almost certainly correct whatever deficiencies are realized in the present system.

Recently, a series of publications have highlighted the importance of the renal sinus and sinus veins in the staging of RCC,[7,8] factors first included in the AJCC staging system in 2002. In a retrospective study, it was recently shown that a significant proportion of cases that die of apparent pT1 disease in fact have renal sinus fat invasion.[9] Therefore, a careful gross examination and adequate sampling of the renal sinus-tumor interface, especially in larger tumors, is strongly recommended.

CLEAR CELL (CONVENTIONAL) RCC

Clear cell RCC comprises approximately 60% to 65% of all renal cortical tumors.[5,10] They typically show tumor cells with clear cytoplasm (because of the abundant intracytoplasmic lipid and glycogen) and an acinar or solid-nested growth pattern, invested by an intricate, arborizing vasculature. The cytoplasmic clarity is especially more common in low-grade tumors. The higher grade tumors less often show pure clear cell cytology, and may contain variable proportions of (or even exclusive) tumor cells with granular/eosinophilic cytoplasm (**Fig. 1**A). In these high-grade areas, a loss of the acinar growth pattern is quite frequent, and such areas are more likely to have solid or sometimes sarcomatoid histology. It is important to look for areas of transition to a lower grade so as to establish the correct diagnosis. The intricate vasculature tends to be retained in most tumors, except in the very high-grade areas with solid or sarcomatoid differentiation. Sarcomatoid differentiation occurs in approximately 5% of these tumors and, as in other subtypes of RCC, is an indicator of high-grade tumor with generally ominous prognosis.[5,11,12] These tumors may take on a papillary or pseudopapillary appearance focally, but this is usually because of degenerative changes rather than true papillae formation.

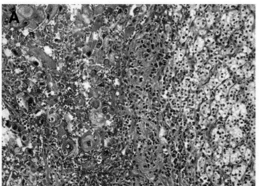 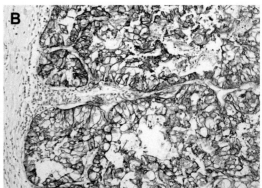

Fig. 1. Clear cell RCC. (*A*) The high-grade areas to the left have large, Fuhrman nuclear grade 4 cytology and non-clear ("granular") cytoplasm. (HE;100×). (*B*) Diffuse and membranous immunoreactivity for carbonic anhydrase IX (CA IX) is characteristic (CA-IX; 100×).

Clear cell RCCs are characterized by the loss of genetic material of the short arm of chromosome 3 (3p) and mutations in the von Hippel-Lindau tumor suppressor (*VHL*) gene.[13–17] In patients with von Hippel-Lindau disease, such losses and mutations are described in virtually all cases. Somatic mutations/promoter hypermethylations in the same region can be found in 75% to 80% of the more common sporadic tumors as well.[18] The product of a normal *VHL* gene, pVHL, is required to target and degrade hypoxia-induced factor (HIF) in normoxemic states. In cells that are hypoxic, or lack pVHL (as in most cases of clear cell RCC), HIF escapes degradation and activates downstream targets, including vascular endothelial growth factor, platelet derived growth factor, glucose transporter 1, and carbonic anhydrase IX (CA IX), among others. The expression of these downstream products at the immunohistochemical level may be used as diagnostic markers of clear cell RCC (**Fig. 1**B) or as targets for novel therapies.[6,19–22] CA IX and HIF-1 immunohistochemical expression has also been reported to be related to prognosis, although large prospective studies evaluating such associations are currently not available.[22–24]

PAPILLARY RCC

Papillary RCC (PRCC) constitute up to 15% of all renal cortical neoplasms. There are at least two distinct types of papillary RCC, both at the morphologic and genetic level, and they appear to have distinct clinical behaviors as well.[25–28] Architecturally, most of these tumors have a papillary, tubular, or tubulo-papillary growth pattern. Some have a solid growth pattern because of compression of the papillary structures, while others show a glomeruloid appearance. The cytoplasm may be amphophilic, eosinophilic, or even partially clear. Papillary RCCs are often multifocal, are frequently associated with papillary adenomas (tumors less than 5 mm in size, by definition) and are the most common RCC type with bilateral disease. Classically, papillary tumors display abundant lipid laden, foamy macrophages within fibrovascular cores, a feature helpful in establishing the correct diagnosis. It needs to be emphasized that correct classification of these tumors requires experience and a detailed review of all available slides.

Some experts feel that the Fuhrman grading scheme is well suited for papillary RCC but others disagree.[10,26,29,30] Delahunt and Eble[25] have suggested a two-tiered system (types 1 and 2) (**Fig. 2**) based on nuclear features and growth pattern characteristics, which has also been accepted in the latest World Health Organization classification. Whether these tumors should be graded and, if so, what system to use remains controversial.

Cytogenetic and molecular studies have revealed distinct findings in PRCC that distinguishes them from other renal epithelial tumors.[31,32] The majority of tumors, particularly type 1, are characterized by trisomy of chromosomes 7 and 17, as well as loss of chromosome Y.[3,31,33–37] Approximately 10% of the sporadic PRCC also show somatic mutations in the *c-MET* gene, a genetic abnormality that is common as a germline mutation in familial cases.[38] Some investigators have suggested that tumors exhibiting trisomy 7/17 only are likely to be benign, whereas those exhibiting additional genetic abnormalities will behave aggressively, a hypothesis that has not been confirmed in the literature. Recently, a group from the National Institutes of Health described mutations in the *fumarate hydratase* gene associated with a subset of type 2 papillary RCC.[4] In most large

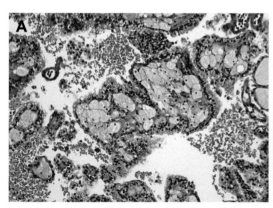 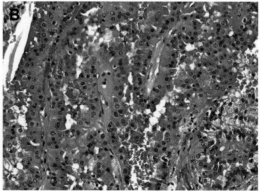

Fig. 2. Variants of papillary RCC. (*A*) Type 1, with low-grade cytology and abundant foamy histiocytes in the cores of the papillae (HE; 100×). (*B*) Type 2, with high-grade nuclei, eosinophilic cytoplasm, and nuclear pseudostratification (HE; 100×).

well-studied series, papillary RCC is a less aggressive tumor than clear cell RCC, with 5-year survival rates of 80% to 85%.[5,29,30,39]

TRANSLOCATION ASSOCIATED RCC

Translocation associated RCC constitute a small group of RCCs that may have a prominent papillary architecture, often associated with clear cell cytology and psammomatous calcifications. However, nested architecture and cells with granular eosinophilic cytoplasm are also common. In general, they tend to present in younger patients, although a series of cases in adults has also recently been described.[40–42] These are often associated with an aggressive behavior, more so in the adults.[42] Most cases are associated with t(X;17) or t(X;1), translocations resulting in the fusion of the *TFE3* gene on Xp11.2 to usually the *ASPL* gene on chromosome17 or *PRCC* on chromosome 1. Both types show strong nuclear immunohistochemical staining with TFE3 antibody. Another subtype seen in children and young adults is characterized by t(6;11) (p21;q12),[43] and it shows strong immunopositivity for transcripton factor TFEB. It is very likely that translocation associated carcinomas were incorrectly classified in the past as unusual variants of clear cell carcinoma, PRCC, or even RCC, unclassified type.

CHROMOPHOBE RCC

Chromophobe RCC, first described in 1985 by Thöenes and colleagues,[1] constitute approximately 6% of renal cortical neoplasms. Because of their cytoplasmic features, many of these tumors may previously have been classified as clear cell or granular RCC. The morphologic features include a solid growth pattern with sheets of cells separated by incomplete fibrovascular septations. Occasionally, tubular, nested or cord-like growth, mimicking renal oncocytoma, may be present. The cells may be predominantly clear (with finely reticulated cytoplasm), eosinophilic, or most often with a mixture of clear and eosinophilic cells. Nuclei usually exhibit widespread hyperchromasia and nuclear membrane irregularity, although such nuclear features may sometimes be only focal. Classically, one sees perinuclear clearing (perinuclear "halo"), corresponding to distended microvesicles—a distinctive ultrastructural feature of chromophobe RCC. Thöenes and colleagues[2] also described an eosinophilic variant that may be confused with oncocytoma (**Fig. 3**A). As in other RCC types, chromophobe RCC with sarcomatoid features is a highly aggressive variant.

Chromophobe RCC are genetically characterized by multiple chromosomal losses, usually affecting chromosomes 1, Y, 6, 10, 13, 17, and 21,[44–47] with resultant hypodiploidy.[48] These tumors have a much better prognosis than clear cell and papillary RCC, with the 5-year disease free survivals of greater than 90%.[29,30,49] Even in metastatic settings, Motzer and colleagues[50] demonstrated that chromophobe carcinomas progress more indolently than other nonclear cell RCCs.

RENAL ONCOCYTOMA

Oncocytomas of the kidney constitute approximately 6% to 9% of renal cortical neoplasms.[5] They are benign neoplasms that require distinction from a number of malignant renal epithelial neoplasms with eosinophilic cytoplasm. Distinction from eosinophilic variant of chromophobe RCC may be particularly difficult for pathologists with less experience. Histologically, oncocytomas are

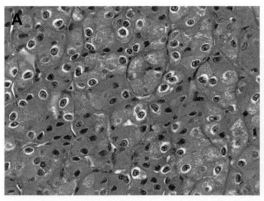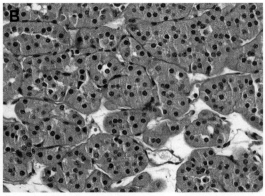

Fig. 3. (*A*) Eosinophilic variant of chromophobe RCC showing nuclear irregularities and perinuclear clearing. (*B*) Renal oncocytoma with abundant pink cytoplasm similar to that in (*A*), but uniform round nuclei and absence of perinuclear halos (HE; 100×).

characterized by cells with deeply eosinophilic cytoplasm arranged in nests, cords, or tubules and with uniform round, vesicular nuclei, often with prominent central nucleoli (**Fig. 3**B).[51,52] Electron microscopy reveals cytoplasm loaded with mitochondria, which is responsible for the cytoplasmic eosinophilia and a mahogany brown gross appearance.[53,54] Uniformity of nuclear features is the rule, although occasional isolated or groups of cells may exhibit marked degenerative-appearing hyperchromasia and pleomorphism. Prominent papillary growth and extensive tumor necrosis are not the features of renal oncocytoma. Likewise, mitotic activity is rarely noted. A central, stellate scar has been considered characteristic; however, such scars can also be seen in other low-grade renal cortical neoplasms. Microscopically, the scar may contain occasional entrapped tumor cells exhibiting focal cytoplasmic clearing. Other than in this scenario, clear cells are not a feature of renal oncocytoma. Tumor cells may infiltrate perirenal soft tissue, and may occasionally be present within small and even the larger vessels. None of these features affect its benign clinical behavior. Although rare questionable reported cases have metastasized,[52] no known case has died of the disease.

Genetically, oncocytomas do not exhibit 3p-, trisomy 7/17, or multiple combined chromosomal losses. They commonly exhibit loss of chromosomes Y and 1, and a few cases have been described with translocations involving chromosome 11.

Recently, the authors have described a group of patients with multiple oncocytic lesions (oncocytosis).[55] Among several characteristic morphologic features, some had a hybrid morphology between oncocytomas and chromophobe RCC, suggesting that these tumors may be genetically or causally related. In fact, there is a hypothesis that chromophobe tumors may represent a genetic/morphologic progression from oncocytoma. It is very likely that many, if not all of those patients, belonged to Birt-Hogg-Dubé (BHD) syndrome families.

COLLECTING DUCT AND MEDULLARY CARCINOMA

Collecting duct (Bellini duct) carcinoma (CDC) is very rare, constituting approximately 1% of renal epithelial tumors. In general, the tumors are centered in the renal medulla, particularly when small, and show marked invasive multinodular growth pattern with desmoplasia, highly atypical cytologic features, and papillary, tubular, solid, or microcystic architecture.[56] The papillae rarely, if ever, contain foamy macrophages, but acute or chronic inflammatory cells may be abundant within the tumor (**Fig. 4**). Characteristically, dysplastic or neoplastic cells may be present within adjacent renal tubules. Cytoplasmic and luminal mucin is frequent. Most show immunoreactivity for carcinoembryogenic antigen, peanut lectin agglutinin, and ulex europaeus agglutinin.[57,58] Cytokeratins 34BE12 and CK 7 may be positive as well.

CDC may present at any age, although it tends to occur in younger patients.[57,59] More than 50% of the patients present with metastatic disease. In a recent large, Japanese series of 81 cases, regional lymph node metastasis was detected in 44% and distant metastasis in another 32%.[59] Most patients die of disease within 3 years of diagnosis.

Another tumor, which some investigators believe to be a particularly aggressive variant of CDC, is the medullary carcinoma.[60–63] It preferentially occurs in young patients with sickle cell trait, hemoglobin SC disease, or very rarely sickle cell disease. Their morphologic features show some overlaps with those seen in CDC and high-grade urothelial tumors of the renal pelvis. Most reported cases had metastatic disease at presentation. The reported mean survivals in the two largest series to date have been 15 weeks and 4 months, respectively.[60,63]

TUBULOCYSTIC CARCINOMA

In the recent past, the morphologic spectrum of collecting was expanded to include some low-grade tumors characterized by a tubulocystic pattern of growth, tumor cells with low-grade nuclei, and mucin production.[64] More recently, the terminology of "tubulocystic carcinoma of the kidney" has been proposed for these tumors.[65,66] They

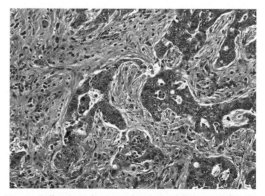

Fig. 4. Collecting duct carcinoma. As is typical for this tumor type, note the high-grade cytology, stromal desmoplasia, and inflammatory cell infiltrate within the stroma and epithelium of the tumor (HE; 100×).

are grossly well-circumscribed. Microscopically, besides the tubulocystic growth pattern, the tumor cells show abundant eosinophilic cytoplasm, and usually round nuclei with prominent nucleoli. However, in the authors' experience, not only do tumors with such pure morphologic features exist, other tumors showing similar histology but admixed with high-grade CDC-like areas are also observed. Therefore, their relationship to collecting duct carcinoma remains to be clarified.

UNCLASSIFIED RCC

Unclassified RCC form up to 6% of all renal epithelial tumors,[5,29] and include renal carcinomas that do not fit into any of the usual subtypes of renal cortical tumors.[67] Thus, tumors of unrecognizable cell or architectural types, or those with apparent composites of the recognized types, are all included in this category. While many of the tumors are of high cytomorphologic grade and aggressive clinical behavior, by definition they are not a pure entity and include many other low-grade and less aggressive tumors.

It is expected that with accumulation of tumors and with more experience gained with them, pathologists will be in a better position to recognize tumors with similar clinicopathologic features within this category. That ability would enable the reclassification of groups of tumors from the unclassified category as distinct entities, which is exemplified by the next few tumor types.

MUCINOUS TUBULAR AND SPINDLE CELL CARCINOMA

Mucinous tubular and spindle cell carcinoma is unique among renal tumors; in spite of showing a spindle cell (low-grade sarcomatoid) component, it usually does not behave in an aggressive manner.[68,69] Of the approximately 100 reported cases in the literature, only 1 has had local lymph node metastasis. This carcinoma predominantly occurs in females, ranging in age from 17 to 78 years (average 53 years). Grossly, it is usually well-circumscribed and located in the renal medulla. Histologically, the tumor is composed of elongated, interconnected tubules, many appearing straight and with slit-like lumina, solid compressed cords, and prominent low-grade spindle cell areas (**Fig. 5**). The nonspindled cells are low cuboidal, showing a small amount of amphophilic to eosinophilic cytoplasm, and low-grade bland-appearing nuclei. Myxoid stroma is present in virtually all cases.[70]

Ultrastructural evaluation done on a few cases shows close resemblance to the normal loop of

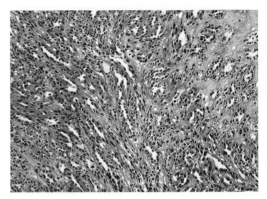

Fig. 5. Mucinous tubular and spindle cell carcinoma. In addition to the more round tubules and myxoid stroma (*left side*), elongated tubules and spindle cells with low-grade nuclei are seen in the right side of the figure (HE; 100×).

Henle.[68,69] Comparative genomic hybridization data available on a few cases shows frequent losses at chromosomes 1, 4q, 6, 8p, 11q, 13, 14 and 15, with gains at 11q, 16q, 17 and 20q. No evidence of VHL deletions, or trisomy 7 and 17 was found by fluorescence in situ hybridization analysis.[69,71]

ACQUIRED CYSTIC DISEASE OF KIDNEY-ASSOCIATED RENAL CELL CARCINOMA

The recently described RCC is associated with end-stage kidneys with acquired cystic disease.[72] Most, but not all, cases occur in patients on dialysis. The tumors are characteristically composed of large eosinophilic cells with prominent nucleoli, inter- and intracellular vacuoles (holes) imparting a vaguely cribriform architecture, and intratumoral oxalate crystals. Architecture is variable and there may be papillary, acinar, tubular, and sheet-like areas in variable proportions. Such architectural features may have led in the past to many of these being considered papillary, clear cell, or even unclassified RCC.[73]

Immunohistochemical staining for α-methylacyl-CoA racemase is strongly positive, whereas CK7 is mostly negative.[72] Some of these tumors behave aggressively, metastasize, and may cause death.

The other group of tumors that, because of their prominent clear cell cytology and often a papillary architecture might sometimes have been considered as unclassified RCC, is the translocation-associated RCC described above.

HEREDITARY FORMS OF RENAL TUMORS

The majority of renal neoplasms are sporadic, although a small percentage may be hereditary, such as the clear cell (conventional) RCCs associated with von Hippel-Lindau syndrome.[74–77] In all forms of inherited renal neoplasms, tumors are more likely to be diagnosed at an early age and are more likely to be multifocal and bilateral.[78] VHL disease is an autosomal dominant syndrome characterized by retinal hemangiomas, clear cell (conventional) RCCs and multiple renal cysts, cerebellar and spinal hemangioblastomas, pheochromocytomas, endocrine pancreatic tumors, and epididymal cystadenomas. The tumor-suppressor *VHL* gene, located at chromosome 3p25, can be inactivated by various mutations, loss of heterozygosity, hypermethylations, or other alterations in VHL modifier genes. Lack of normal VHL protein increases the HIF-1α levels, resulting in overexpression of endothelial growth factors and culminating in a hypervascular state seen in most VHL-related tumors, and possible tumorigenesis. Other familial non-VHL clear cell (conventional) RCC have been reported, most of which involve translocations of chromosome 3 including 3p14 (Fragile Histidine Triad), 3q13.3 and 3q21 genes, while a few others do not involve chromosome 3.[78,79]

Hereditary forms of type 1 PRCC is associated with activating mutations of *c-MET* proto-oncogene at chromosome 7q34.[80] Up-regulation of the gene results in the activation of a tyrosine kinase that is a receptor for hepatocyte growth factor/scatter factor, and is involved in angiogenesis, cellular motility, growth, invasion, and cellular differentiation. The renal tumors with trisomy 7 in this syndrome harbor *c-MET* mutants in two of the chromosome copies.[78] The renal tumors associated with hereditary leiomyomatosis and renal cell carcinoma syndrome are associated with mutations in *fumarate hydratase* (1q42.3-q43) gene, and often—though not always—show features of type 2 PRCC.[81]

Birt-Hogg-Dubé syndrome is another syndrome recently recognized to be related to multifocal and bilateral renal tumors. This autosomal dominant syndrome is characterized by cutaneous lesions (fibrofolliculomas, trichodiscomas, and acrochordons), spontaneous pneumothorax, bronchiectasis, and bronchospasm, colonic neoplasms, and lipomas, all occurring in conjunction with the renal tumors.[82,83] The renal tumors in the authors' experience are renal oncocytomas, chromophobe RCC, or predominantly oncocytic neoplasms displaying hybrid features of both types. A recent study on a large number of renal tumors from patients with BHD syndrome revealed similar findings.[84] The *BHD* gene has been mapped to chromosome 17p12-q11.2, and the exact mode of tumorigenesis is not yet completely elucidated.[83] Of the families identified with familial renal oncocytoma, a number of these have been subsequently found to have BHD syndrome.[78,79] Rarely, a constitutional reciprocal translocation between 8q24.1 and 9q34.3 has been reported in cases of bilateral, multifocal renal oncocytoma.[85]

IMMUNOHISTOCHEMISTRY IN THE DIFFERENTIAL DIAGNOSIS OF RENAL EPITHELIAL TUMORS, AND ITS UTILITY IN LIMITED MATERIAL

Immunohistochemistry is potentially useful to differentiate among renal tumor subtypes, as well as to confirm renal origin at a metastatic site.[5] Numerous antibodies have been used and reported to be of use in both these situations. Unfortunately many of these antibodies are able to discriminate only between better-differentiated tumor subtypes when light microscopic evaluation is sufficient to properly classify the tumor. In situations where the antibodies are most often required, such as high grade or poorly differentiated tumors, the staining characteristics have traditionally been unreliable. However, in our more recent experience some newly available antibodies are more useful in such situations. CA IX appears to be among the most useful in the differential diagnosis of renal cell tumors.[86,87] It shows diffuse and strong membranous reactivity in more than 90% of clear cell RCC, compared with absent or at the most focal, usually perinecrotic positivity in other common subtypes of renal cell tumors.[86,87] Interestingly, this diffuse reactivity is retained even in the sarcomatoid components of most cases of clear cell RCC.[11] The authors find some other antibodies of practical utility in the differential diagnosis of renal cell tumors, including c-kit (CD117), and CK7.[87,88]

Depending on the subtype and the stage of the renal tumor, as well as its expected biologic behavior, clinical comorbidities, and other aspects, multiple therapeutic options, including *in-situ* ablation of the tumor, targeted therapies in a neoadjuvant setting, or even watchful waiting in selected cases are now being offered to patients. In view of these developments, availability of a robust and dependable panel of immunohistochemical stains has become even more important, as pathologists are now frequently being asked to render diagnosis on limited material. Using a select panel of five antibodies—CA IX, CK7, c-kit, racemase, and CD10—the authors recently reported more than 90% diagnostic accuracy on in vivo needle-core biopsies of renal cell tumors (**Table 1**). This indicates that if pathologists are provided with adequate biopsy samples, close attention to cytomorphologic features together with a judicious use

Table 1
Immunohistochemical profile of common renal cortical tumor subtypes using a small, practical panel of antibodies

Antibody	Clear Cell	Papillary	Chromophobe	Oncocytoma
CA IX	++, Diffuse membranous	±, Focal, predominantly perinecrotic and tips of papillae	–	–
CD10	++, Diffuse membranous	+, Focal to diffuse, usually luminal membranous	±, Focal cytoplasmic	–
CK7	–	++	++, Cytoplasmic with peripheral accentuation	–
Racemase	±	++	±, Focal cytoplasmic	±, Focal cytoplasmic
c-kit	–	–	++	+

of immunohistochemistry will allow for an accurate diagnosis in the overwhelming majority of the cases.[88]

In summary, recent advances in the study of renal neoplasms have allowed pathologists to match the morphologic phenotype to the genotype, as well as clinical behavior in a more accurate manner. It has allowed us to do away with entities, such as "granular" and "sarcomatoid" RCC, which we now know do not exist as specific tumor types. Pathologists have also realized that Fuhrman's nuclear grading scheme is applicable to clear cell RCC but its application for other tumor types is debatable and needs further evaluation. Antigen expression within renal tumor subtypes is genetically driven and can be used, to a certain extent, to properly classify tumors. Antigen expression at the cellular level may also of great utility in evaluating targeted therapy, and the pathologist will play an important role in the development, characterization, and evaluation of targeted therapy in these diseases.

REFERENCES

1. Thoenes W, Storkel S, Rumpelt HJ. Human chromophobe cell renal carcinoma. Virchows Arch B Cell Pathol Incl Mol Pathol 1985;48:207–17.
2. Thoenes W, Storkel S, Rumpelt HJ. Histopathology and classification of renal cell tumors (adenomas, oncocytomas and carcinomas). The basic cytological and histopathological elements and their use for diagnostics. Pathol Res Pract 1986;181:125–43.
3. Kovacs G, Wilkens L, Papp T, et al. Differentiation between papillary and nonpapillary renal cell carcinomas by DNA analysis. J Natl Cancer Inst 1989; 81:527–30.
4. Linehan WM, Walther MM, Zbar B. The genetic basis of cancer of the kidney. J Urol 2003;170: 2163–72.
5. Reuter VE, Tickoo SK. Adult renal tumors. In: Mills Carter, Greenson Oberman, Reuter Stoler, editors. Sternberg's diagnostic surgical pathology. 4th edition. Philadelphia: Lippincott Williams & Wilkins; 2004. p. 1955–99.
6. Motzer RJ, Hutson TE, Tomczak P, et al. Sunitinib versus interferon alfa in metastatic renal-cell carcinoma. N Engl J Med 2007;356:115–24.
7. Bonsib SM. Renal veins and venous extension in clear cell renal cell carcinoma. Mod Pathol 2007; 20:44–53.
8. Bonsib SM, Gibson D, Mhoon M, et al. Renal sinus involvement in renal cell carcinomas. Am J Surg Pathol 2000;24:451–8.
9. Thompson RH, Blute ML, Krambeck AE, et al. Patients with pT1 renal cell carcinoma who die from disease after nephrectomy may have unrecognized renal sinus fat invasion. Am J Surg Pathol 2007;31: 1089–93.
10. Reuter VE, Presti JC Jr. Contemporary approach to the classification of renal epithelial tumors. Semin Oncol 2000;27:124–37.
11. Tickoo SK, Alden D, Olgac S, et al. Immunohistochemical expression of hypoxia inducible factor-1alpha and its downstream molecules in sarcomatoid renal cell carcinoma. J Urol 2007;177:1258–63.
12. de Peralta-Venturina M, Moch H, Amin M, et al. Sarcomatoid differentiation in renal cell carcinoma: a study of 101 cases. Am J Surg Pathol 2001;25: 275–84.
13. Kovacs G, Erlandsson R, Boldog F, et al. Consistent chromosome 3p deletion and loss of heterozygosity in renal cell carcinoma. Proc Natl Acad Sci U S A 1988;85:1571–5.

14. Carroll PR, Murty VV, Reuter V, et al. Abnormalities at chromosome region 3p12–14 characterize clear cell renal carcinoma. Cancer Genet Cytogenet 1987;26: 253–9.
15. Nordenson I, Ljungberg B, Roos G. Chromosomes in renal carcinoma with reference to intratumor heterogeneity. Cancer Genet Cytogenet 1988;32: 35–41.
16. Walter TA, Berger CS, Sandberg AA. The cytogenetics of renal tumors. Where do we stand, where do we go? Cancer Genet Cytogenet 1989;43:15–34.
17. Teyssier JR, Ferre D. Chromosomal changes in renal cell carcinoma. No evidence for correlation with clinical stage. Cancer Genet Cytogenet 1990;45: 197–205.
18. Zbar B. Von Hippel-Lindau disease and sporadic renal cell carcinoma. Cancer Surv 1995;25:219–32.
19. Linehan WM. Molecular targeting of VHL gene pathway in clear cell kidney cancer. J Urol 2003;170: 593–4.
20. Pantuck AJ, Zeng G, Belldegrun AS, et al. Pathobiology, prognosis, and targeted therapy for renal cell carcinoma: exploiting the hypoxia-induced pathway. Clin Cancer Res 2003;9:4641–52.
21. Kim HL, Seligson D, Liu X, et al. Using protein expressions to predict survival in clear cell renal carcinoma. Clin Cancer Res 2004;10:5464–71.
22. Bui MH, Seligson D, Han KR, et al. Carbonic anhydrase IX is an independent predictor of survival in advanced renal clear cell carcinoma: implications for prognosis and therapy. Clin Cancer Res 2003; 9:802–11.
23. Bui MH, Visapaa H, Seligson D, et al. Prognostic value of carbonic anhydrase IX and KI67 as predictors of survival for renal clear cell carcinoma. J Urol 2004;171:2461–6.
24. Leibovich BC, Sheinin Y, Lohse CM, et al. Carbonic anhydrase IX is not an independent predictor of outcome for patients with clear cell renal cell carcinoma. J Clin Oncol 2007;25:4757–64.
25. Delahunt B, Eble JN. Papillary renal cell carcinoma: a clinicopathologic and immunohistochemical study of 105 tumors. Mod Pathol 1997;10:537–44.
26. Delahunt B, Eble JN, McCredie MR, et al. Morphologic typing of papillary renal cell carcinoma: comparison of growth kinetics and patient survival in 66 cases. Hum Pathol 2001;32:590–5.
27. Allory Y, Ouazana D, Boucher E, et al. Papillary renal cell carcinoma. Prognostic value of morphological subtypes in a clinicopathologic study of 43 cases. Virchows Arch 2003;442:336–42.
28. Jiang F, Richter J, Schraml P, et al. Chromosomal imbalances in papillary renal cell carcinoma: genetic differences between histological subtypes. Am J Pathol 1998;153:1467–73.
29. Amin MB, Tamboli P, Javidan J, et al. Prognostic impact of histologic subtyping of adult renal epithelial neoplasms: an experience of 405 cases. Am J Surg Pathol 2002;26:281–91.
30. Cheville JC, Lohse CM, Zincke H, et al. Comparisons of outcome and prognostic features among histologic subtypes of renal cell carcinoma. Am J Surg Pathol 2003;27:612–24.
31. Presti JC Jr, Rao PH, Chen Q, et al. Histopathological, cytogenetic, and molecular characterization of renal cortical tumors. Cancer Res 1991;51:1544–52.
32. Yoshida MA, Ohyashiki K, Ochi H, et al. Cytogenetic studies of tumor tissue from patients with nonfamilial renal cell carcinoma. Cancer Res 1986;46:2139–47.
33. Dal Cin P, Gaeta J, Huben R, et al. Renal cortical tumors. Cytogenetic characterization. Am J Clin Pathol 1989;92:408–14.
34. Henn W, Zwergel T, Wullich B, et al. Bilateral multicentric papillary renal tumors with heteroclonal origin based on tissue-specific karyotype instability. Cancer 1993;72:1315–8.
35. Ishikawa I, Shikura N, Ozaki M. Papillary renal cell carcinoma with numeric changes of chromosomes in a long-term hemodialysis patient: a karyotype analysis. Am J Kidney Dis 1993;21:553–6.
36. van den Berg E, van der Hout AH, Oosterhuis JW, et al. Cytogenetic analysis of epithelial renal-cell tumors: relationship with a new histopathological classification. Int J Cancer 1993;55:223–7.
37. de Jong B, Molenaar IM, Leeuw JA, et al. Cytogenetics of a renal adenocarcinoma in a 2-year-old child. Cancer Genet Cytogenet 1986;21:165–9.
38. Schmidt L, Junker K, Nakaigawa N, et al. Novel mutations of the MET proto-oncogene in papillary renal carcinomas. Oncogene 1999;18:2343–50.
39. Tickoo SK, Reuter VE. Subtyping papillary renal cell carcinoma: a clinicopathologic study of 103 cases. Mod Pathol 2001;14:124A.
40. Argani P, Ladanyi M. Translocation carcinomas of the kidney. Clin Lab Med 2005;25:363–78.
41. Argani P, Antonescu CR, Couturier J, et al. PRCC-TFE3 renal carcinomas: morphologic, immunohistochemical, ultrastructural, and molecular analysis of an entity associated with the t(X;1) (p11.2;q21). Am J Surg Pathol 2002;26:1553–66.
42. Argani P, Olgac S, Tickoo SK, et al. Xp11 translocation renal cell carcinoma in adults: expanded clinical, pathologic, and genetic spectrum. Am J Surg Pathol 2007;31:1149–60.
43. Argani P, Lae M, Hutchinson B, et al. Renal carcinomas with the t(6;11) (p21;q12): clinicopathologic features and demonstration of the specific Alpha-TFEB gene fusion by immunohistochemistry, RT-PCR, and DNA PCR. Am J Surg Pathol 2005;29:230–40.
44. Weiss LM, Gelb AB, Medeiros LJ. Adult renal epithelial neoplasms. Am J Clin Pathol 1995;103:624–35.
45. Bugert P, Gaul C, Weber K, et al. Specific genetic changes of diagnostic importance in chromophobe renal cell carcinomas. Lab Invest 1997;76:203–8.

46. Schwerdtle RF, Storkel S, Neuhaus C, et al. Allelic losses at chromosomes 1p, 2p, 6p, 10p, 13q, 17p, and 21q significantly correlate with the chromophobe subtype of renal cell carcinoma. Cancer Res 1996;56:2927–30.

47. Kovacs A, Kovacs G. Low chromosome number in chromophobe renal cell carcinomas. Genes Chromosomes Cancer 1992;4:267–8.

48. Akhtar M, Al-Sohaibani MO, Haleem A, et al. Flow cytometric DNA analysis of chromophobe cell carcinoma of the kidney. J Urol Pathol 1996;4:15–23.

49. Crotty TB, Farrow GM, Lieber MM. Chromophobe cell renal carcinoma: clinicopathological features of 50 cases. J Urol 1995;154:964–7.

50. Motzer RJ, Bacik J, Mariani T, et al. Treatment outcome and survival associated with metastatic renal cell carcinoma of non-clear-cell histology. J Clin Oncol 2002;20:2376–81.

51. Amin MB, Crotty TB, Tickoo SK, et al. Renal oncocytoma: a reappraisal of morphologic features with clinicopathologic findings in 80 cases. Am J Surg Pathol 1997;21:1–12.

52. Perez-Ordonez B, Hamed G, Campbell S, et al. Renal oncocytoma: a clinicopathologic study of 70 cases. Am J Surg Pathol 1997;21:871–83.

53. Tickoo SK, Lee MW, Eble JN, et al. Ultrastructural observations on mitochondria and microvesicles in renal oncocytoma, chromophobe renal cell carcinoma, and eosinophilic variant of conventional (clear cell) renal cell carcinoma. Am J Surg Pathol 2000;24:1247–56.

54. Erlandson RA, Shek TW, Reuter VE. Diagnostic significance of mitochondria in four types of renal epithelial neoplasms: an ultrastructural study of 60 tumors. Ultrastruct Pathol 1997;21:409–17.

55. Tickoo SK, Reuter VE, Amin MB, et al. Renal oncocytosis: a morphologic study of fourteen cases. Am J Surg Pathol 1999;23:1094–101.

56. Srigley JR, Eble JN. Collecting duct carcinoma of kidney. Semin Diagn Pathol 1998;15:54–67.

57. Amin MB, Varma M, Tickoo SK, et al. Collecting duct carcinoma of the kidney. Adv Anat Pathol 1997;4:85–94.

58. Rumpelt HJ, Storkel S, Moll R, et al. Bellini duct carcinoma: further evidence for this rare variant of renal cell carcinoma. Histopathology 1991;18:115–22.

59. Tokuda N, Naito S, Matsuzaki O, et al. Collecting duct (Bellini duct) renal cell carcinoma: a nationwide survey in Japan. J Urol 2006;176:40–3.

60. Davis CJ, Mostofi FK, Sesterhenn IA. Renal medullary carcinoma. The seventh sickle cell nephropathy. Am J Surg Pathol 1995;19:1–11.

61. Avery RA, Harris JE, Davis CJ, et al. Renal medullary carcinoma: clinical and therapeutic aspects of a newly described tumor. Cancer 1996;78:128–32.

62. Adsay NV, deRoux SJ, Sakr W, et al. Cancer as a marker of genetic medical disease: an unusual case of medullary carcinoma of the kidney. Am J Surg Pathol 1998;22:260–4.

63. Swartz MA, Karth J, Schneider DT, et al. Renal medullary carcinoma: clinical, pathologic, immunohistochemical, and genetic analysis with pathogenetic implications. Urology 2002;60:1083–9.

64. MacLennan GT, Farrow GM, Bostwick DG. Low-grade collecting duct carcinoma of the kidney: report of 13 cases of low-grade mucinous tubulocystic renal carcinoma of possible collecting duct origin. Urology 1997;50:679–84.

65. Amin MB, Paraf F, Cheville JC, et al. Tubulocystic carcinoma of the kidney: clinicopathologic analysis of 29 cases of a distinctive rare subtype of renal cell carcinoma (RCC). Lab Invest 2004;84:137A.

66. Yang XJ, Zhou M, Hes O, et al. Tubulocystic carcinoma of the kidney: clinicopathologic and molecular characterization. Am J Surg Pathol 2008;32:177–87.

67. Eble JN, Sauter G, Epstein JI, et al, editors. Tumours of the kidney. WHO classification of tumours. Lyon (France): IARC Press; 2004. p. 10–1.

68. Parwani AV, Husain AN, Epstein JI, et al. Low-grade myxoid renal epithelial neoplasms with distal nephron differentiation. Hum Pathol 2001;32:506–12.

69. Srigley JR, Kapusta L, Reuter V, et al. Phenotypic, molecular and ultrastructural studies of a novel low grade renal epithelial neoplasm possibly related to the loop of Henle. Mod Pathol. 2002;12:182A.

70. Fine SW, Argani P, DeMarzo AM, et al. Expanding the histologic spectrum of mucinous tubular and spindle cell carcinoma of the kidney. Am J Surg Pathol 2006;30:1554–60.

71. Argani P, Netto G, Parwani A. Papillary renal cell carcinoma with low grade spindle cells lining angulated tubules: a mimic of mucinous tubular and spindle cell carcinoma. Mod Pathol 2008;21(Suppl 1):146A.

72. Tickoo SK, dePeralta-Venturina MN, Harik LR, et al. Spectrum of epithelial neoplasms in end-stage renal disease: an experience from 66 tumor-bearing kidneys with emphasis on histologic patterns distinct from those in sporadic adult renal neoplasia. Am J Surg Pathol 2006;30:141–53.

73. Sule N, Yakupoglu U, Shen SS, et al. Calcium oxalate deposition in renal cell carcinoma associated with acquired cystic kidney disease: a comprehensive study. Am J Surg Pathol 2005;29:443–51.

74. Poston CD, Jaffe GS, Lubensky IA, et al. Characterization of the renal pathology of a familial form of renal cell carcinoma associated with von Hippel-Lindau disease: clinical and molecular genetic implications. J Urol 1995;153:22–6.

75. Wagner JR, Linehan WM. Molecular genetics of renal cell carcinoma. Semin Urol Oncol 1996;14:244–9.

76. Bugert P, Kovacs G. Molecular differential diagnosis of renal cell carcinomas by microsatellite analysis. Am J Pathol 1996;149:2081–8.

77. Suzuki H, Ueda T, Komiya A, et al. Mutational state of von Hippel-Lindau and adenomatous polyposis coli genes in renal tumors. Oncology 1997;54:252–7.
78. Bodmer D, van den Hurk W, van Groningen JJ, et al. Understanding familial and non-familial renal cell cancer. Hum Mol Genet 2002;11:2489–98.
79. Takahashi M, Kahnoski R, Gross D, et al. Familial adult renal neoplasia. J Med Genet 2002;39:1–5.
80. Schmidt L, Duh FM, Chen F, et al. Germline and somatic mutations in the tyrosine kinase domain of the MET proto-oncogene in papillary renal carcinomas. Nat Genet 1997;16:68–73.
81. Merino MJ, Torres-Cabala C, Pinto P, et al. The morphologic spectrum of kidney tumors in hereditary leiomyomatosis and renal cell carcinoma (HLRCC) syndrome. Am J Surg Pathol 2007;31:1578–85.
82. Zbar B, Alvord WG, Glenn G, et al. Risk of renal and colonic neoplasms and spontaneous pneumothorax in the Birt-Hogg-Dube syndrome. Cancer Epidemiol Biomarkers Prev 2002;11:393–400.
83. Khoo SK, Giraud S, Kahnoski K, et al. Clinical and genetic studies of Birt-Hogg-Dube syndrome. J Med Genet 2002;39:906–12.
84. Pavlovich CP, Walther MM, Eyler RA, et al. Renal tumors in the Birt-Hogg-Dube syndrome. Am J Surg Pathol 2002;26:1542–52.
85. Teh BT, Blennow E, Giraud S, et al. Bilateral multiple renal oncocytomas and cysts associated with a constitutional translocation (8;9) (q24.1;q34.3) and a rare constitutional VHL missense substitution. Genes Chromosomes Cancer 1998;21:260–4.
86. Al-Ahmadie HA, Alden D, Qin L-X, et al. Carbonic anhydrase IX expression in clear cell renal cell carcinoma: an immunohistochemical study comparing two antibodies. Am J Surg Pathol 2008;32:377–82.
87. Tu JJ, Chen Y-T, Hyjek E, et al. Carbonic anhydrase IX as a highly sensitive and specific marker of clear cell renal cell carcinoma: A comparative immunohistochemical study using a panel of commonly utilized antibodies in the differential diagnosis of renal cell tumors. Mod Pathol 2005;18:169A.
88. Al-Ahmadie HA, Alden D, Olgac S, et al. The role of immunohistochemical evaluation of adult renal cortical tumors on core biopsy: an ex-vivo study. Mod Pathol 2007;20:134A.

Familial and Hereditary Renal Cancer Syndromes

Jonathan A. Coleman, MD

KEYWORDS

- Hereditary kidney cancer • von Hippel-Lindau
- Birt Hogg Dubé
- Hereditary leiomyomatosis renal cell carcinoma
- Hereditary papillary renal carcinoma • VHL

Hereditary kidney cancer and familial renal cancer syndromes comprise an important group of patients in which early screening and careful follow-up of affected individuals and their relatives can positively impact disease-related morbidity and survival. Statistics on the incidence and per capita increase in cases of kidney cancer have been well documented, although not so well understood is the true proportion of patients who have familial cancers. Others have estimated that 3% to 5% of patients who have renal cancer have inherited forms of disease; however, there is evidence that a familial history of renal cancer or associated cancer syndromes may be much more common.[1,2] Several factors may contribute to underreporting, including lack of available complete family history, low clinical suspicion at the time of evaluation, and the limited current understanding of genetically linked cancer syndromes.

Hereditary renal cancers (HRC) may be defined broadly as the finding of a single cancer or constellation of tumors in more than one first- or second-degree family member that may be passed on through germline mutations. Hereditary kidney cancer syndromes that have been identified with known gene mutations include von Hippel-Lindau disease (VHL), hereditary papillary renal cancer (HPRC), Birt-Hogg-Dubé syndrome (BHD), hereditary leiomyomatosis renal cell carcinoma syndrome (HLRCC), and tuberous sclerosis complex (TSC). Several other presumed heritable tumor groups have been observed but no direct mechanistic evidence has been discovered, as in patients who have familial renal oncocytoma, multilocular cystic nephroma and lymphoma.[1] Other hereditary cancer syndromes with increased risk of associated kidney cancer also have been reported, and it is likely that more may exist.

Improved techniques of genetic research have facilitated the relatively recent discovery of the mutations associated with many HRC syndromes. Before identification of the genes responsible, heritable kidney cancer was identified based on the constellation of clinical findings used to define the phenotypic manifestations of the syndrome. These findings still provide the best initial means for evaluating individuals suspected of having hereditary kidney cancer and for screening their relatives.

Screening approaches have been described for many of the known HRC syndromes based on the study of families that have these diseases and the ages at which relevant phenotypic expression may be identified.[3] Effective evaluation and treatment is approached best with a multidisciplinary team of physicians and nurses aware of the syndrome and it management. Often, frequent testing and imaging studies need to be coordinated between services, as do medical and surgical interventions when indicated. Combined approaches to care may help limit the risks to patients associated with the requirements of management, including radiographic exposure and surgical procedures.

Genetic testing, although available and highly reliable, must involve careful discussion of the many factors and consequences that come into play and should be performed by a trained genetic counselor. Many patients are intensely interested in pursuing genetic testing when there is a suspicion of a hereditary basis for their disease, but

Department of Surgery/Urology Division, Weill Cornell Medical College, Memorial Sloan Kettering Cancer Center, Box 12, 1275 York Avenue, NY 10021, USA
E-mail address: colemaj1@mskcc.org

Urol Clin N Am 35 (2008) 563–572
doi:10.1016/j.ucl.2008.07.014

they may not be fully aware of the ethical and legal issues that can be raised. These issues can include the duty to inform relatives, the impact on spousal relationships within the family, and prenatal and infant testing.[4] Many have raised concerns about discrimination in employment or insurance on the basis of a genetically inherited disease, prompting the passage of the Genetic Information Non-discrimination Act by the U.S. Congress in 2007. The expansion of the understanding of the human genome and the search for genetic causes for disease are promising but also are complex and challenging for both the individual and society.

Investigations of patients who have clinical manifestations of HRC syndromes have helped identify genes and associated germline mutations that result in cancerous and benign neoplasms in a variety of organ systems. Variable phenotypic expression within families has been recognized, although the mechanism remains unclear; it is speculated that possible environmental influences or epigenetic mechanisms are at play. Importantly, the finding of cancer genes related to the formation of seemingly unrelated tumors in separate organ systems has helped shed light on the pathogenesis of cancer in a variety of tissues and the common pathways they share.

Although familial forms of kidney cancer affect a limited group of patients, the investigation of these syndromes has had valuable impact on the management of renal cancer. For most major subtypes of renal cortical tumors there is an associated heritable form of the disease identified with a familial cohort. Screening of affected families and careful follow-up has provided a greater understanding of the natural history of these tumors, allowing insight into growth and other characteristics of the different forms of kidney cancer. Somatic mutations in these same genes have been found responsible for a large percentage of sporadic kidney cancers as well, forming the basis for an emerging understanding of the molecular pathogenesis for kidney cancer.

HEREDITARY KIDNEY CANCER SYNDROMES
von Hippel-Lindau Disease

In 1895, Dr. Eugen von Hippel, an ophthalmologist, described a 23-year-old patient who suffered progressive ocular angiomas causing blindness in both eyes. Years later, at the age of 47 years, this same patient developed notable neurologic progression of his disease and died; autopsy findings were reported by Brandt.[5] This report identified brain and ocular hemangioblastomas and pancreatic and renal cysts. Lindau, a Swedish pathologist, later linked the findings of brain,

spinal, and ocular hemangioblastomas as a single disease entity that could also be associated with pancreatic and renal cysts and tumors, which he reported in 1926.[5] The von Hippel-Lindau syndrome was named by Davison in 1936, who described the many manifestations of the disease. The syndrome includes several neoplasms, including brain and ocular hemangioblastomas, endolymphatic sac tumors of the ear, conventional clear cell renal cancer and renal cysts, pheochromocytoma, pancreatic neuroendocrine tumors and cysts, and cysts in the epididymis of the testis in men and of the broad ligament in women. In isolated cases pulmonary cysts have been seen, but as yet these cysts are not considered a part of the syndrome.

Genetics of von Hippel-Lindau disease

Genetic studies have identified the *VHL* gene located on the short arm of chromosome 3 (3p26-25).[6] The *VHL* gene and its product (pVHL) function as a tumor suppressor gene through the regulation of hypoxia-inducible factor 1-alpha (HIF1α) and hypoxia-inducible factor 2-alpha (HIF2α).[7] The VHL protein stabilizes HIF1α and HIF2α by forming a complex with elongin B and C in association with cullin-2.[8,9] Together the pVHL/elongin BC/cullin-2 complex binds to HIF1α and HIF2α and aid in targeting the bound HIF molecule for ubiquitin-mediated proteosomal degradation.[7] Under conditions of hypoxia, or when pVHL is dysfunctional because of mutation (pseudohypoxia), HIF is allowed to regulate several proteins involved in the pathways of angiogenesis and proliferation, including vascular endothelial growth factor, transforming growth factor alpha, and platelet-derived growth factor bets.[10] Mutations in *VHL* lead to dysregulation and overaccumulation of HIF1α and HIF2α, causing activation of pathways for neovascularization and cellular proliferation in target tissues.[11,12]

Inheritance of VHL is an autosomal dominant germline mutation resulting in a heterozygous, highly penetrant form of disease affecting 1 person in 36,000. The development of a second mutation causing deletion of the normal VHL allele leads to tumor formation in affected individuals. More than 300 different types of mutations have been described that involve the three exons of the *VHL* gene.[13,14] Differences in the phenotype associated with *VHL* mutations have been identified and are thought to be related to the location and type of mutation.[13–15] Clustering of certain tumor types from variations in phenotypic expression have been characterized broadly into four main groups (**Table 1**). Type 1 describes VHL kindreds who do not develop pheochromocytomas. In type 2

Table 1
Subtypes of von Hippel-Lindau (VHL) syndrome by phenotype

VHL Group	Phenotype	Genotype Mutations
Type 1	Low risk of pheochromocytoma	Deletions, truncations
Type 2	High risk of pheochromocytoma	Missense substitutions
Type 2a	Hemangiomas, low risk of renal cell carcinoma	—
Type 2b	Hemangiomas, high risk of renal cell carcinoma	—
Type 2c	Pheochromocytoma predominant	—

families, pheochromocytomas are more common; this category may be subdivided further into three subtypes: 2a has low risk for renal cancer, 2b has a high risk for renal cancer, and 2c has pheochromocytoma only.[16] It is unclear how these subtypes relate to forms of mutations in VHL and the resultant variety of seemingly dissimilar tumor types in an isolated number of organ systems.

Clinical features

All individuals who inherit *VHL* gene mutations express some form of the phenotype, although significant variation in the severity of disease can be seen even in families who share the same mutation.[17] Earliest manifestations, particularly ocular and brain tumors, can be seen in children and infants.[18] By age 25 years, most affected individuals have a detectable lesion.[3] Multiorgan involvement often requires the attention and coordination of clinical care by a number of specialties.

Screening and follow-up regimens for patients who have VHL have been described.[3] Ocular evaluation should be performed in neonates and followed annually. Neurologic, otologic, and endocrine evaluation of children should be initiated at age 8 years or earlier for any signs associated with central nervous system involvement or pheochromocytoma including tinnitus, vertigo, symptoms of loss of balance, palpitations, sweating, or frequent headaches. Abdominal imaging with ultrasound is recommended starting at age 8 years to evaluate the kidneys, adrenals, and pancreas. An MRI of the brain and spine is recommended at age 11 years. Routine CT scan imaging usually is initiated at about the age of 18 years and repeated as clinically indicated. When possible, efforts should be made to limit radiation exposure from frequent imaging studies.

Although ocular and central nervous system hemangiomas have been the most common finding and cause of morbidity for patients who have VHL, kidney cancer has been the leading cause of death. Renal lesions, found in 40% of patients who have VHL, typically are multifocal and bilateral with cystic and partly cystic lesions detected (**Fig. 1**). Management strategies focus on preservation of renal function and limiting intervention until solid tumors reach 3 cm in diameter on imaging studies.[19] Nephron-sparing surgery at the time of surgical intervention involves the removal of all appreciable lesions from the kidney with priority given to lesions containing solid components, although an attempt also should be made to remove more simple-appearing cystic lesions (**Fig. 2**). Because patients are at lifetime risk for forming tumors, repeat procedures commonly are necessary and hold a greater likelihood of complications, although reasonable functional outcomes can be obtained.[20,21] Minimally invasive approaches including laparoscopic and robotic partial nephrectomy for multiple tumors and percutaneous ablation procedures have been described with favorable results at experienced centers.[22–24] Long-term outcomes with regard to efficacy and renal function have not been reported.

Pheochromocytomas are detected in type 2 forms of the disease and can pose a significant threat to patients if unrecognized, particularly during surgery for hemangioblastomas where there is risk of severe bleeding. Functional adrenal studies

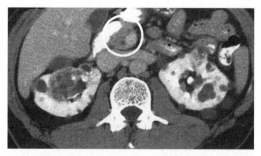

Fig. 1. Axial abdominal CT in a patient who has VHL demonstrating the spectrum of multifocal, bilateral renal cysts and semicystic and solid renal tumors. Small cysts and enhancing neuroendocrine tumor are visible in the uncinate process of the pancreas (*circled*).

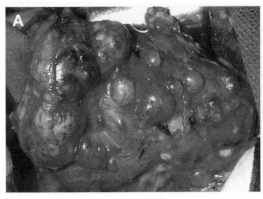
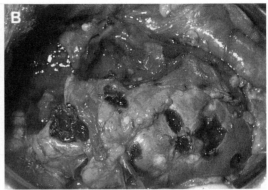

Fig. 2. Operative images of multiple renal cysts and tumors before (*left*) and after (*right*) excision with nephron-sparing techniques to treat all visible sites of disease.

should be performed annually in all patients who have VHL, and it is recommended that meta-iodobenzylguanidine studies be performed in patients who have positive functional studies because of the possibility of extra-adrenal para-gangliomas: these tumors may be multiple and reside in atypical sites including the paravesicle space (**Fig. 3**). Surgical excision using open or lap-aroscopic techniques typically is performed with perioperative adrenergic blockade. Pheochromo-cytomas involving the adrenal gland may be resected safely using partial adrenalectomy approaches to spare a portion of the normal adre-nal tissue and prevent the need for lifelong replacement steroid therapy.[25–27]

Hereditary Papillary Renal Carcinoma

Genetics of hereditary papillary renal carcinoma

Type 1 HPRC has been linked to an activating mutation in the c-Met oncogene on chromosome 7 (7q31).[28] Tumors from patients who have herita-ble and sporadic forms of type 1 papillary renal tumors have demonstrated this defect in c-Met,

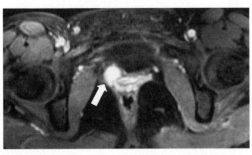

Fig. 3. Axial pelvic MRI of a female patient who has VHL demonstrating extra-adrenal right perivesical pheochromocytoma (*arrow*) at the bladder neck adja-cent to the ureter.

which causes aberrant activity of the intracellular tyrosine kinase domain of the membrane-bound c-Met receptor, producing the cascade of activa-tion of the hepatocyte growth factor/c-Met path-way.[29,30] Germline defects in c-Met have been identified in affected individuals; these defects may be passed on in an autosomal dominant pat-tern with variable penetrance, requiring trisomy of chromosome 7 with duplication of the mutated parental allele.[31,32]

Clinical features

HPRC was described initially in 1994 with further features of the disease discovered through screening and clinical studies of affected kindreds.[32,33] Patients inheriting the mutation show a variable degree of penetrance exhibited by the formation of renal tumors that often are multifocal and bilateral. As far as has been determined, the formation of papillary renal tumors is the only phenotype associated with the muta-tion. Median age of survival for affected members of these families was 52 years. Tumors often were discovered incidentally by radiographic screening.[32]

Management of patients who have HPRC includes genetic counseling and screening within families because of the often insidious nature of these occult tumors. Preferred treatment is surgi-cal excision with nephron-sparing approaches when possible, recognizing that these tumors often are multifocal. There are data suggesting that expectant management for HPRC tumors, allowing growth up to 3 cm in diameter before resection, does not jeopardize long-term survival or risk of metastases.[34]

Birt-Hogg-Dubé Syndrome

Hornstein and Knickenberg[35] were the first to describe a syndrome of perifollicular skin lesions of the face and trunk in three first-degree relatives from two generations suggesting an inherited dermatologic disorder associated with colonic polyposis. In 1977, 2 years after this earlier report, Drs. Birt, Hogg, and Dubé[36] presented their work on dermatologic findings in 15 of 70 family members who developed skin nodules after age 25 years characterizing a genodermatosis consisting of fibrofolliculomas, trichodiscomas, and acrochordons. More recently, the cutaneous findings described by Hornstein and Knickenberg[35] and by Birt and colleagues[36] have been shown to reflect a spectrum of a single dermatopathology resulting from abnormal deposits of folliculin, the BHD gene product.[37–40] Other associated findings now include renal tumors and pulmonary cysts or blebs that can cause spontaneous pneumothoraces.[41–43] A host of other disease processes also have been encountered in patients who have BHD, although inconsistent data have failed to prove an association with the known mutation. These entities include multinodular goiter, medullary thyroid carcinoma, parotid oncocytoma, and colonic polyposis.[39]

Genetics of Birt-Hogg-Dubé syndrome

Linkage studies have identified and localized the BHD gene to chromosome 17 (17p12q11) with inheritance demonstrating an autosomal dominant pattern.[28,44] The BHD gene codes for the folliculin protein which becomes abnormally truncated and accumulates in certain tissues of patients who have BHD gene mutations. Folliculin has been proposed to take part in regulation of the mammalian target of rapamycin pathway through recently described folliculin-interacting protein and 5′-AMP–activated protein kinase.[45] BHD normally is found in a variety of organs including brain, parotid gland, lung, pancreas, breast, prostate, kidney, and skin.[46] Absence of BHD mRNA in renal tumors from patients who have the syndrome supports its role as a tumor suppressor gene.

Clinical features

Before the identification of the gene, diagnosis of BHD was made on clinical findings alone. The classic triad of skin fibrofolliculomas, pulmonary cysts, and renal tumors, as characterized in original screening studies of multigenerational families, defined the phenotype.[37,47] Zbar and colleagues[48] reported on 223 screened members of 33 families with the disease, identifying 98 affected individuals with clinical findings and 13 haplotype carriers. Of the 111 persons who had genetic mutations in BHD, 14% had renal tumors, compared with 2% of the nonaffected family members. Spontaneous

pneumothoraces, seen predominantly in younger family members (< 40 years), were encountered in 23% of individuals who had BHD and in 1% of nonaffected family members. Only a subset of patients were evaluated with high-resolution lung CT scans, which identified lung cysts in 83% of family members who had BHD and in 10% of nonaffected relatives. Importantly, colonic polyps, which had been reported as part of the syndrome, were evaluated and found to have a statistically similar prevalence among family members with and without BHD. A more recent study in 50 new syndromic families demonstrated cutaneous manifestations in 90% of the family members who had BHD and renal tumors in 34% of affected relatives.[49]

Renal tumors found in BHD are not as uniform as those encountered in other HRC syndromes. Tumor histologies include chromophobe tumors, oncocytoma, clear cellcarcinoma, and hybrid oncocytic tumors composed of elements of oncocytoma and chromophobe tumors. The approximate distribution of these cancers was evaluated in 130 tumors from 30 confirmed cases: 50% were hybrid oncocytoma/chromophobe tumors, 34% were chromophobe tumors, 9% were conventional clear cellcarcinoma, 5% were oncocytoma, and 2 5% were papillary tumors.[50] Discordant histology was identified in 80% of patients, with a majority occurring as multifocal and/or bilateral tumors. Mean age at diagnosis in this cohort was 51 years.

Although clinical series suggest that most renal tumors may occur in older patients, significant tumors have been reported in younger patients. A locally invasive oncocytic tumor has been described in a 35-year-old man who developed subsequent pulmonary metastases of similar histology, and clear cell carcinoma has been resected from a patient at age 20 years.[51] Leter and colleagues[52] described a 39-year-old patient who had BHD and a renal tumor of mixed histology, including clear cell components, which developed distant progression resulting in death. These examples emphasize the heterogeneity of renal tumors encountered in BHD that may belie the indolent characteristics often attributed to the oncocytomas and chromophobe renal cancers associated with the disease. Untreated local tumor growth, even for more benign histologies, can result in progression to renal insufficiency and failure. For these reasons, tumors in patients who have BHD should be evaluated closely with nephron-sparing approaches initiated when possible. Intermediate data suggest that, as in patients who have VHL and HPRC, these tumors may be observed safely up to a size of 3 cm before intervention.[34,42]

Hereditary Leiomyomatosis Renal Cell Carcinoma

HLRCC is a rare inherited disorder in which affected individuals are at risk of developing cutaneous and uterine leiomyomas and renal cell carcinoma. Affected HLRCC kindreds are characterized by germline mutation of the Krebs cycle enzyme, fumarate hydratase (FH). Recent studies have suggested that a poorly defined but particularly lethal form of renal cell carcinoma is associated with HLRCC. These tumors initially were described histologically as papillary neoplasms but, because of their aggressive clinical behavior, were classified separately as type 2 papillary tumors or were potentially misclassified as collecting duct tumors.[53] With further experience and more refined characterization of the pathologic features, this nomenclature has been abandoned at experienced centers, and the term "HLRCC renal tumors" is used now.[54]

Genetics of hereditary leiomyomatosis renal cell carcinoma

Genetic alteration in HLRCC has been mapped to a region on chromosome 1 (1q42.3-43) containing 10 exons encoding for FH.[55,56] Germline mutations in the gene may be inherited in an autosomal dominant fashion. Phenotypic expression shows high penetrance for cutaneous leiomyomas and uterine fibromas, leading many early investigators to refer to the syndrome as "multiple cutaneous and uterine leiomyomatosis" or "multiple leiomyomatosis."[55,57] The occurrence of renal tumors among patients who have the syndrome has been estimated at 2% to 21%, a prevalence low enough to prompt some researchers to continue to differentiate between multiple leiomyomatosis and HLRCC although they represent the same disease.[56,58,59] In the syndrome of HLRCC, loss of heterozygosity reveals the tumor suppressor function of the gene, demonstrating impaired enzymatic function of FH with resultant effects in Krebs cycle catabolism.[60] Biallelic loss of FH in several models indicate that aberrant signaling may be mediated through HIF-dependent pathways, suggesting that mechanisms of pseudohypoxia may play a role in tumorigenesis in a similar fashion to VHL.[7,60,61] Reports of clear cell histology with FH mutation in a patient who had HLRCC may support a common mechanism of tumorigenesis through HIF activation.[62,63]

Clinical features

Clinical features of this disease are notable for uterine leiomyomas (fibroids) of significant severity for which, in a recently described series in the United States, as many as 89% of affected women underwent hysterectomy, 44% of them before the age of 30 years.[64] Isolated cases of uterine leiomyosarcomas have been reported. (Ylisaukko 2006) Most patients who have the syndrome harbor some form of cutaneous leiomyoma, although these lesions may be subtle and difficult to identify. These features of cutaneous lesions and a striking familial history for highly symptomatic uterine fibroids are helpful for clinical screening of patients before considering genetic testing that may be impractical or unreliable.

Patients who have renal tumors may exhibit an aggressive, rapidly progressive disease with evidence of advanced stages of metastases despite small primary tumor size.[65,66] The National Cancer Institute reported a series of 19 surgically managed patients who had HLRCC renal tumors; the median age was 39 years. Four of seven patients who had T1 tumors (≤ 7.0 cm) had regional lymph node involvement at the time of initial surgery, and 9 of 19 (49%) had evidence of metastases at the time of initial diagnosis.[67] Based on these observations, careful evaluation and regular follow-up, including annual abdominal imaging studies, is required for patients who have HLRCC. Suspicious renal lesions may appear partly cystic and need more frequent imaging evaluation. Interval growth or change in character may require intervention. The role of nephron-sparing surgery has been questioned in this setting, emphasizing that any surgical approach must be undertaken with care.[67,68] Preoperative positron emission tomography scans may prove beneficial when lymph node or nonlocalized disease is suspected.

Tuberous Sclerosis

An autosomal dominant disorder with renal manifestations, tuberous sclerosis affects as many as 1 person in 6000. TSC typically is characterized by seizures, mental retardation, and the development of hamartomas in multiple organs as a result of mutations in either the TSC1 or TSC2 gene.[69] The gene products hamartin and tuberin together form a protein complex that inhibits activation of the downstream pathways of mammalian target of rapamycin.[70] Aberrant function of the hamartin-tuberin complex through mutation reveals their role as tumor suppressor genes.

TSC1 has been mapped to chromosome 9 (9q34), and TSC2 is found on chromosome 16 (16p13.3).[71–73] Similar to other heritable syndromes, TSC may express a spectrum of severity depending on the type and location of the mutation. Differences in the phenotype have been linked to mutations in either TSC1 or TSC2 with more severe manifestations of the syndrome,

Table 2
Biologic basis of hereditary kidney tumor syndromes: comparison of described hereditary renal tumor syndromes with biologic and clinical correlates

Syndrome	Gene/Protein	Function	Pathway[a]	Phenotype
VHL	3p25/pVHL	Tumor suppressor	HIF	Central nervous system/ocular hemangioblastoma Endolymphatic sac tumors Pheochromocytoma Pancreatic neuroendocrine tumors Clear cell renal cell carcinoma
HPRC	7q31/c-Met tyrosine kinase domain	Oncogent	Hepatocyte growth factor /c-Met	Papillary type 1 renal cell carcinoma
BHD	17p12/folliculin	Tumor suppressor	Mammalian target of rapamycin	Fibrofolliculomas Pulmonary blebs Chromophobe/ oncocytoma/clear cell renal cell carcinoma
HLRCC	1q42.3/fumarase	Tumor suppressor	HIF	Skin leiomyoma Uterine leiomyoma/ sarcoma HLRCC renal cancer
TSC	TSC1 9q34TSC2 16p13.3 tubulin/ hamartin	Tumor suppressor	Mammalian target of rapamycin	Angiomyolipoma Clear cell renal cell carcinoma

[a] Putative primary pathway for mechanism of action.

including mental retardation and renal lesions, highly associated with mutations in *TSC2*.[74] Renal manifestations seen in TSC include renal angiomyolipomas, cysts, and clear cell carcinoma. In a series of 490 patients reported by Sancak and colleagues,[75] *TSC2* mutations were significantly associated with renal cysts, angiomyolipomas, and mental retardation. Rakowski and colleagues[76] reported on renal manifestations seen in 167 patients who had TSC and noted the presence of renal lesions in 58% of these patients. Of the patients who had renal lesions, 85% had angiomyolipomas, 45% had cysts, and 4% had clear cell carcinoma.

events underlying tumorigenesis in patients who have HRC and elucidating the downstream alterations resulting from these events, the mechanisms by which such processes can be blocked or reversed are being revealed slowly (**Table 2**). The discovery of these same mutations and involved pathways in nonrenal tumors and sporadic forms of cancer has helped usher in the era of molecular therapeutics and alternative management strategies for the treatment of kidney cancer. Awareness of and familiarity with known HRC syndromes surely will lead to the detection of new cancer syndromes and will broaden the understanding of cancer biology.

SUMMARY

The investigation of hereditary kidney cancer syndromes has uncovered the tremendous gains to be made in merging genetics research with clinical medicine. Through understanding the primary

REFERENCES

1. Zbar B, Glenn G, Merino M, et al. Familial renal carcinoma: clinical evaluation, clinical subtypes and risk of renal carcinoma development. J Urol 2007;177(2):461–5 [discussion: 465].

2. Rini BI, Campbell SC, Rathmell WK. Renal cell carcinoma. Curr Opin Oncol 2006;18(3):289–96.

3. Lonser RR, Glenn GM, Walther M, et al. von Hippel-Lindau disease. Lancet 2003;361(9374):2059–67.

4. Offit K, Thom P. Ethical and legal aspects of cancer genetic testing. Semin Oncol 2007;34(5):435–43.

5. Molino D, Sepe J, Anastasio P, et al. The history of von Hippel-Lindau disease. J Nephrol 2006; 19(Suppl 10):S119–23.

6. Seizinger BR, Rouleau GA, Ozelius LJ, et al. Von Hippel-Lindau disease maps to the region of chromosome 3 associated with renal cell carcinoma. Nature 1988;332(6161):268–9.

7. Isaacs JS, Jung YJ, Mole DR, et al. HIF overexpression correlates with biallelic loss of fumarate hydratase in renal cancer: novel role of fumarate in regulation of HIF stability. Cancer Cell 2005;8(2):143–53.

8. Pause A, Lee S, Worrell RA, et al. The von Hippel-Lindau tumor-suppressor gene product forms a stable complex with human CUL-2, a member of the Cdc53 family of proteins. Proc Natl Acad Sci U S A 1997;94(6):2156–61.

9. Lonergan KM, Iliopoulos O, Ohh M, et al. Regulation of hypoxia-inducible mRNAs by the von Hippel-Lindau tumor suppressor protein requires binding to complexes containing elongins B/C and Cul2. Mol Cell Biol 1998;18(2):732–41.

10. Bratslavsky G, Sudarshan S, Neckers L, et al. Pseudohypoxic pathways in renal cell carcinoma. Clin Cancer Res 2007;13(16):4667–71.

11. Linehan WM, Vasselli J, Srinivasan R, et al. Genetic basis of cancer of the kidney: disease-specific approaches to therapy. Clin Cancer Res 2004; 10(18 Pt 2):6282S–9S.

12. Kaelin WG Jr. The von Hippel-Lindau tumor suppressor protein and clear cell renal carcinoma. Clin Cancer Res 2007;13(2 Pt 2):680s–4s.

13. Gallou C, Chauveau D, Richard S, et al. Genotype-phenotype correlation in von Hippel-Lindau families with renal lesions. Hum Mutat 2004;24(3):215–24.

14. Ong KR, Woodward ER, Killick P, et al. Genotype-phenotype correlations in von Hippel-Lindau disease. Hum Mutat 2007;28(2):143–9.

15. Wong WT, Agron E, Coleman HR, et al. Genotype-phenotype correlation in von Hippel-Lindau disease with retinal angiomatosis. Arch Ophthalmol 2007; 125(2):239–45.

16. Chen F, Kishida T, Yao M, et al. Germline mutations in the von Hippel-Lindau disease tumor suppressor gene: correlations with phenotype. Hum Mutat 1995;5(1):66–75.

17. Maranchie JK, Afonso A, Albert PS, et al. Solid renal tumor severity in von Hippel Lindau disease is related to germline deletion length and location. Hum Mutat 2004;23(1):40–6.

18. Wong WT, Agron E, Coleman HR, et al. Clinical characterization of retinal capillary hemangioblastomas in a large population of patients with von Hippel-Lindau disease. Ophthalmology 2008;115(1):181–8.

19. Duffey BG, Choyke PL, Glenn G, et al. The relationship between renal tumor size and metastases in patients with von Hippel-Lindau disease. J Urol 2004;172(1):63–5.

20. Bratslavsky G, Liu JJ, Johnson AD, et al. Salvage partial nephrectomy for hereditary renal cancer: feasibility and outcomes. J Urol 2008;179(1):67–70.

21. Herring JC, Enquist EG, Chernoff A, et al. Parenchymal sparing surgery in patients with hereditary renal cell carcinoma: 10-year experience. J Urol 2001; 165(3):777–81.

22. Hwang JJ, Walther MM, Pautler SE, et al. Radio frequency ablation of small renal tumors: intermediate results. J Urol 2004;171(5):1814–8.

23. Coleman J, Singh A, Pinto P, et al. Radiofrequency-assisted laparoscopic partial nephrectomy: clinical and histologic results. J Endourol 2007;21(6): 600–5.

24. Rogers CG, Singh A, Blatt AM, et al. Robotic partial nephrectomy for complex renal tumors: surgical technique. Eur Urol 2008;53(3):514–23.

25. Baghai M, Thompson GB, Young WF Jr, et al. Pheochromocytomas and paragangliomas in von Hippel-Lindau disease: a role for laparoscopic and cortical-sparing surgery. Arch Surg 2002;137(6): 682–9.

26. Diner EK, Franks ME, Behari A, et al. Partial adrenalectomy: the National Cancer Institute experience. Urology 2005;66(1):19–23.

27. Nambirajan T, Leeb K, Neumann HP, et al. Laparoscopic adrenal surgery for recurrent tumours in patients with hereditary phaeochromocytoma. Eur Urol 2005;47(5):622–6.

28. Schmidt L, Duh FM, Chen F, et al. Germline and somatic mutations in the tyrosine kinase domain of the MET proto-oncogene in papillary renal carcinomas. Nat Genet 1997;16(1):68–73.

29. Dharmawardana PG, Giubellino A, Bottaro DP. Hereditary papillary renal carcinoma type I. Curr Mol Med 2004;4(8):855–68.

30. Choi JS, Kim MK, Seo JW, et al. MET expression in sporadic renal cell carcinomas. J Korean Med Sci 2006;21(4):672–7.

31. Fischer J, Palmedo G, von Knobloch R, et al. Duplication and overexpression of the mutant allele of the MET proto-oncogene in multiple hereditary papillary renal cell tumours. Oncogene 1998;17(6):733–9.

32. Zbar B, Glenn G, Lubensky I, et al. Hereditary papillary renal cell carcinoma: clinical studies in 10 families. J Urol 1995;153(3 Pt 2):907–12.

33. Zbar B, Tory K, Merino M, et al. Hereditary papillary renal cell carcinoma. J Urol 1994;151(3):561–6.

34. Grubb RL, Corbin NS, Choyke P, et al. Analysis of 3-cm tumor size threshold for intervention in patients with Birt-Hogg-Dubé and hereditary papillary renal

cancer [abstract 980]. San Antonio (TX): American Urological Association National Conference; 2005.

35. Hornstein OP, Knickenberg M. Perifollicular fibromatosis cutis with polyps of the colon—a cutaneo-intestinal syndrome sui generis. Arch Dermatol Res 1975; 253(2):161–75.

36. Birt AR, Hogg GR, Dube WJ. Hereditary multiple fibrofolliculomas with trichodiscomas and acrochordons. Arch Dermatol 1977;113(12):1674–7.

37. van Steensel MA, Verstraeten VL, Frank J, et al. Novel mutations in the BHD gene and absence of loss of heterozygosity in fibrofolliculomas of Birt-Hogg-Dube patients. J Invest Dermatol 2007; 127(3):588–93.

38. Schulz T, Ebschner U, Hartschuh W. Localized Birt-Hogg-Dube syndrome with prominent perivascular fibromas. Am J Dermatopathol 2001;23(2):149–53.

39. Adley BP, Smith ND, Nayar R, et al. Birt-Hogg-Dube syndrome: clinicopathologic findings and genetic alterations. Arch Pathol Lab Med 2006;130(12): 1865–70.

40. De la Torre C, Ocampo C, Doval IG, et al. Acrochordons are not a component of the Birt-Hogg-Dube syndrome: does this syndrome exist? Case reports and review of the literature. Am J Dermatopathol 1999;21(4):369–74.

41. Nickerson ML, Warren MB, Toro JR, et al. Mutations in a novel gene lead to kidney tumors, lung wall defects, and benign tumors of the hair follicle in patients with the Birt-Hogg-Dube syndrome. Cancer Cell 2002;2(2):157–64.

42. Pavlovich CP, Grubb RL 3rd, Hurley K, et al. Evaluation and management of renal tumors in the Birt-Hogg-Dube syndrome. J Urol 2005;173(5):1482–6.

43. Toro JR, Pautler SE, Stewart L, et al. Lung cysts, spontaneous pneumothorax, and genetic associations in 89 families with Birt-Hogg-Dube syndrome. Am J Respir Crit Care Med 2007;175(10):1044–53.

44. Khoo SK, Bradley M, Wong FK, et al. Birt-Hogg-Dube syndrome: mapping of a novel hereditary neoplasia gene to chromosome 17p12-q11.2. Oncogene 2001;20(37):5239–42.

45. Baba M, Hong SB, Sharma N, et al. Folliculin encoded by the BHD gene interacts with a binding protein, FNIP1, and AMPK, and is involved in AMPK and mTOR signaling. Proc Natl Acad Sci U S A 2006;103(42):15552–7.

46. Warren MB, Torres-Cabala CA, Turner ML, et al. Expression of Birt-Hogg-Dube gene mRNA in normal and neoplastic human tissues. Mod Pathol 2004; 17(8):998–1011.

47. Vincent A, Farley M, Chan E, et al. Birt-Hogg-Dube syndrome: a review of the literature and the differential diagnosis of firm facial papules. J Am Acad Dermatol 2003;49(4):698–705.

48. Zbar B, Alvord WG, Glenn G, et al. Risk of renal and colonic neoplasms and spontaneous pneumothorax

in the Birt-Hogg-Dube syndrome. Cancer Epidemiol Biomarkers Prev 2002;11(4):393–400.

49. Toro JR, Wei MH, Glenn G, et al. BHD mutations, clinical and molecular genetic investigations of Birt-Hogg-Dube Syndrome: a new series of 50 families and a review of published reports. J Med Genet 2008;45(6):321–31.

50. Pavlovich CP, Walther MM, Eyler RA, et al. Renal tumors in the Birt-Hogg-Dube syndrome. Am J Surg Pathol 2002;26(12):1542–52.

51. Khoo SK, Giraud S, Kahnoski K, et al. Clinical and genetic studies of Birt-Hogg-Dube syndrome. J Med Genet 2002;39(12):906–12.

52. Leter EM, Koopmans AK, Gille JJ, et al. Birt-Hogg-Dube syndrome: clinical and genetic studies of 20 families. J Invest Dermatol 2008;128(1):45–9.

53. Kiuru M, Launonen V. Hereditary leiomyomatosis and renal cell cancer (HLRCC). Curr Mol Med 2004;4(8):869–75.

54. Merino MJ, Torres-Cabala C, Pinto P, et al. The morphologic spectrum of kidney tumors in hereditary leiomyomatosis and renal cell carcinoma (HLRCC) syndrome. Am J Surg Pathol 2007; 31(10):1578–85.

55. Alam NA, Bevan S, Churchman M, et al. Localization of a gene (MCUL1) for multiple cutaneous leiomyomata and uterine fibroids to chromosome 1q42.3-q43. Am J Hum Genet 2001;68(5):1264–9.

56. Alam NA, Olpin S, Rowan A, et al. Missense mutations in fumarate hydratase in multiple cutaneous and uterine leiomyomatosis and renal cell cancer. J Mol Diagn 2005;7(4):437–43.

57. Tomlinson IP, Alam NA, Rowan AJ, et al. Germline mutations in FH predispose to dominantly inherited uterine fibroids, skin leiomyomata and papillary renal cell cancer. Nat Genet 2002;30(4):406–10.

58. Barker KT, Spendlove HE, Banu NS, et al. No evidence for epigenetic inactivation of fumarate hydratase in leiomyomas and leiomyosarcomas. Cancer Lett 2006;235(1):136–40.

59. Hodge JC, Morton CC. Genetic heterogeneity among uterine leiomyomata: insights into malignant progression. Hum Mol Genet 2007;16(Spec No 1): R7–13.

60. Pollard PJ, Briere JJ, Alam NA, et al. Accumulation of Krebs cycle intermediates and over-expression of HIF1alpha in tumours which result from germline FH and SDH mutations. Hum Mol Genet 2005; 14(15):2231–9.

61. Pollard PJ, Spencer-Dene B, Shukla D, et al. Targeted inactivation of fh1 causes proliferative renal cyst development and activation of the hypoxia pathway. Cancer Cell 2007;11(4):311–9.

62. Lehtonen HJ, Blanco I, Piulats JM, et al. Conventional renal cancer in a patient with fumarate hydratase mutation. Hum Pathol 2007; 38(5):793–6.

63. Sudarshan S, Linehan WM, Neckers L. HIF and fumarate hydratase in renal cancer. Br J Cancer 2007;96(3):403–7.

64. Toro JR, Nickerson ML, Wei MH, et al. Mutations in the fumarate hydratase gene cause hereditary leiomyomatosis and renal cell cancer in families in North America. Am J Hum Genet 2003;73(1):95–106.

65. Launonen V, Vierimaa O, Kiuru M, et al. Inherited susceptibility to uterine leiomyomas and renal cell cancer. Proc Natl Acad Sci U S A 2001;98(6): 3387–92.

66. Refae MA, Wong N, Patenaude F, et al. Hereditary leiomyomatosis and renal cell cancer: an unusual and aggressive form of hereditary renal carcinoma. Nat Clin Pract Oncol 2007;4(4):256–61.

67. Grubb RL 3rd, Franks ME, Toro J, et al. Hereditary leiomyomatosis and renal cell cancer: a syndrome associated with an aggressive form of inherited renal cancer. J Urol 2007;177(6):2074–9 [discussion: 2079–80].

68. Sudarshan S, Pinto PA, Neckers L, et al. Mechanisms of disease: hereditary leiomyomatosis and renal cell cancer—a distinct form of hereditary kidney cancer. Nat Clin Pract Urol 2007;4(2):104–10.

69. Al-Saleem T, Wessner LL, Scheithauer BW, et al. Malignant tumors of the kidney, brain, and soft tissues in children and young adults with the tuberous sclerosis complex. Cancer 1998;83(10): 2208–16.

70. Nellist M, Sancak O, Goedbloed M, et al. Functional characterisation of the TSC1-TSC2 complex to assess multiple TSC2 variants identified in single families affected by tuberous sclerosis complex. BMC Med Genet 2008;9(1):10.

71. Harris RM, Carter NP, Griffiths B, et al. Physical mapping within the tuberous sclerosis linkage group in region 9q32-q34. Genomics 1993;15(2):265–74.

72. Povey S, Burley MW, Attwood J, et al. Two loci for tuberous sclerosis: one on 9q34 and one on 16p13. Ann Hum Genet 1994;58(Pt 2):107–27.

73. Janssen B, Sampson J, van der Est M, et al. Refined localization of TSC1 by combined analysis of 9q34 and 16p13 data in 14 tuberous sclerosis families. Hum Genet 1994;94(4):437–40.

74. Au KS, Williams AT, Roach ES, et al. Genotype/phenotype correlation in 325 individuals referred for a diagnosis of tuberous sclerosis complex in the United States. Genet Med 2007;9(2):88–100.

75. Sancak O, Nellist M, Goedbloed M, et al. Mutational analysis of the TSC1 and TSC2 genes in a diagnostic setting: genotype–phenotype correlations and comparison of diagnostic DNA techniques in tuberous sclerosis complex. Eur J Hum Genet 2005;13(6): 731–41.

76. Rakowski SK, Winterkorn EB, Paul E, et al. Renal manifestations of tuberous sclerosis complex: incidence, prognosis, and predictive factors. Kidney Int 2006;70(10):1777–82.

Molecular Biology of Renal Cortical Tumors

Tobias Klatte, MD, Allan J. Pantuck, MD*

KEYWORDS
• HIF • VEGF • Raf • mTOR • Therapy • VHL

Renal cell carcinoma (RCC) accounts for approximately 3% of all adult malignancies. The incidence of RCC has been steadily increasing; in 2008, over 50,000 Americans will be newly diagnosed with RCC and over 12,000 will die of the disease.[1] The clinical management of RCC is rapidly evolving along with our understanding of the disease process. Historically, RCC was regarded as a single entity. Today, RCC is more accurately recognized as a family of cancers that results from distinct genetic abnormalities that have unique morphologic features but is uniformly derived from renal tubular epithelium. The current World Health Organization classification distinguishes clear cell, papillary, chromophobe, collecting duct, medullary, and unclassified RCC and other rare entities.[2] Advances in genetics and molecular biology have provided insight into the genetic alterations underlying the various renal cortical tumor types and the subsequent downstream molecular pathways involved in their tumorigenesis. These recognized differences reflect a greater sophistication in tumor analysis based on cytology, histology, genetic aberrations, glycogen content, electron microscopy of cytoplasmic microvesicles, and immunohistochemistry of intermediate filament proteins. For example, the discovery of the von Hippel-Lindau (VHL) tumor suppressor gene and the hypoxia-induced pathway in clear cell RCC has provided a valuable substrate for application of new strategies for diagnosis, patient selection, and targeted therapy.[3] This article briefly reviews the major genetic alterations underlying our current understanding of renal cortical tumors, addresses the crucial biologic pathways that become altered in the various RCC subtypes (**Fig. 1**), and gives some consideration to how an understanding of these key molecular receptors and ligands has permitted the rational and evidence-based development of pharmaceutic agents capable of specifically targeting key steps in these pathways.

HEREDITARY KIDNEY CANCER

Hereditary kidney cancer accounts for approximately 3% to 5% of RCC cases. Four well-described forms are distinguished, including VHL, hereditary papillary RCC (HPRCC), hereditary leiomyomatosis RCC (HLRCC), and Birt-Hogg-Dubé (BHD). These hereditary RCC forms are associated with specific, characteristic histologic subtypes. Principally, mutations can be "loss-of-function mutations" in tumor suppressor genes and "gain-of-function-mutations" in proto-oncogenes, which are then called oncogenes.

Research regarding hereditary clear cell RCC has led to the identification of a relevant gene locus on the short arm of chromosome 3.[4–6] This loss-of-function-mutation led to the assumption of the existence of a tumor suppressor gene, and subsequently, further research led to the identification of the VHL gene.[7] VHL is an hereditary cancer syndrome in which affected individuals have a high risk for the development of tumors in multiple organs, including cerebellar and spinal hemangioblastomas, retinal angiomas, pancreatic neuroendocrine tumors, pheochromocytoma, and bilateral, multifocal clear cell RCC.[8] Loss of VHL also occurs in about 50% of the sporadic clear cell RCCs.[9] VHL loss is strongly linked with activation of the hypoxia-induced pathway, which is discussed further later.

Department of Urology, Room B7-298 CHS, Box 951738, David Geffen School of Medicine, University of California–Los Angeles, Los Angeles, CA 90095-1738, USA
* Corresponding author.
E-mail address: apantuck@mednet.ucla.edu (A.J. Pantuck).

Urol Clin N Am 35 (2008) 573–580
doi:10.1016/j.ucl.2008.07.006

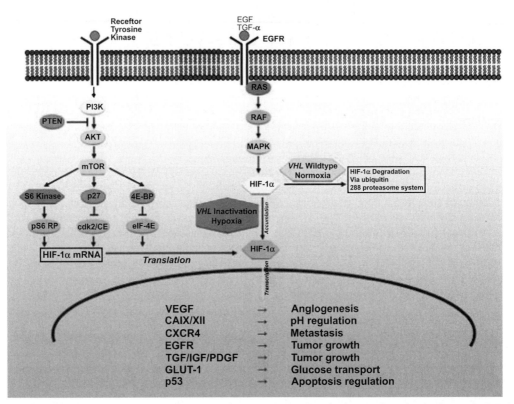

Fig.1. Crucial pathways involved in RCC biology and tumorigenesis (see further explanation in the text). CAIX/XII, carbonic anhydrase IX/XII; CXCR4, the chemokine receptor fusin; 4E-BP, eukaryotic initiation factor 4E binding protein; EGFR, epidermal growth factor receptor; eIF-4E, eukaryotic initiation factor 4E; HIF-1α, hypoxia-inducible factor 1α; GLUT-1, glucose transporter 1; IGF, insulin-like growth factor; MAPK, mitogen-activated protein kinase; mTOR, mammalian target of rapamycin; PDGF, platelet-derived growth factor; PI3K, phosphatidylinositol 3-kinase; PTEN, phosphatase and tensin homolog; TGF, transforming growth factor; VEGF, vascular endothelial growth factor.

Two hereditary forms of papillary RCC are distinguished: HPRCC and HLRCC.[8] The incidence of these hereditary forms of papillary RCC is low, and almost all cases seen by urologists are sporadic tumors.[10] HPRCC is a rare autosomal dominant syndrome associated with type 1 papillary RCC, which is caused by a gain-of-function mutation of the *MET* proto-oncogene on chromosome 7q, which encodes a transmembrane receptor (c-Met) that interacts with hepatocyte growth factor (HGF).[11,12] An early- and a late-onset phenotype of HPRCC have been described.[13,14] Mutations in the *MET* proto-oncogene are also observed in a small proportion of patients who have sporadic papillary RCC. HLRCC is caused by a mutation of the fumarate hydratase gene, leading to cutaneous and uterine leiomyomas (50% of the affected women have had a hysterectomy by age 30 years) and an aggressive type 2 papillary RCC.[8] About 50% of the affected patients present with nodal or distant metastases.[15] Accumulation of fumarate leads to activation of the hypoxia-induced pathway, because

fumarate is a very potent competitive inhibitor of hypoxia-inducible factor (HIF) prolyl hydroxylase.[8] Thus, increased expression of HIF-1, HIF-2, and glucose transporter 1 (GLUT-1) have been observed in HLRCC.[16]

The BHD syndrome is a genodermatosis characterized by cutaneous fibrofolliculomas, pulmonary cysts, spontaneous pneumothoraces, and an increased risk for multiple or bilateral RCCs.[17,18] BHD-associated histologic subtypes comprise chromophobe RCC (33%), hybrid chromophobe-oncocytic RCC (50%), clear cell RCC (9%), and oncocytoma (5%). The *BHD* gene is located on the short arm of chromosome 17 and has the characteristics of a tumor suppressor gene. Mutation or loss of the somatic allele of the *BHD* gene was detected in approximately 70% of BHD-associated renal tumors.[19]

HYPOXIA-INDUCED PATHWAY

The hypoxia-inducible pathway plays a key role in regulation of angiogenesis, glucose transport, glycolysis, pH control, epithelial proliferation, cell migration, and apoptosis of RCC, and is responsible for the ability of cancers to adapt to a hypoxic microenvironment. HIF-1 mediates responses to changes in tissue oxygenation by serving as a transcription factor.[20,21] HIF-1 was identified and purified as a nuclear factor that was induced in hypoxic cells and bound to hypoxia response element (HRE) of the erythropoietin gene.[22,23] HIF-1 is a heterodimer and consists of a constitutively expressed HIF-1β subunit and a HIF-1α subunit, the latter of which is controlled at the biosynthetic and posttranslational levels. The helix-loop-helix and the PER-ARNT-SIM (PAS) domains mediate heterodimer formation between the two subunits. In addition, HIF-2α can dimerize with HIF-1β and mediate HRE-dependent transcriptional activity.[24-28] In clear cell RCC, it has been suggested that HIF-2α activation may favor tumor proliferation and growth. A progressive switch to a HIF-2α response may occur during carcinogenesis.[29] This switch may be due to an antisense transcript of HIF-1α, which has been reported to be highly expressed in clear cell RCC.[30] A third member of the HIF-α subunit family, HIF-3α/inhibitory PAS protein, appears to function as an inhibitor and to negatively regulate transcriptional responses to hypoxia.[31]

HIF-1α expression increases with decreasing oxygen concentration, whereas HIF-1β is constitutively expressed.[32] Under normoxic conditions, tumor cells continuously synthesize, ubiquitinate, and degrade HIF-1α protein.[33-35] In addition, HIF-1α expression is controlled at the posttranslational level by hypoxia through the VHL protein.[34] The first 154 residues of VHL comprise the β domain, which interacts with HIF-1α or HIF-2α. Residues 155 to 213 of VHL comprise the α domain, which interacts with elongin C. An E3 ubiquitin–protein ligase complex consisting of VHL, elongin C, elongin B, CUL2, and RBX1 targets HIF-1α for ubiquitination and proteasomal degradation.[36] Under normoxic conditions, the interaction of VHL with HIF-1α or HIF-2α depends on the hydroxylation of the HIF-α subunit at two proline residues (Pro402, Pro564) by prolyl hydroxylases that utilize oxygen as a substrate.[37] Under hypoxic conditions, the unhydroxylated form of HIF-1α does not bind to VHL; therefore, it is not degraded by the ubiquitin-proteasome. Instead, it migrates into the nucleus, dimerizes with HIF-1β, and binds to HREs within hypoxia-inducible genes and activates their transcription. Another hypoxia-sensing region of HIF-1α is called the carboxy-terminal transactivation domain (CTAD). CTAD binds transcriptional coactivators p300 and CREB-binding protein (CBP) and activates transcription of genes under hypoxic conditions.[38] Hydroxylation of an asparaginyl residue in CTAD by factor-inhibiting HIF-1 during normoxic conditions down-regulates the function of the HIF-α transactivation domain by preventing recruitment of p300 and CBP.[21,39] In addition to hypoxia, inactivation of the VHL tumor suppressor gene leads to defective ubiquitination of HIF and subsequently to accumulation of HIF-1α, even in the absence of hypoxia.[34,36] VHL mutation or gene loss occurs in about 50% to 60% of sporadic clear cell RCC, suggesting a major impact of the VHL-HIF axis in clear cell RCC tumorigenesis.[9,36,40]

HIF-α dysregulation results in transcriptional activation of downstream hypoxia-inducible genes, which encode for growth and angiogenic factors such as vascular endothelial growth factor (VEGF), platelet-derived growth factor (PDGF), transforming growth factor α, and erythropoietin.[41] Genes encoding for enzymes that are involved in glucose uptake and metabolism (such as GLUT-1) and pH regulation (such as carbonic anhydrase IX [CAIX]) and matrix metalloproteinases are also activated by HIF-1 dysregulation. In addition, loss of VHL leads to (1) HIF-1–dependent inhibition of the CDH1 gene, which encodes E-cadherin, responsible for epithelial cell–cell adhesion and maintenance of tissue architecture,[42,43] and (2) activation of the MET proto-oncogene,[44] which encodes HGF receptor. In addition, loss of VHL leads to up-regulation of the chemokine receptor CXCR4 (also known as fusin), which plays a role in metastatic spread.[45]

Stimuli other than hypoxia and VHL loss can also induce HIF-1 activation and, subsequently, transcription of hypoxia-inducible genes. For example, signaling by way of the HER2/neu or type I insulin-like growth factor (IGF-I) receptor tyrosine kinase induces HIF-1 expression by an oxygen-independent mechanism.[46-48] IGF-I–induced HIF-1α synthesis depends on the mammalian target of rapamycin (mTOR)[49] and the mitogen-activated protein kinase pathways, further described in the following paragraphs.[47] Other growth factors, such as epidermal growth factor (EGF) and a dysfunctional phosphatase and tensin homolog deleted on chromosome 10 (PTEN) tumor suppressor gene, also increase HIF-1α expression through this signal transduction pathway.[49] In addition to growth factors, prostaglandin E2, thrombin, angiotensin II, 5-hydroxytryptamine, acetylcholine, and some nitric oxide donors can induce HIF-1 activation under normoxic conditions.[50-53]

MAMMALIAN TARGET OF RAPAMYCIN PATHWAY (PHOSPHATIDYLINOSITOL 3-KINASE/PROTEIN KINASE B PATHWAY)

The mTOR pathway has a central role in the regulation of cell growth, and increasing evidence suggests its dysregulation in cancer.[54] Receiving input from multiple signals, the pathway stimulates protein synthesis by phosphorylating key translational regulators such as S6 kinase. The mTOR pathway also contributes to many other critical cellular functions, including protein degradation and angiogenesis.

Signaling through the mTOR pathway begins with activation of membrane-bound receptor tyrosine kinases by circulating growth factor ligands. Their activation leads to autophosphorylation of tyrosine residues in the receptor and transphosphorylation of adaptor proteins. Activation of phosphatidylinositol 3-kinase (PI3K) subsequently occurs on binding of the src homology (SH2) domains to specific phosphotyrosine residues on the activated receptor or associated adaptor proteins. This causes the translocation of the enzyme to the membrane and results in activation of the p110 catalytic unit.[55,56] Subsequently, activated PI3K phosphorylates phosphatidylinositol-4-phosphate to phosphatidylinositol-3,4-biphosphate and phosphatidylinositol-4,5-biphosphate (PIP_2) to phosphatidylinositol-3,4,5-triphosphate (PIP_3).

Subsequent signaling from PI3K is mainly mediated through the recruitment of serine/threonine kinases Akt and PDK1.[57] Akt is relocated from the cytoplasm to the inner surface of the plasma membrane. On binding to PIP3, Akt undergoes conformation changes that allow the phosphorylation by PDK1 at Thr308 in the activation loop. Subsequent phosphorylation at Ser473 results in full Akt activation,[58] which translocates to the cytosol and nucleus where it phosphorylates its substrates. Akt promotes cell survival by inhibiting the proapoptotic activity of BAD and caspase-9 and by activating several antiapoptotic proteins such as IκB kinase and cyclic AMP response element binding protein.[59,60] Inhibition of glycogen synthase kinase-3, p21Cip1, and p27Kip1, and decreased proteolytic degradation of cyclin D1 promote cell cycle progression through the G1/S phase.[61,62]

mTOR is a downstream target of Akt that plays a critical role in the cell cycle progression from the G1 to the S phase. Activation of mTOR by Akt occurs through inactivation of the tuberous sclerosis complex (TSC). Unphosphorylated TSC2 (tuberin) is bound to TSC1 (hamartin) in a complex that blocks mTOR activation. This complex is disrupted when TSC2 is phosphorylated by Akt, relieving the Rheb GAP activity of TSC2 and allowing Rheb to bind ATP. In the presence of ATP, Rheb switches GDP to GTP and subsequently activates mTOR.[63] The major downstream targets of mTOR are the translational components ribosomal S6 kinase 1 (S6K1) and eukaryotic initiation factor 4E (eIF4E)-binding protein 1 (4E-BP1). Activation of S6K1 enhances the translation of mRNAs containing the 50-terminal oligopyrimidine tract, whereas phosphorylation of 4E-BP allows the release of eIF4E that facilitates mRNA binding to the 40S ribosomal subunit.[64] Thus, mTOR stimulates the translation of proteins required for the cell cycle progression from the G1 to the S phase.

PI3K signaling is terminated by degradation of PIP3, which can be mediated by two different phosphatases. SH2-containing inositol phosphatase dephosphorylates PIP_3 at position D5 and thereby produces phosphatidylinositol-3,4-biphosphat,[65] whereas PTEN removes the phosphate group at position D3, thereby converting PIP_3 back to PIP_2.[66] PTEN function is frequently impaired due to deletions or mutations, resulting in constitutive activation of Akt and upregulation of the mTOR pathway.

RAS/RAF/MEK/EXTRACELLULAR SIGNAL-REGULATED KINASE PATHWAY

The Ras/Raf/MEK/extracellular signal-regulated kinase (ERK) signaling pathway is an important mediator of tumor cell proliferation and angiogenesis. It plays a central role in regulating cell growth by transmitting signals from tyrosine kinase receptors such as EGF receptor, HER-2, VEGF receptor, PDGF receptor, and MET to the nucleus. Genes encoding for proteins involved in this pathway are frequently mutated in cancers.[67] Aberrant signaling and activation of this pathway leads to increased cell survival, cell cycle progression, proliferation, angiogenesis, invasion and metastasis, inhibition of apoptosis, and resistance to radiation and chemotherapy.[68]

Signaling starts by binding of a ligand to one the four erbB proteins, the most prominent of which is the erbB1 (EGF receptor). After binding of the ligands, the receptor becomes phosphorylated on tyrosine residues, allowing the Ras protein to bind GTP and to become active. Receptor binding is followed by activation of Raf kinase, which phosphorylates and activates MEK, which phosphorylates and activates ERK1/2, which phosphorylates several substrates involved in many cellular responses, including translation and transcription of important proteins such as S6 kinase.[68,69]

UBIQUITIN-PROTEASOME PATHWAY

Ubiquitin is a 9-KD protein that can activate proteins and target them for degradation by way of the 26S proteasome. Proteasomal degradation is a critical component of numerous cellular processes, including cell cycle regulation and antigen presentation.[70,71] Aberrations of ubiquitination have been linked with a wide variety of diseases, including cancer. Protein ubiquitination is accomplished by coordinated reaction with three enzymes: E1 (ubiquitin-activating enzyme), E2 (ubiquitin-conjugating enzyme), and the substrate-specific E3 (ubiquitin-ligase). The target protein has to be labeled with at least four ubiquitin monomers before it is recognized by the 26S proteasome,[72] which is the site for ATP-dependent degradation[73-75] and is composed of two major subunits, 20S and 19S. The 20S subunit is the core of the 26S proteasome and is made up of four heptameric protein rings. The 19S regulatory subunit assembles at each pore of the 20S subunit to form the 26S proteasome. On translocation into the proteasome, the target protein is degraded proteolytically. The 19S and the 20S subunit are necessary for correct proteolytic activity of the proteasome.[72,76]

THERAPEUTIC TARGETS

Unraveling the molecular pathways underlying RCC has permitted the design and development of agents specifically targeting these pathways, a process that is currently revolutionizing the medical management of RCC and making it a paradigm for the targeted therapy of solid malignancies. Numerous drugs are now available for the systemic therapy of RCC that interfere with certain targets of the previously described pathways. For example, sorafenib is a multikinase inhibitor that was initially described as a Raf kinase inhibitor but also targets VEGF receptor and PDGF receptor β. Sorafenib has been shown to be effective in phase II and III trials and is now approved for the treatment of advanced RCC.[77,78] Another multityrosine kinase inhibitor, sunitinib, inhibits VEGF receptor and PDGF receptor β, and showed a response rate of 31% in patients who had metastatic RCC, leading to prolongation of progression-free survival compared with interferon-α.[79] The monoclonal anti-VEGF antibody bevacizumab also led to improvement of progression-free survival.[80,81] The mTOR inhibitor temsirolimus (CCI-779) prolonged overall survival among patients who had metastatic RCC and poor prognosis.[82] Other inhibitors of mTOR, such as everolimus (RAD001), are currently being explored in clinical trials, as are antibodies and receptor tyrosine kinase inhibitors capable of inhibiting the c-Met pathway, a strategy that may have particular applicability to type I papillary RCC subtype. Targeting EGF receptor with erlotinib has been explored in RCC in combination with bevacizumab but did not provide additional clinical benefit compared with bevacizumab alone.[83] Targeting CAIX with an anti-CAIX antibody in 35 patients who had metastatic RCC showed a clinical benefit in 8 patients (23%), including 3 partial responses and 5 disease stabilizations.[84] Because CAIX is a ubiquitous transmembrane protein expressed by most clear cell RCCs, efforts are underway to develop imaging modalities based on CAIX binding. Finally, episodic reports indicate that the proteasome inhibitor bortezomib may be efficient for systemic therapy of metastatic RCC.[85]

SUMMARY

The last 10 years have witnessed a dramatic evolution in our understanding of RCC biology, which has led to the development of novel medical therapies and revolutionized the approach to RCC clinical management. This review considers the genetic basis of RCC and the molecular mechanisms of the hypoxia-induced pathway, the mTOR pathway, the ERK pathway, and the ubiquitin-proteasome pathway. All these molecular pathways are involved in RCC biology, tumorigenesis, and progression, and serve as the source of new rational treatment strategies based on the design of small molecule inhibitors directed against their targets.

REFERENCES

1. Jemal A, Siegel R, Ward E, et al. Cancer statistics. CA Cancer J Clin 2008;58(2):71–96.
2. Lopez-Beltran A, Scarpelli M, Montironi R, et al. 2004 WHO classification of the renal tumors of the adults. Eur Urol 2006;49(5):798–805.
3. Lam JS, Leppert JT, Figlin RA, et al. Role of molecular markers in the diagnosis and therapy of renal cell carcinoma. Urology 2005;66(5 Suppl):1–9.
4. Cohen AJ, Li FP, Berg S, et al. Hereditary renal-cell carcinoma associated with a chromosomal translocation. N Engl J Med 1979;301(11):592–5.
5. Kovacs G, Brusa P, deRiese W. Tissue-specific expression of a constitutional 3;6 translocation: development of multiple bilateral renal-cell carcinomas. Int J Cancer 1989;43(3):422–7.
6. Pathak S, Strong LC, Ferrell RE, et al. Familial renal cell carcinoma with a 3;11 chromosome translocation limited to tumor cells. Science 1982;217(4563):939–41.

7. Latif F, Tory K, Gnarra J, et al. Identification of the von Hippel-Lindau disease tumor suppressor gene. Science 1993;260(5112):1317–20.

8. Linehan WM, Pinto PA, Srinivasan R, et al. Identification of the genes for kidney cancer: opportunity for disease-specific targeted therapeutics. Clin Cancer Res 2007;13(2 Pt 2):671s–9s.

9. Patard JJ, Trinh QD, Karakiewicz PI, et al. Low CAIX expression and absence of VHL gene mutation are associated with tumor aggressiveness and poor survival in patients with renal cell carcinoma (RCC). J Urol (Suppl) 2007;77(4):[abstract 216].

10. Méjean A, Hopirtean V, Bazin JP, et al. Prognostic factors for the survival of patients with papillary renal cell carcinoma: meaning of histological typing and multifocality. J Urol 2003;170(3):764–7.

11. Fischer J, Palmedo G, von Knobloch R, et al. Duplication and overexpression of the mutant allele of the MET proto-oncogene in multiple hereditary papillary renal cell tumours. Oncogene 1998;17(6):733–9.

12. Zhuang Z, Park WS, Pack S, et al. Trisomy 7-harbouring non-random duplication of the mutant MET allele in hereditary papillary renal carcinomas. Nat Genet 1998;20(1):66–9.

13. Schmidt L, Junker K, Weirich G, et al. Two North American families with hereditary papillary renal carcinoma and identical novel mutations in the MET proto-oncogene. Cancer Res 1998;58(8):1719–22.

14. Schmidt LS, Nickerson ML, Angeloni D, et al. Early onset hereditary papillary renal carcinoma: germline missense mutations in the tyrosine kinase domain of the MET proto-oncogene. J Urol 2004;172(4 Pt 1):1256–61.

15. Grubb RL III, Franks ME, Toro J, et al. Hereditary leiomyomatosis and renal cell cancer: a syndrome associated with an aggressive form of inherited renal cancer. J Urol 2007;177(6):2074–9.

16. Isaacs JS, Jung YJ, Mole DR, et al. HIF overexpression correlates with biallelic loss of fumarate hydratase in renal cancer: novel role of fumarate in regulation of HIF stability. Cancer Cell 2005;8(2):143–53.

17. Birt AR, Hogg GR, Dube WJ. Hereditary multiple fibrofolliculomas with trichodiscomas and acrochordons. Arch Dermatol 1977;113(12):1674–7.

18. Pavlovich CP, Grubb RL III, Hurley K, et al. Evaluation and management of renal tumors in the Birt-Hogg-Dube syndrome. J Urol 2005;173(5):1482–6.

19. Vocke CD, Yang Y, Pavlovich CP, et al. High frequency of somatic frameshift BHD gene mutations in Birt-Hogg-Dube-associated renal tumors. J Natl Cancer Inst 2005;97(12):931–5.

20. Ivan M, Kaelin WG Jr. The von Hippel-Lindau tumor suppressor protein. Curr Opin Genet Dev 2001;11(1):27–34.

21. Lando D, Peet DJ, Whelan DA, et al. Asparagine hydroxylation of the HIF transactivation domain: a hypoxic switch. Science 2002;295(5556):858–61.

22. Semenza GL, Wang GL. A nuclear factor induced by hypoxia via de novo protein synthesis binds to the human erythropoietin gene enhancer at a site required for transcriptional activation. Mol Cell Biol 1992;12(12):5447–54.

23. Wang GL, Semenza GL. Purification and characterization of hypoxia-inducible factor 1. J Biol Chem 1995;270(3):1230–7.

24. Atzpodien J, Kuchler T, Wandert T, et al. Rapid deterioration in quality of life during interleukin-2- and alpha-interferon-based home therapy of renal cell carcinoma is associated with a good outcome. Br J Cancer 2003;89(1):50–4.

25. Ema M, Taya S, Yokotani N, et al. A novel bHLH-PAS factor with close sequence similarity to hypoxia-inducible factor 1alpha regulates the VEGF expression and is potentially involved in lung and vascular development. Proc Natl Acad Sci U S A 1997;94(9):4273–8.

26. Hogenesch JB, Chan WK, Jackiw VH, et al. Characterization of a subset of the basic-helix-loop-helix-PAS superfamily that interacts with components of the dioxin signaling pathway. J Biol Chem 1997;272(13):8581–93.

27. Jiang BH, Rue E, Wang GL, et al. DNA binding, and transactivation properties of hypoxia-inducible factor 1. J Biol Chem 1996;271(30):17771–8.

28. Tian H, McKnight SL, Russell DW. Endothelial PAS domain protein 1 (EPAS1), a transcription factor selectively expressed in endothelial cells. Genes Dev 1997;11(1):72–82.

29. Mandriota SJ, Turner KJ, Davies DR, et al. HIF activation identifies early lesions in VHL kidneys: evidence for site-specific tumor suppressor function in the nephron. Cancer Cell 2002;1(5):459–68.

30. Thrash-Bingham CA, Tartof KD. aHIF: a natural antisense transcript overexpressed in human renal cancer and during hypoxia. J Natl Cancer Inst 1999;91(2):143–51.

31. Makino Y, Kanopka A, Wilson WJ, et al. Inhibitory PAS domain protein (IPAS) is a hypoxia-inducible splicing variant of the hypoxia-inducible factor-3alpha locus. J Biol Chem 2002;277(36):32405–8.

32. Jiang BH, Semenza GL, Bauer C, et al. Hypoxia-inducible factor 1 levels vary exponentially over a physiologically relevant range of O2 tension. Am J Physiol 1996;271(4 Pt 1):C1172–1180.

33. Huang LE, Gu J, Schau M, et al. Regulation of hypoxia-inducible factor 1alpha is mediated by an O2-dependent degradation domain via the ubiquitin-proteasome pathway. Proc Natl Acad Sci U S A 1998;95(14):7987–92.

34. Maxwell PH, Wiesener MS, Chang GW, et al. The tumour suppressor protein VHL targets hypoxia-

inducible factors for oxygen-dependent proteolysis. Nature 1999;399(6733):271–5.

35. Salceda S, Caro J. Hypoxia-inducible factor 1alpha (HIF-1alpha) protein is rapidly degraded by the ubiquitin-proteasome system under normoxic conditions. Its stabilization by hypoxia depends on redox-induced changes. J Biol Chem 1997;272(36): 22642–7.

36. Ohh M, Park CW, Ivan M, et al. Ubiquitination of hypoxia-inducible factor requires direct binding to the beta-domain of the von Hippel-Lindau protein. Nat Cell Biol 2000;2(7):423–7.

37. Schofield CJ, Ratcliffe PJ. Oxygen sensing by HIF hydroxylases. Nat Rev Mol Cell Biol 2004;5(5): 343–54.

38. Ruas JL, Poellinger L, Pereira T. Role of CBP in regulating HIF-1-mediated activation of transcription. J Cell Sci 2005;118(Pt 2):301–11.

39. Mahon PC, Hirota K, Semenza GL. FIH-1: a novel protein that interacts with HIF-1alpha and VHL to mediate repression of HIF-1 transcriptional activity. Genes Dev 2001;15(20):2675–86.

40. Linehan WM, Walther MM, Zbar B. The genetic basis of cancer of the kidney. J Urol 2003;170(6 Pt 1): 2163–72.

41. Pantuck AJ, Zeng G, Belldegrun AS, et al. Pathobiology, prognosis, and targeted therapy for renal cell carcinoma: exploiting the hypoxia-induced pathway. Clin Cancer Res 2003;9(13): 4641–52.

42. Esteban MA, Tran MG, Harten SK, et al. Regulation of E-cadherin expression by VHL and hypoxia-inducible factor. Cancer Res 2006;66(7):3567–75.

43. Krishnamachary B, Zagzag D, Nagasawa H, et al. Hypoxia-inducible factor-1-dependent repression of E-cadherin in von Hippel-Lindau tumor suppressor-null renal cell carcinoma mediated by TCF3, ZFHX1A, and ZFHX1B. Cancer Res 2006;66(5): 2725–31.

44. Pennacchietti S, Michieli P, Galluzzo M, et al. Hypoxia promotes invasive growth by transcriptional activation of the MET protooncogene. Cancer Cell 2003;3(4):347–61.

45. Staller P, Sulitkova J, Lisztwan J, et al. Chemokine receptor CXCR4 downregulated by von Hippel-Lindau tumour suppressor pVHL. Nature 2003; 425(6955):307–11.

46. Feldser D, Agani F, Iyer NV, et al. Reciprocal positive regulation of hypoxia-inducible factor 1alpha and insulin-like growth factor 2. Cancer Res 1999;59(16): 3915–8.

47. Fukuda R, Hirota K, Fan F, et al. Insulin-like growth factor 1 induces hypoxia-inducible factor 1-mediated vascular endothelial growth factor expression, which is dependent on MAP kinase and phosphatidylinositol 3-kinase signaling in colon cancer cells. J Biol Chem 2002;277(41):38205–11.

48. Laughner E, Taghavi P, Chiles K, et al. HER2 (neu) signaling increases the rate of hypoxia-inducible factor 1alpha (HIF-1alpha) synthesis: novel mechanism for HIF-1-mediated vascular endothelial growth factor expression. Mol Cell Biol 2001;21(12): 3995–4004.

49. Zhong H, Chiles K, Feldser D, et al. Modulation of hypoxia-inducible factor 1alpha expression by the epidermal growth factor/phosphatidylinositol 3-kinase/PTEN/AKT/FRAP pathway in human prostate cancer cells: implications for tumor angiogenesis and therapeutics. Cancer Res 2000;60(6):1541–5.

50. Hirota K, Fukuda R, Takabuchi S, et al. Induction of hypoxia-inducible factor 1 activity by muscarinic acetylcholine receptor signaling. J Biol Chem 2004;279(40):41521–8.

51. Kasuno K, Takabuchi S, Fukuda K, et al. Nitric oxide induces hypoxia-inducible factor 1 activation that is dependent on MAPK and phosphatidylinositol 3-kinase signaling. J Biol Chem 2004;279(4):2550–8.

52. Pagé EL, Robitaille GA, Pouyssegur J, et al. Induction of hypoxia-inducible factor-1alpha by transcriptional and translational mechanisms. J Biol Chem 2002;277(50):48403–9.

53. Richard DE, Berra E, Pouyssegur J. Nonhypoxic pathway mediates the induction of hypoxia-inducible factor 1alpha in vascular smooth muscle cells. J Biol Chem 2000;275(35):26765–71.

54. Sarbassov DD, Ali SM, Sabatini DM. Growing roles for the mTOR pathway. Curr Opin Cell Biol 2005; 17(6):596–603.

55. Cantley LC. The phosphoinositide 3-kinase pathway. Science 2002;296(5573):1655–7.

56. Luo J, Manning BD, Cantley LC. Targeting the PI3K-Akt pathway in human cancer: rationale and promise. Cancer Cell 2003;4(4):257–62.

57. Fresno Vara JA, Casado E, de CJ, et al. PI3K/Akt signalling pathway and cancer. Cancer Treat Rev 2004;30(2):193–204.

58. Nicholson KM, Anderson NG. The protein kinase B/Akt signalling pathway in human malignancy. Cell Signal 2002;14(5):381–95.

59. Datta SR, Brunet A, Greenberg ME. Cellular survival: a play in three Akts. Genes Dev 1999;13(22): 2905–27.

60. Downward J. PI 3-kinase, Akt and cell survival. Semin Cell Dev Biol 2004;15(2):177–82.

61. Chang F, Lee JT, Navolanic PM, et al. Involvement of PI3K/Akt pathway in cell cycle progression, apoptosis, and neoplastic transformation: a target for cancer chemotherapy. Leukemia 2003;17(3):590–603.

62. Liang J, Slingerland JM. Multiple roles of the PI3K/PKB (Akt) pathway in cell cycle progression. Cell Cycle 2003;2(4):339–45.

63. Manning BD, Cantley LC. United at last: the tuberous sclerosis complex gene products connect the phosphoinositide 3-kinase/Akt pathway to

mammalian target of rapamycin (mTOR) signalling. Biochem Soc Trans 2003;31(Pt 3):573–8.

64. Hay N, Sonenberg N. Upstream and downstream of mTOR. Genes Dev 2004;18(16):1926–45.

65. Damen JE, Liu L, Rosten P, et al. The 145-kDa protein induced to associate with Shc by multiple cytokines is an inositol tetraphosphate and phosphatidylinositol 3,4,5-triphosphate 5-phosphatase. Proc Natl Acad Sci U S A 1996;93(4):1689–93.

66. Cantley LC, Neel BG. New insights into tumor suppression: PTEN suppresses tumor formation by restraining the phosphoinositide 3-kinase/AKT pathway. Proc Natl Acad Sci U S A 1999;96(8):4240–5.

67. Eisenmann KM, VanBrocklin MW, Staffend NA, et al. Mitogen-activated protein kinase pathway-dependent tumor-specific survival signaling in melanoma cells through inactivation of the proapoptotic protein Bad. Cancer Res 2003;63(23):8330–7.

68. Sridhar SS, Hedley D, Siu LL. Raf kinase as a target for anticancer therapeutics. Mol Cancer Ther 2005; 4(4):677–85.

69. Kohno M, Pouyssegur J. Pharmacological inhibitors of the ERK signaling pathway: application as anticancer drugs. Prog Cell Cycle Res 2003;5:219–24.

70. Koepp DM, Harper JW, Elledge SJ. How the cyclin became a cyclin: regulated proteolysis in the cell cycle. Cell 1999;97(4):431–4.

71. Rock KL, Goldberg AL. Degradation of cell proteins and the generation of MHC class I-presented peptides. Annu Rev Immunol 1999;17:739–79.

72. Thrower JS, Hoffman L, Rechsteiner M, et al. Recognition of the polyubiquitin proteolytic signal. EMBO J 2000;19(1):94–102.

73. Arrigo AP, Tanaka K, Goldberg AL, et al. Identity of the 19S 'prosome' particle with the large multifunctional protease complex of mammalian cells (the proteasome). Nature 1988;331(6152):192–4.

74. Hough R, Pratt G, Rechsteiner M. Ubiquitin-lysozyme conjugates. Identification and characterization of an ATP-dependent protease from rabbit reticulocyte lysates. J Biol Chem 1986;261(5):2400–8.

75. Voges D, Zwickl P, Baumeister W. The 26S proteasome: a molecular machine designed for controlled proteolysis. Annu Rev Biochem 1999;68:1015–68.

76. Glickman MH, Rubin DM, Coux O, et al. A subcomplex of the proteasome regulatory particle required for ubiquitin-conjugate degradation and related to the COP9-signalosome and eIF3. Cell 1998;94(5):615–23.

77. Escudier B, Eisen T, Stadler WM, et al. Sorafenib in advanced clear-cell renal-cell carcinoma. N Engl J Med 2007;356(2):125–34.

78. Ratain MJ, Eisen T, Stadler WM, et al. Phase II placebo-controlled randomized discontinuation trial of sorafenib in patients with metastatic renal cell carcinoma. J Clin Oncol 2006;24(16):2505–12.

79. Motzer RJ, Hutson TE, Tomczak P, et al. Sunitinib versus interferon alfa in metastatic renal-cell carcinoma. N Engl J Med 2007;356(2):115–24.

80. Escudier B, Pluzanska A, Koralewski P, et al. Bevacizumab plus interferon alfa-2a for treatment of metastatic renal cell carcinoma: a randomised, double-blind phase III trial. Lancet 2007;370(9605):2103–11.

81. Yang JC, Haworth L, Sherry RM, et al. A randomized trial of bevacizumab, an anti-vascular endothelial growth factor antibody, for metastatic renal cancer. N Engl J Med 2003;349(5):427–34.

82. Hudes G, Carducci M, Tomczak P, et al. Temsirolimus, interferon alfa, or both for advanced renal-cell carcinoma. N Engl J Med 2007;356(22):2271–81.

83. Bukowski RM, Kabbinavar FF, Figlin RA, et al. Randomized phase II study of erlotinib combined with bevacizumab compared with bevacizumab alone in metastatic renal cell cancer. J Clin Oncol 2007; 25(29):4536–41.

84. Bleumer I, Oosterwijk E, Oosterwijk-Wakka JC, et al. A clinical trial with chimeric monoclonal antibody WX-G250 and low dose interleukin-2 pulsing scheme for advanced renal cell carcinoma. J Urol 2006;175(1):57–62.

85. Ronnen EA, Kondagunta GV, Motzer RJ. Medullary renal cell carcinoma and response to therapy with bortezomib. J Clin Oncol 2006;24(9):e14.

Epidemiology, Clinical Staging, and Presentation of Renal Cell Carcinoma

G. Joel DeCastro, MD, MPH*, James M. McKiernan, MD

KEYWORDS

- Renal cell carcinoma • Epidemiology

Renal cell carcinoma (RCC) accounts for 3% of all cancer diagnoses in the United States.[1] In 2007 there were approximately 51,200 new cases of RCC, and an estimated 12,900 deaths. When compared with 1971, these numbers represent a fivefold increase in new cases and a twofold increase in mortality.[2] In fact, the incidence of RCC has been steadily increasing since the early 1980s, from approximately 7.1 per 100,000 to 10.9 in 2002.[3]

The reasons behind this rise are multiple. The primary reason relates to the increased availability and use of abdominal imaging in the American health care system during the past 2 decades.[4] As a result, more renal masses are being diagnosed incidentally—that is, in the absence of symptoms typically associated with RCC.[5-7] In 1970 approximately 10% of RCCs were detected incidentally, compared with more than 60% in 1998.[8-11]

This shift in clinical presentation has had an important effect on the number of renal cancers detected as well as on the characteristics of the newly diagnosed lesions. The features of incidentally detected tumors tend to differ from symptomatic lesions in several respects. Incidentally detected renal masses tend to be smaller than their symptomatic counterparts.[7,12] Accordingly, the average size of diagnosed RCC masses has decreased significantly over the past 2 decades. In a review of the Memorial Sloan Kettering experience, Lee and colleagues[13] described the mean RCC tumor size at diagnosis in 1989 to be 7.8 cm, decreasing to 5.3 cm in 1998. Similarly,

Hollingsworth and colleagues[3] found that the rise in incidence of RCC between 1983 and 2002 (7.1 to 10.8 per 100,000) was mostly a result of tumors 4 cm or smaller in diameter.

CHANGES IN STAGE AT PRESENTATION

Incidentally detected RCC tends to be lower stage and more likely to be localized than symptomatic lesions at diagnosis.[8,12] Luciani and colleagues[8] examined over 1,000 consecutive patients who presented with RCC at a single institution between 1982 and 1997. Consistent with other studies, the proportion of tumors detected incidentally rose rapidly during this period (from 13% to 59%). At the same time, the proportion of clinical stage T1-T2 tumors increased from 49% to 74%, while the percentage of patients with M1 disease decreased from 20% to 10%. Similar patterns have been noted for pathologic stage. At Memorial Sloan Kettering, the proportion of renal tumors that were stage pT1 in 1989 was 4%, versus 22% in 2000.[13] However, since the hospital-based patient samples in these studies are composed mainly of patients who are at least being considered for surgery, they are likely to be biased toward those with lower stage, and thus resectable, disease.[11] Interpretation of this data as evidence of a downward stage migration of RCC may therefore be inaccurate.

Whereas small, localized renal masses are responsible for most incident cases today, the incidence of *all* stages of RCC, including advanced

Department of Urology, Columbia University/New York Presbyterian Hospital, Atchley Pavillion, 11th floor, 161 Fort Washington Avenue, New York, NY 10032, USA
* Corresponding author.
E-mail address: gjd16@columbia.edu (G.J. DeCastro).

Urol Clin N Am 35 (2008) 581–592
doi:10.1016/j.ucl.2008.07.005
0094-0143/08/$ – see front matter © 2008 Elsevier Inc. All rights reserved.

and metastatic disease, is on the rise. Hock and colleagues[14] compared incidence rates of RCC between 1973 to 1985 and 1986 to 1998 using the SEER (Surveillance Epidemiology and End Results) cancer registry. They found that localized disease rose by an annual 3.7% (95% CI 3.2–4.2), regional disease by 1.9% (95% CI 1.2–2.6), and distant metastatic disease by 0.68 (95% CI 0.1–1.3). Similarly findings have been echoed by other authors.[4]

CHANGES IN DEMOGRAPHICS

In addition to changes in disease characteristics at presentation, significant changes have been noted in the demographics of RCC. There continues to be a strong gender preponderance, with men accounting for two-thirds of RCC diagnoses and deaths.[15,16] Luciani and colleagues[8] found that the mean age of patients presenting with RCC has increased from a mean of 57 years in 1982 to 63 years in 1997. When restricted to incidentally detected tumors only, they found that mean age at detection increased to 64 years. More recently, the SEER cancer registry reported that median age at diagnosis between 2000 and 2004 was 65 years.[17] The causes for this shift in age at diagnosis are unclear. It may in part be the result of increased exposure to the health care system owing to a greater number of comorbidities as a patient ages.[8]

Race has also emerged as an important factor in the epidemiology of RCC. Using the SEER cancer registry, Vaishampayan and colleagues[18] found that between 1975 and 1998, incidence rates among blacks increased by 4.5% compared with 2.9% in whites. Similarly, Chow and colleagues[4] estimated the RCC incidence among white men between 1975 and 1995 to be 2.3%, compared with 3.9% in black men. During the same period white women had a 3.1% annual increase, while the rate in black women increased by 4.9% per year.

The reason why blacks have had a higher incidence rate of RCC during the past 2 decades is uncertain. There is no evidence that RCC in this population is being disproportionately detected via increased use of abdominal imaging. The underlying reason for this disparity is therefore likely to involve changes in the affected population itself.[18] For example, it is possible that there is increased exposure within this population to risk factors associated with RCC. As described in more detail later in this article, established risk factors for RCC such as obesity and hypertension affect the black population disproportionately.

Racial disparities have also been observed in mortality rates from RCC. The study by Vaishampayan and colleagues[18] found that between 1975 and 1998, the median disease-specific survival for all stages of RCC for blacks was 47 months, compared with 53 months for whites. When limited to those patients 60 years of age and younger with localized disease, the disparity in median survival rates between the two groups increased: 190 and 259 months, respectively (P < .01). In other words, the survival difference between black and white patients seems to be amplified in younger cohorts with less severe disease. Similar findings have been cited by other authors.[19]

Again, reasons for this difference are unclear. Racial disparities in cancer rates and outcomes exist for multiple solid organ neoplasms, including prostate and bladder cancer. However, while the poorer outcomes in bladder cancer can be in part explained by more advanced stage at presentation, racial disparities in survival for RCC are greatest among younger patients with localized disease.[18,20] Delayed presentation is therefore not a sufficient explanation for this phenomenon, and requires further study. With the exception of renal medullary carcinoma, predisposition to more malignant histologies in the black population do not seem to be borne out in the literature.[21]

In an analysis of the SEER cancer registry, Berndt and colleagues[22] examined the treatment patterns between blacks and whites diagnosed with RCC. They found that after adjusting for known disease- and patient-specific variables affecting surgical candidacy, blacks were less likely to undergo nephrectomy than whites (relative risk [RR] 0.93, 95% CI 0.9–0.96). Survival was significantly worse for blacks, although the disparity was reduced after controlling for comorbidities. It is therefore possible that the worse prognosis in blacks diagnosed with RCC can be partly explained by the increased prevalence of significant comorbidities in this population, as well as by their lower rate of surgical intervention.

MORTALITY RATES

Excellent 5-year survival rates have been reported for the small, localized masses that comprise the majority of newly diagnosed renal tumors today. Tsui and colleagues found that incidentally detected tumors were more likely to be smaller, lower stage, and lower grade than symptomatic lesions. Accordingly, 5-year disease-free survival (DFS) rates were 85.3% and 62.5%, respectively.

In their review of 4,000 patients who underwent nephrectomy between 1984 and 1999, Patard and colleagues[7] found that at 73 months DFS was 93% for incidentally detected tumors and 59% for symptomatic lesions. Similarly, Pantuck and colleagues[23] found a doubling of 5-year DFS rates for patients with RCC between the time periods of 1963 to 1973 and 1982 to 1992. They postulate that this improvement was mostly the result of an increasing proportion of smaller, incidentally detected tumors included in the analyses.

While the disease characteristics may have changed over the past 2 decades, aggressive treatment remains the standard for incident renal tumors. Between 1983 and 2002, the incidence of renal surgery increased from 0.9 to 3.6 per 100,000, mostly for tumors 4 cm or smaller.[3] Whether this is an appropriate extension of aggressive therapy remains to be determined.

In a review of the SEER cancer registry, Chow and colleagues[4] found that despite the increasing proportion of localized, incidentally detected RCCs, mortality rates continue to rise. This documented rise in mortality is likely to be in part the result of the concomitant increase in all stages of RCC, including advanced disease. But if the increasing incidence of RCC is primarily a result of smaller, localized tumors, and these are being addressed with effective surgical treatments, why have overall mortality rates not decreased? If these localized masses are being detected early in their progression before they advance and cause mortality, why has their treatment not effected a decrease in advanced disease and in disease-specific mortality? This "treatment disconnect" is the subject of much debate.[3,24]

As argued by Parsons and colleagues,[24] if the increase in overall incidence of RCC is primarily a result of the detection of earlier stages of the disease, we would expect a "screening effect" similar to that noted for prostate-specific antigen and prostate cancer. Namely, over a period of time, disease-specific mortality should decrease. However, the incidence of advanced disease continues to rise, as do mortality rates. This therefore begs the question of what risk these small, incidental masses truly represent, and therefore what constitutes appropriate therapy.

First, the conclusions about mortality rates that can be made from improved 5-year DFS statistics are limited, as this measure may not ultimately translate into decreased mortality. Using the SEER cancer registry, Welch and colleagues[25] found that the 5-year DFS rates for 20 selected malignancies all increased between 1950 and 1995. However, eventual mortality decreased for only 12 of 20 cancers during the same time period, and increased for the remainder. They concluded that improvements in 5-year DFS may not translate into eventual decreases in mortality, but may instead be affected by changes in diagnostic patterns.[25] Part of this explanation stems from the phenomenon of lead-time bias: in the case of RCC, smaller tumors being diagnosed and recognized earlier than in the past may give an artificial increase in survival time without affecting eventual mortality rates.[24,26] However, this presumes that a large percentage of these asymptomatic, incidentally detected renal masses are destined to progress. At this time there is insufficient evidence to suggest that this is true.

The increasing mortality rates and incidence of advanced stages of RCC represent a challenge to our current treatment paradigm for small, incidentally detected renal masses. It is possible that many of these lesions are unlikely to progress to advanced stages, or to result in mortality. This possibility, combined with an independently rising incidence of advanced disease, may provide part of the explanation as to why overall mortality rates for RCC are increasing. Examining the biology and natural course of incidentally detected renal masses may help in clarifying this dilemma. Therefore, in the absence of prospective clinical trials, observations taken from retrospective, active surveillance programs may provide meaningful insight into this issue.

In 2006, Chawla and colleagues[26] performed a meta-analysis of 234 renal lesions with a mean diameter of 2.6 cm followed on active surveillance at 10 institutions. At a mean follow-up of 34 months, the mean growth rate was estimated as 0.28 cm per year. Pathology was available in 46% of the cases, of which 92% (120 of 131) were confirmed as RCC variants. Within the subgroup of patients with documented RCC, a mean growth rate of 0.40 cm per year was observed. Development of metastases was seen in 1% of lesions (3 of 286) during follow-up. This review of the available world literature on surveillance of small solid renal lesions provides valuable insight into why the detection of these indolent lesions has not led to a demonstrable decrease in mortality from this disease.

In an analysis of a prospectively collected database of 482 renal masses resected between 2001 and 2005, Schachter and colleagues[27] found that of those lesions 4 cm or smaller in diameter (n = 228), 26% were benign, compared with 8% of lesions larger than 4 cm (n = 254). Similarly, in a large-scale study of more than 2,700 nephrectomy specimens, there was an inverse relationship between tumor size and benign histology: of tumors smaller than 1 cm, 46% were benign, versus 6% of those 7 cm or larger.[28] Similar patterns have been reported by other authors.[29] These findings suggest that many of the small masses that comprise the majority of incident RCCs today are more likely to be benign. However, more research is needed into the natural course of these cancers before clinical guidelines can be suggested.

RISK FACTORS
Smoking

There are myriad risk factors that have been linked to the development of RCC.[30–32] Smoking, obesity, and hypertension are the three most well-established factors associated with RCC. A recent review by Vineis and colleagues[33] revealed a relative risk of 1.5 to 2.0 for development of RCC in persons who smoke 20 or more cigarettes daily. Similarly, a cohort study of more than 350,000 Swedish men found a significantly increased risk of RCC in individuals with any smoking history.[34] More recently, a meta-analysis by Hunt and colleagues[35] in 2005 reviewed 19 case-control studies and 5 cohort studies (**Fig. 1**). In their comparison of "ever" versus "never" smokers, they found that the relative risk for RCC in smokers was 1.39 (95% CI 1.27–1.5). Among men, the relative risk was 1.54 (1.42–1.68), and in women 1.22 (1.09–1.36). There was also a significant dose-dependent effect, with relative risk increasing in those smoking more than 20 cigarettes per day compared with fewer than 10. In men, the relative risk was 2.03 (95% CI 1.51–2.74) versus 1.6 (95% CI 1.21–2.12). In women this dose-effect was less salient: 1.58 (95% CI 1.14–2.2) compared with 0.98 (95% CI 0.71–1.35). The authors explained this gender-based difference by the "maturity" of smoking patterns, that is, men are likely to have been smoking for a longer period of time than women.

Smoking cessation significantly decreased the relative risk of RCC after 10 years compared with those who had quit less than 10 years ago, but this difference was noted only in men (RR 1.75, 95% CI 1.41–2.18 versus 1.21, 95% CI 0.86–1.7). Similarly, Parker and colleagues[36] found that the risk of RCC decreased with increasing number of years after quitting smoking. After controlling for age, sex, body mass index (BMI), hypertension, and pack-years of smoking, for those having quit for 30 years or longer versus fewer than 30 years there was a 50% decrease in risk of developing RCC (odds ratio [OR] = 0.5, 95% CI 0.3–0.8).

Obesity

Obesity has long been considered an important risk factor for developing RCC. In the previously cited study, Chow and colleagues[34] divided patients into three groups based on increasing BMI. They found that those in the middle group had a 60% greater risk of developing RCC than those in the lower group, while the risk in the highest BMI group doubled (*P* < .01). In a recent large-scale study, 2 million Norwegian men and women were followed for a mean of 23 years between

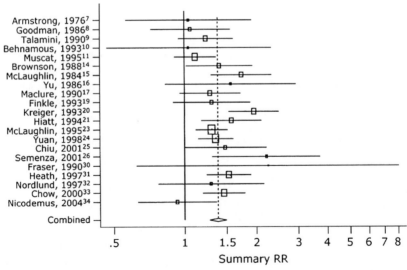

Fig. 1. Forrest plot for estimated RR for ever smokers Q-test for heterogeneity (*P* = .083). (*From* Hunt JD, van der Hel OL, McMillan GP, Boffetta P, Brennan P. Renal cell carcinoma in relation to cigarette smoking: meta-analysis of 24 studies. Int J Cancer 2005;114(1):101–8; with permission.)

1963 and 2001.[37] The calculated relative risk per unit of BMI for both men and women was 1.05 (95% CI 1.04–1.06). Compared with men of normal weight, men with a BMI of 35 to 39 had a relative risk of 1.89 (95% CI 1.22–2.94), increasing to 2.76 (95% CI 0.89–8.56) for a BMI of 40 or greater. In a more recent review of the literature, Calle and Kaaks[38] noted that compared with individuals with normal weight, the relative risk of developing RCC for persons with a BMI of 25 to 30 was 1.5, and 2.5 for those with BMI 30 or greater. The authors calculate that the population-attributable fraction of being overweight to the development of RCC in the United States is more than 30%.

The prevalence of obesity in the United States has increased dramatically over the past 3 decades. In 1980 approximately 15% of American adults were estimated to be obese, as defined by a BMI of 30 or greater. This estimate has more than doubled to 33% in 2004.[39] This trend must be considered when discussing the increasing incidence of RCC in the United States that has been largely attributed to abdominal imaging. As a well-established risk factor for RCC, the "epidemic" of obesity in the United States may help explain the rising incidence of all stages of RCC.

Multiple mechanisms of how obesity may be related to the development of RCC have been proposed. Researchers have pointed to the endocrine and metabolic role of adipose tissue.[38] Consequently, obesity may lead to increased release of adipokines such as free fatty acids and tumor necrosis factor-α. Together with the hyperinsulinemia and increased bioavailability of insulin-like growth factor-1 associated with obesity, these adipokines may lead to increased cell proliferation, decreased apoptosis, and tumorigenesis. As proposed by Gago-Dominguez and colleagues,[40] lipid peroxidation of proximal renal tubules may be carcinogenic, and increased lipid bioavailability in obese individuals may predispose them to RCC.

Hypertension

Multiple studies have demonstrated the association between hypertension and RCC. Chow and colleagues[34] noted a positive trend in RCC risk with increasing diastolic and systolic blood pressure. As shown in **Table 1**, compared with individuals with diastolic blood pressures less than 70 mm Hg, those with values higher than 90 mm Hg had a doubled risk of developing RCC. Similarly, compared with patients with a systolic blood pressure of less than 120 mm Hg, those with a value higher than 150 mm Hg had a 60% higher risk of RCC. In this same study, no association was found between blood pressure values and the risk of renal pelvis

cancer, which has a distinct histology and clinical course from RCC.

Grossman and colleagues[41] performed a meta-analysis using 13 case-control and longitudinal studies, each demonstrating an association between RCC and hypertension. The pooled adjusted odds ratio for hypertensive patients was 1.75 (95% CI 1.6–1.9). A large-scale, 20-year prospective study in Hawaii found a positive association between hypertension and RCC, even after adjusting for age, smoking, alcohol, and obesity.[42] The duration of diagnosed hypertension has also been found to be correlated with development of RCC.[43]

The incidence of hypertension has been increasing in the United States, with variations between 3% and 18% per year depending on age, gender, ethnicity, and body size.[44] The highest increases have been observed in blacks. According to the National Health Examination Survey, the prevalence of hypertension among this group in 1960 was 42.5%, compared with 28.3% in white men.[45] While this disparity diminished between 1960 and 1990, it has again increased since 1999.[46] The increase in hypertension rates in the United States may help to explain why the incidence of RCC has been rising, especially within the black community.

CLINICAL STAGING

The goal of any staging system is to combine available data about malignant disease to make accurate prognoses, as well as to assist in choosing appropriate treatment modalities and determine eligibility of patients for clinical trials. For the past 3 decades the TNM (tumor-node-metastases) staging system has been widely applied to RCC. Instituted in 1974 by the International Union Against Cancer[47] and the American Joint Committee on Cancer (AJCC), the TNM system has since undergone three major revisions, each time incorporating new data with the goal of improving its prognostic accuracy.

In 1987, the size cut-off between T1 and T2 was established as 2.5 cm, but was later demonstrated to have poor prognostic value.[48] In 1997, the size cut-off for T2 disease was increased to 7 cm, thereby improving the prognostic utility of the system (**Table 2**).[49,50]

In 2002, the T1 stage was divided into T1a and T1b substages, separated by a size cut-off of 4 cm.[51] This change was largely prompted by the increasing use of nephron-sparing surgery. Hafez and colleagues[52] examined 485 patients who underwent partial nephrectomy, and found that patients with tumors 4 cm or smaller in diameter

Table 1
Relative risk of RCC and renal-pelvic cancer among men according to smoking status, body mass index, and blood pressure

Variable	No. Men in Cohort (n = 362,992)	Follow-up Person-Year	Renal-Cell Cancer		Renal-Pelvis Cancer	
			No. Men with Cancer	Relative Risk (95% CI)	No. Men with Cancer	Relative Risk (95% CI)
Smoking status						
Nonsmoker	148,206	2,129,536	180	1.0 (ref)	18	1.0 (ref)
Former smoker	51,638	909,630	145	1.3 (1.0–1.6)	19	1.6 (0.9–3.1)
Current smoker	138,332	2,289,228	334	1.6 (1.3–1.9)	82	3.5 (2.1–5.8)
Unknown	25,816	455,494	100	1.6 (1.2–2.0)	17	2.6 (1.3–5.0)
Body mass index						
≤20.75	45,073	705,242	32	1.0 (ref)	15	1.0 (ref)
20.75–21.90	45,131	707,289	46	1.2 (0.7–1.8)	8	0.4 (0.2–1.0)
21.91–22.85	45,057	710,225	43	0.9 (0.6–1.5)	13	0.6 (0.3–1.3)
22.86–23.80	46,516	741,832	78	1.4 (0.9–2.1)	13	0.5 (0.2–1.1)
23.81–24.76	44,916	720,615	107	1.6 (1.1–2.4)	22	0.8 (0.4–1.5)
24.77–25.95	45,987	744,218	102	1.3 (0.8–1.9)	23	0.7 (0.4–1.5)
25.96–27.75	45,499	735,804	156	1.7 (1.1–2.7)	22	0.6 (0.3–1.1)
≥27.76	45,813	718,663	195	1.9 (1.3–2.7)	20	0.5 (0.2–1.0)
P for trend	—	—	—	<.001	—	.25
Diastolic blood pressure						
<70 mm Hg	40,407	540,097	12	1.0 (ref)	6	1.0 (ref)
70–79 mm Hg	110,461	1,695,116	96	1.4 (0.8–2.5)	22	0.6 (0.2–1.5)
80–89 mm Hg	139,998	2,317,216	273	1.7 (0.9–3.0)	49	0.6 (0.2–1.4)
90–99 mm Hg	57,060	974,597	272	2.1 (1.2–3.9)	46	0.7 (0.3–1.8)
100–109 mm Hg	11,627	187,114	78	2.3 (1.2–4.4)	10	0.6 (0.2–1.9)
≥110 mm Hg	4,439	69,748	28	2.2 (1.1–4.5)	3	0.6 (0.1–2.4)
P for trend	—	—	—	<.001	—	.74
Systolic blood pressure						
<120 mm Hg	39,010	554,138	28	1.0 (ref)	11	1.0 (ref)
120–129 mm Hg	100,884	1,561,807	103	1.1 (0.7–1.7)	28	0.8 (0.4–1.7)
130–139 mm Hg	108,165	1,754,399	192	1.5 (1.0–2.2)	29	0.6 (0.3–1.2)
140–149 mm Hg	67,661	1,122,128	168	1.4 (0.9–2.1)	27	0.6 (0.3–1.3)
150–159 mm Hg	27,361	458,505	124	1.6 (1.1–2.4)	20	0.7 (0.3–1.5)
≥160 mm Hg	20,911	332,911	144	1.7 (1.1–2.6)	21	0.7 (0.3–1.5)
P for trend	—	—	—	.007	—	.91

All models included age, smoking status, body-mass index (the weight in kilograms divided by the square of the height in meters), and diastolic blood pressure. CI denotes confidence interval.
Data from Chow WH, Gridley G, Fraumeni JF Jr., Jarvholm B. Obesity, hypertension, and the risk of kidney cancer in men. N Engl J Med 2000;343(18):1305–11.

had significantly better 5-year survival than those with tumors larger patients with than 4 cm. However, given that this study did not directly compare nephron-sparing to radical surgery, it was not designed to make any conclusions regarding surgical therapies. In fact, multiple studies have since found that tumors between 4 and 7 cm in diameter can be safely treated with partial nephrectomy, as long as they are anatomically amenable and that negative margins can be obtained.[53–55] Therefore, it is likely that the differences in survival observed in the Hafez study stemmed from inherent characteristics of larger masses rather than the choice of surgical therapy.[48]

However, the Hafez study did demonstrate a significant difference in survival based on the 4-cm

Table 2
Revisions of TNM staging for RCC

		TNM 1987[48]	TNM 1997[49]	TNM 2002[51]
Extent of Disease	T1	Restricted to kidney, ≤2.5 cm	Restricted to kidney, ≤7 cm	—
	T1a	—	—	Restricted to kidney, ≤4 cm
	T1b	—	—	Restricted to kidney, 4 cm–7 cm
	T2	Restricted to kidney, >2.5 cm	Restricted to kidney, >7 cm	Restricted to kidney, >7 cm
	T3a	Invading adrenal gland or perinephric fat within Gerota's fascia	Invading adrenal gland or perinephric fat within Gerota's fascia	Invading adrenal gland or perinephric fat within Gerota's fascia
	T3b	Extension into renal vein	Extension into renal vein or IVC below diaphragm	Extension into renal vein or IVC below diaphragm
	T3c	Extension into IVC below diaphragm	Extension into the IVC above the diaphragm	Extension into the IVC above the diaphragm or invasion into its wall
	T4	Extension beyond Gerota's fascia	Extension beyond Gerota's fascia	Extension beyond Gerota's fascia
	T4a	Extension into IVC above diaphragm	—	—
Nodal Status	Nx	Lymph nodes not assessed	Lymph nodes not assessed	Lymph nodes not assessed
	N0	No regional lymph node involvement	No regional lymph node involvement	No regional lymph node involvement
	N1	Single regional lymph node involved, ≤2 cm	Single regional lymph node involved	Single regional lymph node involved
	N2	Single regional lymph node involved, 2–5 cm	>1 regional lymph node involved	>1 regional lymph node involved
	N3	Single regional lymph node involved, >5 cm	—	—
Metastases	Mx	Distant metastases not assessed	Distant metastases not assessed	Distant metastases not assessed
	M0	No distant metastases	No distant metastases	No distant metastases
	M1	Distant metastases present	Distant metastases present	Distant metastases present

IVC, inferior vena cava; RCC, renal cell carcinoma; TNM, tumor-node-metastases.

cut-off, and this was subsequently incorporated into the TNM system in 2002. A multi-institutional study of more than 2,200 patients undergoing either radical or partial nephrectomy confirmed a significant difference in 5- and 10-year DFS between T1a, T1b, and T2 subgroups.[56] Other recent studies have also confirmed these findings.[56,57]

During the past several years, multiple researchers have attempted to fine-tune the size cut-off within the T1 substage, as well as between T1 and T2.[58–60] Ficarra and colleagues[59] found that using 5.5 cm to distinguish between T1a and T1b was more prognostically accurate for DFS than 4 cm. Similarly, a study from the Mayo Clinic found that a 5-cm cut-off was more predictive of DFS.[58] These marginal differences in proposed size cut-offs underline the importance of primary tumor size as well as the fact that size is a *continuous* variable that is predictive of survival.

The T2 stage is presently defined as any tumor greater than 7 cm in diameter with no extension beyond the kidney. It appears that at least for clear-cell RCC, tumors greater than 7 cm in diameter have a preponderance of extra-renal extension (ie, T3), thereby making the T2 stage a relative rarity in this subset.[61] In a review of 120 patients, Bonsib[61] found that 85% of tumors 4 cm or smaller in diameter were limited to the kidney (ie, T1a), and only 32% of those between 4 and 7 cm (ie, T1b). Of tumors larger than 7 cm in diameter, only 3% were localized to the kidney, and thus staged as T2. Nevertheless, within the T2 stage, there is increasing data indicating that not all organ-confined tumors larger than 7 cm carry the same risk.[62,63] Frank and colleagues[63] examined 544 patients who underwent radical nephrectomy for T2 RCC. With a median follow-up of almost 4 years, and after adjusting for the presence of regional and distant metastases, they found that tumors under 10 cm in diameter had a lower risk disease-specific mortality than larger lesions. Similarly, an international study that included more than 700 patients found that tumors less than 11 cm in diameter carried 5- and 10-year DFS rates of 73% and 65%, respectively, and 57% and 49% for tumors larger than 11 cm ($P < .001$).[62] The role of tumor size as an independent predictor of survival persisted on multivariate analysis.

The T3a category has engendered the most controversy, owing largely to its inclusion of various degrees of invasiveness and extension into one substage. At present, T3a describes any tumor that extends into the perinephric or renal sinus fat, or into the ipsilateral adrenal gland. While perinephric fat invasion is diagnosed on pathologic examination, extension into the ipsilateral adrenal gland can often be visualized on preoperative imaging. It is therefore difficult to separate the controversies regarding the T3a substage into clinical and pathologic arguments. Nevertheless, the main controversy regarding the T3a substage concerns the implied notion that extension into perinephric and renal sinus fat represents a similar risk level as adrenal invasion.[48]

A recent study from Columbia University demonstrated that T2 tumors had worse DFS than those staged as pT3a, that is, tumor size larger than 7 cm was a more important prognostic factor than the presence or absence of perinephric fat invasion.[64] With a median follow-up of 31 months, DFS at 5 years for patients with T2 and T3a disease was 68% and 85%, respectively, leading to the conclusion that tumor extension beyond the renal capsule is not as important as tumor size. Similarly, in a review of almost 1,800 patients Siemer and colleagues[65] found no independent prognostic value for perinephric fat involvement. Similar conclusions have been made by other researchers.[64] These findings call into question whether there is any prognostic significance to including perinephric fat invasion in a staging system.

The inclusion of ipsilateral adrenal involvement with the other features of T3a disease has also been criticized.[66] First, adrenal involvement in the absence of extension beyond Gerota's fascia is rare. In their prospective analysis of 128 nephrectomies for clinical stage T1 to T3b (N0M0) disease, Kletscher and colleagues[67] found that the incidence of ipsilateral adrenal involvement was less than 2%. Other studies have echoed these results.[68]

More important, however, is that adrenal involvement appears to be associated with significantly worse outcome than perinephric or renal sinus fat involvement.[65] Han and colleagues[69] noted that after radical nephrectomy, median survival and 5-year DFS for patients with ipsilateral adrenal gland involvement was 12.5 months and 0%, respectively, compared with 36 months and 36% for T3a patients with no adrenal involvement. This difference held in multivariate analysis controlling for grade and nodal status. Interestingly, they also found that the DFS of patients with adrenal involvement was statistically equivalent to that for patients with T4 disease.

Tumor extension into the venous system is not uncommon in newly diagnosed patients, with up to 9% having involvement of either the renal vein or vena cava.[70] The 2002 TNM system separates venous thrombus involvement into two categories: T3b includes thrombus extending into the renal vein and up to the inferior vena cava (IVC) below the diaphragm; and T3c describes tumors with thrombus in the IVC above the diaphragm. Findings by Moinzadeh and Libertino[71] argued against this separation. With a mean follow-up of 60 months, they found that 10-year survival of patients with renal vein involvement was 66%, versus 29% in patients with involvement of the infra-diaphragmatic IVC. Given this distinct difference in survival, separating T3b disease into two groups may be justified.

In an attempt to address some of the perceived deficiencies of the TNM staging system, new prognostic tools have been proposed that incorporate additional information. Lam and colleagues[66] recently reviewed the literature on the prognostic significance of variables not included in the TNM system, including tumor grade, histologic subtype, the presence of sarcomatoid features, tumor necrosis, collecting system invasion, and patient performance status. Each of these variables has been found to be associated with prognosis. As a result, some argue that a more comprehensive staging system should be used as a complement to the TNM system.

Nomograms are quantitative tools that provide percentage estimates of survival or recurrence based on both clinical and/or pathologic variables. Nomograms for RCC have a history dating back 20 years, when Elson and colleagues[72] classified patients based partly on Eastern Cooperative Oncology Group (ECOG) status. Since then, there have been several attempts to create more comprehensive and prognostically useful nomograms.

Kattan and colleagues[73] included tumor size, histology, and the presence or absence of symptoms at presentation into their nomogram, resulting in an accurate prognosticator of 5-year DFS. However, whereas past studies have shown a significant difference in survival between incidentally detected and symptomatic tumors,[12] the significance of symptoms does not seem to hold on multivariate analysis controlling for tumor size, stage, and grade.[74] In addition to symptoms, Frank and colleagues have devised the Stage, Size, Grade, Necrosis (SSIGN) staging system for clear-cell carcinoma, which also appears to provide accurate estimates of DFS at 5 years.

The UCLA Integrated Staging System (UISS) incorporates TNM, grade, and ECOG status. Using this data, it stratifies patients into five subgroups according to 2- and 5-ear DFS estimates.[75] The UISS has been found to be a more accurate predictor of risk for developing metastases.[76] A recent study by Cindolo and colleagues[77] compared the predictive accuracy of four prognostic models, including the Kattan and UISS nomograms. Their results suggest that the Kattan model was the most accurate for predicting survival.

SUMMARY

The increasing incidence of renal cell carcinoma over the past 2 decades can be in part explained by the expanding use of abdominal imaging. As a result, the vast majority of incident renal cancers today are small, localized, and asymptomatic. However, the well-documented rise in *all* stages of RCC, including advanced and metastatic disease, calls into question the nature of these asymptomatic lesions. The expected "screening effect" of detecting RCC when it is small and localized, with subsequent decreases in disease-specific mortality, has not been observed. In fact, disease-specific mortality is actually rising, especially in the black community.

The question of what these asymptomatic lesions represent is important. Since effective surgical therapies have not decreased overall mortality rates from RCC, we must question our present treatment paradigm of these incidentally detected cancers. Evidence from available active surveillance protocols provides some insight into the natural course of these masses, but the evidence is as of yet insufficient to establish clinical standards. As a result, the treatment of incidentally detected masses using aggressive, extirpative therapies remains the norm, but with more minimally invasive options as well as energy ablative therapies being increasingly employed.

Racial disparities in the incidence of RCC may be in part explained by the preponderance of two well-established risk factors for RCC in the black population. Multiple studies have shown that both hypertension and obesity are indeed associated with RCC, although the exact mechanism of the relationship has yet to be elucidated. Blacks are particularly affected by these risk factors, which may help to explain the increasing incidence of RCC in this population. Effective interventions aimed at reducing obesity, hypertension, and smoking—especially in the most vulnerable populations—may help to reduce the incidence of RCC in the future.

REFERENCES

1. Jemal A, Siegel R, Ward E, et al. Cancer statistics, 2007. CA Cancer J Clin 2007;57:43–66.
2. Silverberg E, Holleb AI. Cancer statistics, 1971. CA Cancer J Clin 1971;21:13–31.
3. Hollingsworth JM, Miller DC, Daignault S, et al. Rising incidence of small renal masses: a need to reassess treatment effect. J Natl Cancer Inst 2006; 98(18):1331–4.

4. Chow WH, Devesa SS, Warren JL, et al. Rising incidence of renal cell cancer in the United States. JAMA 1999;281:1628–31.

5. Homma Y, Kawabe K, Kitamura T, et al. Increased incidental detection and reduced mortality in renal cancer—recent retrospective analysis at eight institutions. Int J Urol 1995;2(2):77–80.

6. Bretheau D, Koutani A, Lechevallier E, et al. A French national epidemiologic survey on renal cell carcinoma. Oncology Committee of the Association Francaise d'Urologie. Cancer 1998;82(3):538–44.

7. Patard JJ, Rodriguez A, Rioux-Leclercq N, et al. Prognostic significance of the mode of detection in renal tumours. BJU Int 2002;90(4):358–63.

8. Luciani LG, Cestari R, Tallarigo C. Incidental renal cell carcinoma—age and stage characterization and clinical implications: study of 1092 patients. Urology 2000;56(1):58–62.

9. Konnak JW, Grossman HB. Renal cell carcinoma as an incidental finding. J Urol 1985;134(6):1094–6.

10. Skinner DG, Colvin RB, Vermillion CD, et al. Diagnosis and management of renal cell carcinoma A clinical and pathologic study of 309 cases. Cancer 1971;28(5):1165–77.

11. Jayson M, Sanders H. Increased incidence of serendipitously discovered renal cell carcinoma. Urology 1998;51(2):203–5.

12. Tsui KH, Shvarts O, Smith RB, et al. Prognostic indicators for renal cell carcinoma: a multivariate analysis of 643 patients using the revised 1997 TNM staging criteria. J Urol 2000;163(4):1090–5.

13. Lee CT, Katz J, Shi W, et al. Surgical management of renal tumors 4 cm or less in a contemporary cohort. J Urol 2000;163(3):730–6.

14. Hock LM, Lynch J, Balaji KC. Increasing incidence of all stages of kidney cancer in the last 2 decades in the United States: an analysis of surveillance, epidemiology and end results program data. J Urol 2002;167(1):57–60.

15. Parkin CM, Whelan SL, Ferlay J, et alIn: Cancer incidence in five continents, Vol VIII. Lyon (France): International Agency for Research on Cancer; 2002.

16. Aron M, Nguyen MM, Stein RJ, et al. Impact of gender in renal cell carcinoma: an analysis of the SEER database. Eur Urol 2008;54(1):133–40.

17. Ries LAG, Harkins D, Krapcho M, et al. SEER cancer statistics review, 1975–2004. Available at: http://seer.cancer.gov/csr/1975_2004/. Accessed February 1, 2008.

18. Vaishampayan UN, Do H, Hussain M, et al. Racial disparity in incidence patterns and outcome of kidney cancer. Urology 2003;62(6):1012–7.

19. Tripathi RT, Heilbrun LK, Jain V, et al. Racial disparity in outcomes of a clinical trial population with metastatic renal cell carcinoma. Urology 2006;68(2):296–301.

20. Ries LAG, Kosary CL, Hankey BF, et al. SEER cancer statistics review, 1973–1996. Available at: http://seer.cancer.gov/csr/1973_1996. Accessed February 1, 2008.

21. Davis CJJ, Mostofi FK, Sesterhenn IA. Renal medullary carcinoma. The seventh sickle cell nephropathy. Am J Surg Pathol 1995;19(1):1–11.

22. Berndt SI, Carter HB, Schoenberg MP, et al. Disparities in treatment and outcome for renal cell cancer among older black and white patients. J Clin Oncol 2007;25(24):3589–95.

23. Pantuck AJ, Zisman A, Belldegrun AS. The changing natural history of renal cell carcinoma. J Urol 2001;166(5):1611–23.

24. Parsons JK, Schoenberg MS, Carter HB. Incidental renal tumors: casting doubt on the efficacy of early intervention. Urology 2001;57(6):1013–5.

25. Welch HG, Schwartz LM, Woloshin S. Are increasing 5-year survival rates evidence of success against cancer? JAMA 2000;284(16):2975–8.

26. Chawla SN, Crispen PL, Hanlon AL, et al. The natural history of observed enhancing renal masses: meta-analysis and review of the world literature. J Urol 2006;175(2):425–31.

27. Schachter LR, Cookson MS, Chang SS, et al. Second prize: frequency of benign renal cortical tumors and histologic subtypes based on size in a contemporary series: what to tell our patients. J Endourol 2007;21(8):819–23.

28. Frank I, Blute ML, Cheville JC, et al. Solid renal tumors: an analysis of pathological features related to tumor size. J Urol 2003;170(6 Pt 1):2217–20.

29. Duchene DA, Lotan Y, Cadeddu JA, et al. Histopathology of surgically managed renal tumors: analysis of a contemporary series. Urology 2003;62(5):827–30.

30. Collins S, McKiernan J, Landman J. Update on the epidemiology and biology of renal cortical neoplasms. J Endourol 2006;20(12):975–85.

31. Lipworth L, Tarone RE, McLaughlin JK. The epidemiology of renal cell carcinoma. J Urol 2006;176(6):2353–8.

32. Murai M, Oya M. Renal cell carcinoma: etiology, incidence and epidemiology. Curr Opin Urol 2004;14(4):229–33.

33. Vineis P, Alavanja M, Buffler P, et al. Tobacco and cancer: recent epidemiological evidence. J Natl Cancer Inst 2004;96(2):99–106.

34. Chow WH, Gridley G, Fraumeni JF Jr, et al. Obesity, hypertension, and the risk of kidney cancer in men. N Engl J Med 2000;343(18):1305–11.

35. Hunt JD, van der Hel OL, McMillan GP, et al. Renal cell carcinoma in relation to cigarette smoking: meta-analysis of 24 studies. Int J Cancer 2005;114(1):101–8.

36. Parker AS, Cerhan JR, Janney CA, et al. Smoking cessation and renal cell carcinoma. Ann Epidemiol 2003;13(4):245–51.

37. Bjorge T, Tretli S, Engeland A. Relation of height and body mass index to renal cell carcinoma in two

million Norwegian men and women. Am J Epidemiol 2004;160(12):1168–76.

38. Calle EE, Kaaks R. Overweight, obesity and cancer: epidemiological evidence and proposed mechanisms. Nat Rev Cancer 2004;4(8):579–97.

39. Ogden CL, Carroll MD, Curtin LR, et al. Prevalence of overweight and obesity in the United States, 1999–2004. JAMA 2006;295(13):1549–55.

40. Gago-Dominguez M, Castelao JE, Yuan J-M, et al. Lipid peroxidation: a novel and unifying concept of the etiology of renal cell carcinoma. Cancer Causes Control 2002;13(3):287–93.

41. Grossman E, Messerli FH, Boyko V, et al. Is there an association between hypertension and cancer mortality? Am J Med 2002;112(6):479–86.

42. Grove JS, Nomura A, Severson RK, et al. The association of blood pressure with cancer incidence in a prospective study. Am J Epidemiol 1991;134(9):942–7.

43. Fraser GE, Phillips RL, Beeson WL. Hypertension, antihypertensive medication and risk of renal carcinoma in California Seventh-day Adventists. Int J Epidemiol 1990;19(4):832–8.

44. Hajjar I, Kotchen JM, Kotchen TA. Hypertension: trends in prevalence, incidence, and control. Annu Rev Public Health 2006;27:465–90.

45. Burt VL, Cutler JA, Higgins M, et al. Trends in the prevalence, awareness, treatment, and control of hypertension in the adult US population. Data from the health examination surveys, 1960–1991. Hypertension 1995;26:60–9.

46. Glover MJ, Greenlund KJ, Ayala C, et al. Racial/ethnic disparities in prevalence, treatment, and control of hypertension—United States, 1992–2002. MMWR Morb Mortal Wkly Rep 2005;54:7–9.

47. Harmer M. TNM classification of malignant tumors. 3rd edition. Geneva (Switzerland): International Union Against Cancer; 1974.

48. Howard GE, Wood CG. Staging refinements in renal cell carcinoma. Curr Opin Urol 2006;16(5):317–20.

49. Guinan P, Sobin LH, Algaba F, et al. TNM staging of renal carcinoma: workgroup No. 3. Cancer 1997;80(5):992–3.

50. Ficarra V, Novara G, Galfano A, et al. Neoplasm staging and organ-confined renal cell carcinoma: a systematic review. Eur Urol 2004;46(5):559–64.

51. Green FL, Page D, Morrow M. AJCC cancer staging manual. 6th edition. New York: Springer; 2002.

52. Hafez KS, Fergany AF, Novick AC. Nephron sparing surgery for localized renal cell carcinoma: impact of tumor size on patient survival, tumor recurrence and TNM staging. J Urol 1999;162(6):1930–3.

53. Leibovich BC, Blute ML, Cheville JC, et al. Nephron sparing surgery for appropriately selected renal cell carcinoma between 4 and 7 cm results in outcome similar to radical nephrectomy. J Urol 2004;171(3):1066–70.

54. Patard JJ, Shvarts O, Lam JS, et al. Safety and efficacy of partial nephrectomy for all T1 tumors based on an international multicenter experience. J Urol 2004;171(6 Pt 1):2181–5.

55. Mitchell RE, Gilbert SM, Murphy AM, et al. Partial nephrectomy and radical nephrectomy offer similar cancer outcomes in renal cortical tumors 4 cm or larger. Urology 2006;67(2):260–4.

56. Ficarra V, Schips L, Guillè F, et al. Multiinstitutional European validation of the 2002 TNM staging system in conventional and papillary localized renal cell carcinoma. Cancer 2005;104(5):968–74.

57. Salama ME, Guru K, Stricker H, et al. pT1 substaging in renal cell carcinoma: validation of the 2002 TNM staging modification of malignant renal epithelial tumors. J Urol 2005;173(5):1492–5.

58. Cheville JC, Blute ML, Zincke H, et al. Stage pT1 conventional (clear cell) renal cell carcinoma: pathological features associated with cancer specific survival. J Urol 2001;166(2):453–6.

59. Ficarra V, Guille F, Schips L, et al. Proposal for revision of the TNM classification system for renal cell carcinoma. Cancer 2005;104(10):2116–23.

60. Zisman A, Pantuck AJ, Chao D, et al. Reevaluation of the 1997 TNM classification for renal cell carcinoma: T1 and T2 cutoff point at 4.5 rather than 7 cm better correlates with clinical outcome. J Urol 2001;166(1):54–8.

61. Bonsib SM. T2 clear cell renal cell carcinoma is a rare entity: a study of 120 clear cell renal cell carcinomas. J Urol 2005;174(4 Pt 1):1199–202.

62. Klatte T, Patard JJ, Goel RH, et al. Prognostic impact of tumor size on pT2 RCC: an international multicenter experience. J Urol 2007;178(1):35–40.

63. Frank I, Blute ML, Leibovich BC, et al. pT2 Classification for renal cell carcinoma. Can its accuracy be improved? J Urol 2005;173(2):380–4.

64. Murphy AM, Gilbert SM, Katz AE, et al. Re-evaluation of the tumour-node-metastasis staging of locally advanced renal cortical tumours: absolute size (T2) is more significant than renal capsular invasion (T3a). BJU Int 2005;95(1):27–30.

65. Siemer S, Lehmann J, Loch A, et al. Current TNM classification of renal cell carcinoma evaluated: revising stage T3a. J Urol 2005;173(1):33–7.

66. Lam JS, Shvarts O, Leppert JT, et al. Renal cell carcinoma 2005: new frontiers in staging, prognostication and targeted molecular therapy. J Urol 2005;173(6):1853–62.

67. Kletscher BA, Qian J, Bostwick DG, et al. Prospective analysis of the incidence of ipsilateral adrenal metastasis in localized renal cell carcinoma. J Urol 1996;155(6):1844–6.

68. Tsui KH, Shvarts O, Barbaric Z, et al. Is adrenalectomy a necessary component of radical nephrectomy? UCLA experience with 511 radical nephrectomies. J Urol 2000;163(2):437–41.

69. Han KR, Bui MH, Pantuck AJ, et al. TNM T3a renal cell carcinoma: adrenal gland involvement is not the same as renal fat invasion. J Urol 2003;169(3): 899–903.

70. Hatcher PA, Anderson EE, Paulson DF, et al. Surgical management and prognosis of renal cell carcinoma invading the vena cava. J Urol 1991;145(1):20–3.

71. Moinzadeh A, Libertino JA. Prognostic significance of tumor thrombus level in patients with renal cell carcinoma and venous tumor thrombus extension. Is all T3b the same? J Urol 2004;171(2 Pt 1):598–601.

72. Elson PJ, Witte RS, Trump DL. Prognostic factors for survival in patients with recurrent or metastatic renal cell carcinoma. Cancer Res 1988;48(24 Pt 1):7310–3.

73. Kattan MW, Reuter V, Motzer RJ, et al. A postoperative prognostic nomogram for renal cell carcinoma. J Urol 2001;166(1):63–7.

74. Shvarts O, Lam JS, Kim HL, et al. Staging of renal cell carcinoma: current concepts. BJU Int 2005; 95(Suppl 2):8–13.

75. Zisman A, Pantuck AJ, Dorey F, et al. Improved prognostication of renal cell carcinoma using an integrated staging system. J Clin Oncol 2001; 19(6):1649–57.

76. Zisman A, Pantuck AJ, Wieder J, et al. Risk group assessment and clinical outcome algorithm to predict the natural history of patients with surgically resected renal cell carcinoma. J Clin Oncol 2002; 20(23):4559–66.

77. Cindolo L, Patard JJ, Chiodini P, et al. Comparison of predictive accuracy of four prognostic models for nonmetastatic renal cell carcinoma after nephrectomy: a multicenter European study. Cancer 2005; 104(7):1362–71.

Contemporary Radiologic Imaging of Renal Cortical Tumors

Ariadne M. Bach, MD[a],[*], Jingbo Zhang, MD[b]

KEYWORDS

- Renal cortical tumor • Renal cancer • Renal cell carcinoma
- Renal mass • Kidney cancer • Clear cell carcinoma
- Papillary • Chromophobe • Oncocytoma
- Magnetic resonance imaging (MR)
- Computed tomography (CT) • Ultrasound (US)

The renal cortical tumors are a family of neoplasms that are subdivided into benign and malignant neoplasm based on the Heidelberg classification, which more accurately predicts the metastatic potential of the tumor.[1] The malignant renal parenchymal tumors include the clear cell renal carcinoma, papillary renal cell carcinoma, chromophobe renal cell carcinoma, collecting duct (Bellini duct) carcinoma, and a small number of unclassified tumors. The benign renal parenchymal tumors include renal oncocytoma, metanephric adenoma, metanephric adenofibroma, and papillary renal cell adenoma.

The different renal cortical tumors are associated with different disease progression and metastatic potential.[2-5] The conventional clear cell carcinomas have the greatest metastatic potential, whereas papillary and chromophobe carcinomas are associated with less metastatic potential.[5] The oncocytoma is virtually benign.

DETECTION

CT is considered the modality of choice for detection and diagnosis of renal cortical tumors. MR imaging and ultrasonography (US) are problem-solving tools or are used in patients who have contraindications to IV contrast. The improvement in radiologic imaging has led to a great increase in the detection and earlier diagnosis of renal cortical tumors.[6-9] Currently greater than 70% of tumors are discovered incidentally and are generally small, with a median tumor size of less than or equal to 5 cm.[6,7,9] Up to 20% of the suspicious renal cortical tumors detected may be benign (such as oncocytoma, angiomyolipoma [AML], or complex cyst).[7]

Renal US is not considered a useful screening modality because small lesions can be easily missed.[10] CT detects more and smaller renal masses than does US but the two modalities are comparable in characterizing 1- to 3-cm lesions.[11] Although renal sonography may not be the best method for generalized primary screening it may still be beneficial in secondary screening in a more selected patient population, such as the elderly asymptomatic population.[12]

Unfortunately, currently imaging has limited criteria for diagnosing the specific type renal cortical tumor without operative resection. This article specifically focuses on the techniques and roles of CT, US, and MR imaging in the evaluation of renal cortical tumors. The specific renal cortical neoplasms discussed in this article are clear cell renal carcinoma, papillary renal cell carcinoma, chromophobe renal cell carcinoma, renal oncocytoma, and AML.

[a] Department of Radiology, Memorial Sloan Kettering Cancer Center, Rockefeller Outpatient Pavilion, 160 East 53rd Street, Radiology-8th floor, New York, NY 10022, USA
[b] Department of Radiology, Memorial Sloan Kettering Cancer Center, 1275 York Avenue, New York, NY 10021, USA
* Corresponding author.
E-mail address: bacha@mskcc.org (A.M. Bach).

Urol Clin N Am 35 (2008) 593–604
doi:10.1016/j.ucl.2008.07.012

CT Scan

A specific renal protocol is ordered to work up a known or suspected renal lesion. At our institution, a CT scan dedicated for evaluation of a renal mass typically consists of three imaging series: precontrast, corticomedullary phase, and late nephrographic/early excretory phase.[13–15] Precontrast images are used for identification of calcifications and fat, and to provide a baseline density Hounsfield unit (HU) measurement for evaluating the degree and pattern of enhancement in cystic or solid renal masses.[15] Nonionic intravenous (IV) contrast is injected through an IV line. Corticomedullary images are used for the identification of the renal lesion and assessment of lesion vascularity, renal vascular anatomy, and tumor involvement of venous structures.[13] They are probably the most informative for lesion characterization. Not all renal tumors are well identified during the corticomedullary phase and the images obtained during a later phase of enhancement (ie, the nephrographic or excretory phase) are included for the detection of renal masses, especially those of smaller size.[16–19] These excretory phase images are also helpful for identification of anatomic abnormalities or tumor involvement of the renal collecting system.[13] High accuracy (sensitivity up to 100%, specificity up to 95%) has been reported in the detection of renal cortical tumors using proper technique.[19]

The key features in characterizing a renal lesion on CT are: cystic versus solid, enhancement (attenuation change from the noncontrast to the contrast-enhanced images), margins, presence and type of calcification, and the presence of fat. There are strict CT criteria in characterizing a lesion as "simple" and therefore a benign cyst. The cyst must be well marginated, nonenhancing, homogeneous low attenuation (0–20 HU), and have a thin smooth wall. If the lesion on the precontrast study has measurements greater than 20 HU it is not a simple cyst and may represent a complex cyst or a mass. A contrast-enhanced study must be performed to evaluate for enhancement.

Enhancement was considered a change of 10 HU after IV contrast when CT was first introduced and on the single detector scanner. Now with the advancement in CT technology and the use of multidetectors the assessment of enhancement is more complicated. One common pitfall in characterizing renal lesions by CT is the presence of pseudo-enhancement in renal cysts on contrast-enhanced CT images. This finding is believed to be attributable to volume averaging and beam-hardening effects, and the degree of pseudo-enhancement is greater in smaller renal cysts.[20–26] A change of more than 15 HU is considered by some to indicate enhancement.[21,27] Others consider a change of 10 to 20 HU to be indeterminate and in need of further evaluation.[28] Enhancement must be unequivocal because it implies that the lesion has a blood supply, is solid, and is considered a renal cortical tumor after the additional imaging features are considered. For lesions with indeterminate enhancement and in those patients for whom IV contrast is contraindicated US or MR imaging can be performed.

Generally speaking the presence of calcifications in a solid renal mass indicates malignancy.[29] Calcification in a complex cyst with no enhancing soft tissue elements is not concerning for malignancy.[30]

The presence of macroscopic fat implies benignity and the presence of an AML. Fat is diagnosed on the precontrast images. A low-density area, preferably within the center of the lesion, is selected by a region of interest and the HU are measured. If the HU are −10 or less, then fat can be confidentially identified (**Fig. 1**).[31] The fatty component needs to be in the center of the renal lesion. Large renal cortical lesions can grow and engulf the perirenal and sinus fat. Alternatively extrarenal lesions can grow centrally and invade the renal cortex giving the impression that the lesion is renal cortical in origin when it is not. As the name implies, a renal cortical tumor has its epicenter/origin from the renal cortex. An important role of imaging is to correctly identify the origin/location of a tumor. On imaging we look for a claw or beak sign of normal-appearing renal cortex at the periphery of the mass that indicates that the mass is renal cortical in origin. There are some caveats that need to be remembered. There have been reports of fat-containing renal cell carcinoma.[32–36] Most have contained calcification. Renal cell cancer can rarely contain fat and no calcification.[35,36] It is recommended that renal masses containing both fat and calcification should be considered malignant.

Exophytic lesions are significantly more likely than central lesions to be the less aggressive non–clear cell tumors and clear cell tumors are more likely to be central, implying that the exophytic lesion has a better prognosis.[37] Central renal lesions may be urothelial in origin and it is important to alert the clinician of this possibility because this may affect management.

The renal veins and the inferior vena cava (IVC) are an important part of the evaluation in a patient who has a suspected renal malignancy. A thrombus involving the renal vein or IVC in a patient who has malignant renal tumor may represent tumor thrombus, blood clot, or both (**Fig. 2**). The

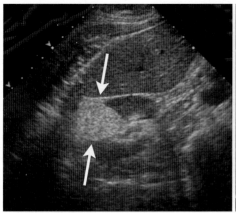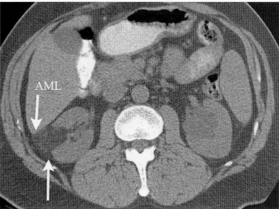

Fig.1. A 55-year-old man who has prostate cancer and incidentally discovered renal angiomyolipoma indicated by arrows. CT demonstrates the mass to have a HU of −59, consistent with fat. The mass is very echogenic on US.

presence of enhancement within the thrombus indicates tumor thrombus, whereas bland thrombus would not enhance after contrast administration.

Solid renal cortical tumors

Enhancement is important in the characterization of solid renal cortical tumor.

A study at our institution by one of the authors (JZ) demonstrated that 90% of the clear cell cancers were hypervascular and heterogenous, 75% were of the papillary type and were hypovascular, and chromophobe often demonstrated moderate enhancement. A mixed enhancement pattern was most predictive of clear cell.[38]

Clear cell carcinoma tends to be hypervascular and heterogeneous (**Fig. 3**).[38–42] Clear cell carcinomas demonstrate peritumoral vascularity more frequently than other malignant renal tumors of similar size.[43]

Papillary renal cell cancer is typically hypovascular and homogeneous (**Fig. 4**).[38,42]

The chromophobe is more variable in appearance. It may demonstrate moderate enhancement.[38] The spoke-wheel–like enhancement with a central scar has been described as an important imaging feature.[44]

Oncocytomas may overlap with renal cell carcinoma in imaging features and degree of enhancement.[38,39,45] Classic angiographic findings for oncocytoma are a spoke-wheel pattern, a homogeneous tumor blush, and a sharp, smooth rim.[46] But none of these findings are specific and a renal cell carcinoma may have any or all of the classic findings.[46] The diagnosis of oncocytoma may be suggested if a central stellate scar is identified on CT within an otherwise homogenous tumor.[47]

The presence of macroscopic fat is characteristic of an AML. AML may present without evidence

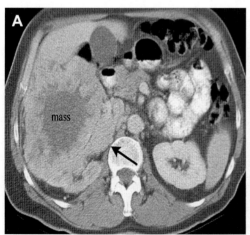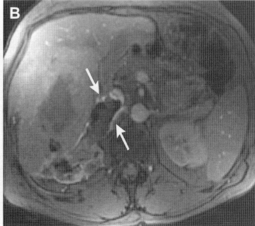

Fig. 2. A 57-year-old man who has 10 × 14 cm right renal clear cell invading the right renal vein and extending into the IVC. (*A*) CT demonstrates mass and arrow indicates the thrombus. (*B*) MR image with arrows pointing out the tumor thrombus in the renal vein and IVC.

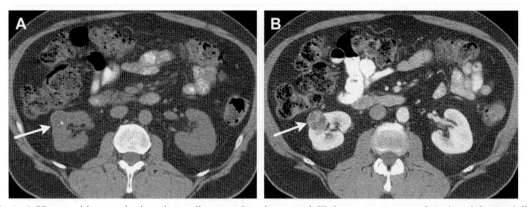

Fig. 3. A 55-year-old man who has clear cell cancer. Renal protocol CT demonstrates an enhancing right partially cystic mass with minimal calcification. The mass enhances from 16 (*A*, noncontrast CT) to 60 HU (*B*, postcontrast CT).

of macroscopic fat—the so-called "AML with minimal fat."[48,49] AMLs have been described as being homogeneously high attenuation on the unenhanced study and demonstrated homogeneous enhancement.[48,49] Overlap has been reported with renal cancer.[38,48] Small (≤3 cm) homogeneously enhancing renal masses on CT may be an AML with minimal fat or renal cell carcinoma.[50]

Cystic renal cortical tumors

The Bosniak Classification system grades the cystic renal masses based on CT findings for the likelihood of malignancy.[51] Category 1 lesions are simple cysts. Category 2 lesions are benign minimally complex cysts that may contain thin septations with calcification. Category 2F lesions are more complex cysts with increase septations and calcification and require follow-up. Category 3 lesions are indeterminate masses with thick irregular walls and may contain calcification. When any solid enhancing component is present,

the cystic renal mass is graded as Bosniak category 4 and considered malignant. The presence of nodular or septal enhancement has been shown to have the highest sensitivity for predicting malignancy with good to moderate interobserver agreement.[52]

Ultrasound

US is an important tool in the evaluation of the renal cortical tumor. It can characterize a renal lesion as cystic or solid. When a lesion is described as cystic it is important to indicate if the lesion is a simple cyst and therefore benign, or a complex cyst and a possible surgical lesion. A simple cyst is anechoic: without echoes and black on the images. A simple cyst has a thin imperceptible wall, posterior enhancement, round or oval shape, and is avascular. If the cyst does not fulfill all the criteria of a simple cyst then it is complex, and the possibility of a cystic renal carcinoma may need to be considered depending on

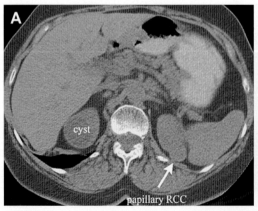
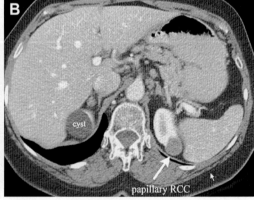

Fig. 4. A 64-year-old woman who has a papillary renal cell carcinoma in the upper pole of the left kidney. Cyst is imaged in the upper pole of the right kidney. (*A*) Noncontrast CT. (*B*) Postcontrast CT.

the sonographic features. Features on US suggestive of a malignant cystic lesion include a thickened (>2 mm) cystic wall, numerous septations, thickened or nodular septations (>2 mm), irregular or central calcifications, and the presence of flow in the septations or cystic wall on Doppler imaging. If any suspicious features are present correlation with other imaging modalities, such as CT and MR imaging, is recommended. Rarely a benign cyst can become complex in the setting of hemorrhage or infection, and could mimic a complex cystic lesion. In that setting comparison with prior imaging and history is critical.

Most renal cortical tumors on US are solid and described by their echogenicity. The terms used to describe the echogenicity are anechoic, isoechoic, hypoechoic, and hyperechoic. A simple cyst is anechoic. The renal cortical tumors may be hyperechoic, isoechoic, or hypoechoic relative to the normal renal cortex (**Fig. 5**). A hyperechoic mass has more echoes and is brighter/lighter than the normal/adjacent renal cortex. An isoechoic lesion is the same as the adjacent renal parenchyma and the hypoechoic mass has fewer echoes and is darker. Cystic areas and calcifications may be present.

All solid renal masses on US usually need to be evaluated with a renal protocol CT for the presence of fat. If fat is present in a noncalcified lesion on CT then in most cases an AML can be diagnosed. AML is typically intensely echoic and can cause acoustic shadowing.[53] Every echogenic mass in the kidney must be further evaluated with a renal protocol CT to confirm the presence of fat (see **Fig. 1**). Up to one third of small renal cell cancers (<3 cm in diameter) can be markedly hyperechoic and mimic AML. Two percent of the renal cancers larger than 3 cm can be markedly echogenic.[54] Alternatively, not all AMLs are hyperechoic and some are only diagnosed after surgical excision.

Attempts have been made to differentiate renal cortical tumors into the different histologic subtypes based on US characteristics. Papillary renal cell carcinomas tend to be hypoechoic or isoechoic but some may also be hyperechoic.[55]

Work has been done in US using Doppler imaging, which allows for assessment of vascular flow.[56] A recent study from our institution indicates that vascular flow within a renal mass, identified by color or power Doppler, is strongly associated with conventional clear cell carcinoma (**Fig. 6**).[57] Contrast-enhanced US has been found to be useful in the diagnosis of renal cortical tumors and in the detection of tumor blood flow in hypovascular renal masses.[58] Contrast-enhanced US has also been useful in classifying renal cystic lesions into the Bosniak classification.[59]

US and cross-sectional imaging modalities (CT and MR) complement each other in the characterization of renal lesions. In the subgroup of patients whose renal lesions are indeterminate on US, a dedicated renal protocol CT or MR imaging may help further characterize the lesion.[60] Conversely, US may prove useful for renal lesions that are considered indeterminate on CT.

US may also assist in the preoperative evaluation of renal cortical tumors. Renal US is requested by the urologists as a template for the intraoperative US. It assists in the selection of the proper surgical technique and determining if a partial nephrectomy can be attempted. Because of its multiplanar capability US can demonstrate important landmarks and planes of sections that can be duplicated in the operating room.

MR Imaging

MR imaging has distinct advantages over other imaging modalities in the detection and staging of renal neoplasms, because of its intrinsic high soft tissue contrast and direct multiplanar imaging capabilities.[61] In addition, pseudo-enhancement artifacts that frequently afflict CT examinations are typically not present on MR images. MR

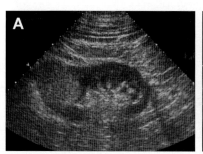 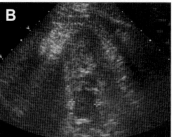 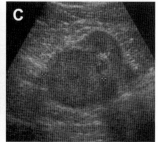

Fig. 5. Spectrum of solid renal cortical tumors on US. (*A*) 5-cm hyperechoic oncocytoma. (*B*) Transverse US image of the left kidney demonstrates a 1.9-cm hypoechoic papillary renal cell carcinoma indicated by calipers. (*C*) 5-cm isoechoic right renal oncocytoma indicated by calipers.

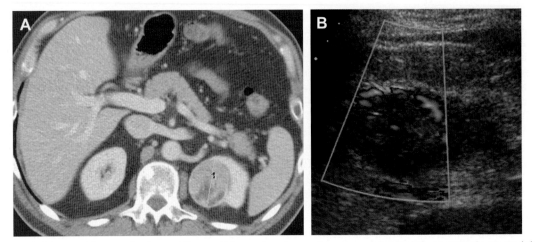

Fig. 6. A 62-year-old man who has a 4.6-cm solid vascular clear cell carcinoma in the left upper pole on CT (*A*). (*B*) US demonstrates flow in the mass on color Doppler.

imaging may be used, therefore, to definitively determine the presence or absence of contrast enhancement in a renal mass that poses as a diagnostic problem on CT.[62] Compared with US, MR imaging is not as operator dependent, nor is its image quality as susceptible to the patient's body habitus. There are certain limitations to MR imaging, however, because of its relatively long acquisition time, greater cost, and thus limited access. In addition, MR imaging used to be considered safe in patients who had renal failure because gadolinium-based contrast agents were believed to be renally excreted yet nonnephrotoxic. MR imaging was often performed as the modality of choice for patients who had renal dysfunction yet needed contrast-enhanced cross-sectional imaging. Unfortunately, an association between

administration of gadolinium-based contrast agents and nephrogenic systemic fibrosis, a rare but potentially disabling or even fatal sequela, has been recently established in patients who had renal failure undergoing MR imaging.[63,64] In patients who have moderate to severe renal dysfunction, therefore, the current recommendation is that administration of gadolinium-based contrast agents should be performed with caution and alternative imaging modalities should be considered.

A modern MR imaging protocol aimed at evaluating renal masses typically includes the following breath-hold sequences: (1) a T1-weighted in- and opposed-phase gradient echo sequence, which is helpful in identifying macroscopic and microscopic fat in a renal mass (**Fig. 7**);[65]

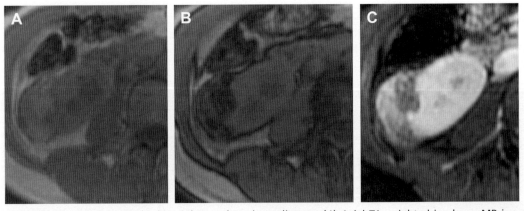

Fig. 7. A 30-year-old woman who has right renal angiomyolipoma. (*A*) Axial T1-weighted in-phase. MR image demonstrates a right renal mass containing areas of T1 hyperintensity. (*B*) Axial T1-weighted opposed-phase MR image demonstrates drop-off of signal in the T1 hyperintense areas, indicating the presence of microscopic fat. (*C*) Axial T1-weighted fat-saturated contrast-enhanced MR image demonstrates heterogeneous enhancement in the right renal mass.

(2) a T2-weighted half-Fourier single shot fast spin echo sequence in axial or coronal planes, which is useful for evaluating the overall anatomy, renal collecting system, and the complexity of a cystic renal lesion; and (3) a dynamic contrast-enhanced T1-weighted fat-suppressed sequence for evaluation of the presence and pattern of enhancement in a renal mass.[66] For the dynamic contrast-enhanced images, three-dimensional fast spoiled gradient echo sequences are typically performed[66,67] before and after contrast administration during the arterial, corticomedullary, and nephrographic phases.[66,68] Multiplanar reconstruction may be performed if necessary to better delineate the spatial relationship of the renal mass to adjacent anatomic structures. If necessary, a dedicated MR angiography sequence may be performed in the coronal plane during the arterial phase for better visualization of accessory renal vessels and facilitation of surgical planning. Coronal images may also be obtained during the excretory phase (often with administration of diuretics), from which maximum-intensity projection images can then be obtained to produce intravenous pyelogram–like images. For patients who cannot cooperate with breath-hold instructions, alternative T1-weighted sequences may need to be explored to reduce respiratory motion–related artifacts. For example, a two-dimensional T1-weighted MR sequence with an inversion recovery pulse followed by a long echo train may provide T1-weighted soft tissue contrast and shortened acquisition time to reduce image blur. The T2-weighted half-Fourier single shot fast spin echo sequences are more robust and less susceptible to motion artifacts, and can typically provide diagnostic images even in non–breath-hold patients.

MR imaging is useful in the detection and differentiation of cystic and solid renal lesions,[69] with accuracy comparable or superior to that of CT.[70] MR imaging may function as an excellent tool for initial diagnosis and posttreatment follow-up in patients who have renal tumors. MR imaging is known to be reliable for evaluation of small renal masses,[71,72] in which case CT can be problematic because of pseudo-enhancement. In addition, because of its multiplanar capability, MR imaging may be superior to CT for determining the origin of a renal mass.

Solid renal tumors are typically isointense or slightly hypointense on T1-weighted images,[69,73] although some renal tumors may contain hemorrhage or a lipid component and demonstrate T1 hyperintensity.[74] Clear cell carcinomas may contain intracellular lipids and demonstrate focal or diffuse signal loss on opposed-phase images, which does not necessarily indicate AML.[66,75,76] Renal cortical tumors tend to be mildly hyperintense[73] on T2-weighted images and demonstrate variable enhancement on dynamic contrast-enhanced images (**Fig. 8**).[69] Simple cysts, on the other hand, are hypointense on T1- and hyperintense on T2-weighted images. Although some complex cysts may demonstrate a higher T1 signal and lower T2 signal because of hemorrhage, debris, or proteinaceous material, there should be no enhancement in cysts after administration of contrast. Identification of the presence of contrast enhancement is essential in evaluating a renal mass. Generally speaking, any non–fat-containing solid tumor or any cystic lesion containing measurable enhancing soft tissue components (such as mural nodules, thickened septations, or cystic walls) is suggestive of a renal neoplasm and likely needs to be managed surgically.[28,62,70,77–79] It has been reported that the optimal percentage of enhancement threshold for distinguishing cysts from solid tumors on MR imaging is 15% when measurement is performed 2 to 4 minutes after administration of contrast material.[78] This threshold may be achieved with quantitative analysis of enhancement with signal intensity measurements.[78] Qualitative analysis of enhancement with image subtraction is equally accurate,

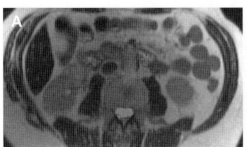
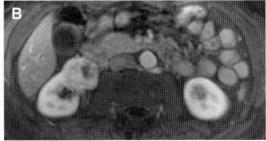

Fig. 8. A 58-year-old man who has right renal clear cell carcinoma. (*A*) Axial T2-weighted single-shot fast spin echo MR image demonstrates a mildly T2-hyperintense mass in the right kidney. (*B*) Axial T1-weighted fat-saturated contrast-enhanced MR image demonstrates heterogeneous enhancement in the renal mass.

particularly in the setting of masses that are hyper-intense on unenhanced MR images.[62] Similar to those seen on CT, three patterns of enhancement have been observed in renal cell carcinomas on MR imaging: predominantly peripheral, heterogeneous, and homogeneous.[69] A classification system based on MR imaging feature analysis using certain imaging characteristics, such as lesion size, peripheral versus central location of the renal lesion, the T2 signal intensity and degree of enhancement of the lesion, the presence of subvoxel fat on chemical shift imaging, the presence of intratumoral necrosis, retroperitoneal vascular collaterals, renal vein thrombosis, and so forth, was recently proposed to help predict the histologic type and nuclear grade of renal masses.[80]

CT and MR imaging perform similarly in classifying most cystic renal masses.[81] In some cases, however, MR images may depict additional septa, thickening of the wall or septa, or enhancement, which may lead to an upgraded Bosniak cyst classification and affect case management.[81]

In addition to the routine MR sequences, diffusion weighted imaging (DWI) is worth discussing because it is an MR imaging technique that was originally established in neuroimaging but has recently gained great interest among investigators in the field of body imaging. DWI measures the Brownian motion of water molecules in biologic tissues, which has been shown to be inversely proportional to cellular density,[82] presumably because increased cellular density limits water diffusion in the interstitial space. The apparent diffusion coefficient (ADC), a quantitative parameter measured from DWI, has been shown to have the potential of differentiating high-grade and low-grade brain gliomas[83,84] and providing incremental value to MR spectroscopy in distinguishing between brain abscesses and necrotic brain tumors.[85] The use of DWI in body imaging is technically challenging, because this technique is generally sensitive to motion and susceptibility and limited in signal-to-noise ratio. Its application in abdominal imaging has been limited. With recent advances in MR technology and faster, more robust sequences, better image quality can be obtained, and DWI has shown great potential for abdominal imaging in several recent investigations.[86–88] For example, DWI was shown to be useful for differentiating focal hepatic lesions,[89–92] and for evaluating diffuse hepatic parenchymal abnormalities, such as cirrhosis.[93] A few studies have been performed to investigate the role of DWI in the evaluation of renal function in native[94–97] and transplanted kidneys.[98] In addition, studies have shown that DWI may differentiate hydronephrosis from pyonephrosis.[99,100] Experience using DWI in characterizing local renal lesions, especially renal masses, has been limited to date.

One preliminary study aimed to investigate the potential role of DWI in the characterization of renal tumors showed that renal lesions with different tissue contents may have different diffusion characteristics.[101] Solid tumor tissue has lower ADC values than necrotic or cystic tumor tissue, whereas necrotic or cystic tumor tissue has lower ADC values than benign cysts. This distinction is important for differentiating benign cysts from extensively necrotic or cystic tumors that may demonstrate little or no contrast enhancement and an imaging appearance similar to a complex benign renal cystic lesion on conventional MR images. In addition, it seems that the T1 signal intensity of a lesion affects the lesion's ADC value. For example, T1 hyperintense cysts have lower ADC values than T1 hypointense cysts, and T1 hyperintense necrotic or cystic tumor areas have lower ADC values than their T1 hypointense counterparts. The T1 characteristics of a lesion may need to be taken into account, therefore, when ADC values are interpreted in an attempt to evaluate a disease process. When both ADC values and T1 features are considered, the benign cysts can be differentiated from necrotic or cystic tumors with only a small overlap in ADC values.[101]

STAGING

The sensitivity of CT for detection of regional lymph node metastases is reported to be as high as 95%.[102] False-positive findings up to 58% have been reported when a size criterion of 1.0 cm is used for determining nodal metastasis, however.[102]

The most common metastatic sites from malignant renal cortical tumors are the lung, bone, brain, liver, and mediastinum.[103] With improved imaging, renal tumors are being detected incidentally in greater numbers at smaller sizes and earlier stages, and distant metastases are unlikely in these patients.

IMAGING FOLLOW-UP

At our institution the renal US is frequently the first imaging obtained following renal surgery. CT of the chest, abdomen, and pelvis is the modality of choice for detection of local recurrence and distant metastases. In patients allergic to iodinated contrast, gadolinium-enhanced MR imaging of the abdomen and pelvis may be performed. Recurrences occur in the lung, bone, nephrectomy site, brain, liver, and the contralateral kidney.[104]

SUMMARY

CT with IV contrast is the imaging modality of choice for detecting, evaluating, and following the patient who has a renal cortical tumor. Certain imaging features and enhancement patterns on CT may help differentiate different subtypes of renal tumors. MR imaging and US function as valuable problem-solving tools or for detection and evaluation if IV contrast cannot be used. Imaging follow-up is important in the identification of tumor recurrence.

REFERENCES

1. Kovacs G, Akhtar M, Beckwith BJ, et al. The Heidelberg classification of renal cell tumours. J Pathol 1997;183(2):131–3.
2. Beck SD, Patel MI, Snyder ME, et al. Effect of papillary and chromophobe cell type on disease-free survival after nephrectomy for renal cell carcinoma. Ann Surg Oncol 2004;11(1):71–7.
3. Eble JN, Bonsib SM. Extensively cystic renal neoplasms: cystic nephroma, cystic partially differentiated nephroblastoma, multilocular cystic renal cell carcinoma, and cystic hamartoma of renal pelvis. Semin Diagn Pathol 1998;15(1):2–20.
4. McKiernan J, Yossepowitch O, Kattan MW, et al. Partial nephrectomy for renal cortical tumors: pathologic findings and impact on outcome. Urology 2002;60(6):1003–9.
5. Motzer RJ, Bacik J, Mariani T, et al. Treatment outcome and survival associated with metastatic renal cell carcinoma of non-clear-cell histology. J Clin Oncol 2002;20(9):2376–81.
6. Russo P. Renal cell carcinoma: presentation, staging, and surgical treatment. Semin Oncol 2000; 27(2):160–76.
7. Russo P. Renal tumors: developing understanding leads to developments in surgical treatment. BJU Int 2006;97:9–10.
8. Smith SJ, Bosniak MA, Megibow AJ, et al. Renal cell carcinoma: earlier discovery and increased detection. Radiology 1989;170(3 Pt 1):699–703.
9. Russo P. Localized renal cell carcinoma. Curr Treat Options Oncol 2001;2(5):447–55.
10. Warshauer DM, McCarthy SM, Street L, et al. Detection of renal masses: sensitivities and specificities of excretory urography/linear tomography, US, and CT. Radiology 1988;169(2):363–5.
11. Jamis-Dow CA, Choyke PL, Jennings SB, et al. Small (≤3-cm) renal masses: detection with CT versus US and pathologic correlation. Radiology 1996;198(3):785–8.
12. Malaeb BS, Martin DJ, Littooy FN, et al. The utility of screening renal ultrasonography: identifying renal cell carcinoma in an elderly asymptomatic population. BJU Int 2005;95(7):977–81.
13. Kauczor HU, Schwickert HC, Schweden F, et al. Bolus-enhanced renal spiral CT: technique, diagnostic value and drawbacks. Eur J Radiol 1994; 18(3):153–7.
14. Sheth S, Scatarige JC, Horton KM, et al. Current concepts in the diagnosis and management of renal cell carcinoma: role of multidetector ct and three-dimensional CT. Radiographics 2001; 21(Spec No):S237–54.
15. Schreyer HH, Uggowitzer MM, Ruppert-Kohlmayr A. Helical CT of the urinary organs. Eur Radiol 2002;12(3):575–91.
16. Yuh BI, Cohan RH, Francis IR, et al. Comparison of nephrographic with excretory phase helical computed tomography for detecting and characterizing renal masses. Can Assoc Radiol J 2000;51(3): 170–6.
17. Szolar DH, Kammerhuber F, Altziebler S, et al. Multiphasic helical CT of the kidney: increased conspicuity for detection and characterization of small (< 3-cm) renal masses. Radiology 1997; 202(1):211–7.
18. Birnbaum BA, Jacobs JE, Ramchandani P. Multiphasic renal CT: comparison of renal cysts during contrast-enhanced CT. AJR Am J Roentgenol 2000;174(2):493–8.
19. Kopka L, Fischer U, Zoeller G, et al. Dual-phase helical CT of the kidney: value of the corticomedullary and nephrographic phase for evaluation of renal lesions and preoperative staging of renal cell carcinoma. AJR Am J Roentgenol 1997; 169(6):1573–8.
20. Birnbaum BA, Maki DD, Chakraborty DP, et al. Renal cyst pseudoenhancement: evaluation with an anthropomorphic body CT phantom. Radiology 2002;225(1):83–90.
21. Birnbaum BA, Hindman N, Lee J, et al. Renal cyst pseudoenhancement: influence of multidetector CT reconstruction algorithm and scanner type in phantom model. Radiology 2007;244:767–75.
22. Coulam CH, Sheafor DH, Lefer RA, et al. Evaluation of pseudoenhancement of renal cysts during contrast-enhanced CT. AJR Am J Roentgenol 2000; 174(2):493–8.
23. Bae KT, Heiken JP, Siegel CL, et al. Renal cysts: is attenuation artifactually increased on contrast-enhanced CT images? Radiology 2000;216(3): 792–6.
24. Heneghan JP, Spielmann AL, Sheafor DH, et al. Pseudoenhancement of simple renal cysts: a comparison of single and multidetector helical CT. J Comput Assist Tomogr 2002;26(1):90–4.
25. Gokan T, Ohgiya Y, Munechika H, et al. Renal cyst pseudoenhancement with beam hardening effect on CT attenuation. Radiat Med 2002;20(4):187–90.

26. Abdulla C, Kalra MK, Saini S, et al. Pseudoenhancement of simulated renal cysts in a phantom using different multidetector CT scanners. AJR Am J Roentgenol 2002;179(6):1473–6.

27. Hartman DS, Choyke PL, Hartman MS. Renal imaging. A practical approach to the cystic renal mass. Radiographics 2004;24:S101–15.

28. Israel GM, Bosniak MA. How I do it: evaluating renal masses. Radiology 2005;236:441–50.

29. Daniel WW, Hartman GW, Witten DM, et al. Calcified renal mass: a review of ten years experience at the Mayo Clinic. Radiology 1972;103:503–8.

30. Israel GM, Bosniak MA. Calcification in cystic renal masses: is it important in diagnosis? Radiology 2003;226:47–52.

31. Sherman JL, Hartman DS, Friedman AC, et al. Angiomyolipoma: computed tomographic-pathologic correlation of 17 cases. AJR Am J Roentgenol 1981;137:1221–6.

32. Helenon O, Merran S, Paraf F, et al. Unusual fat-containing tumors of the kidney: a diagnostic dilemma. Radiographics 1997;17(1):129–44.

33. Helenon O, Chretien Y, Paraf F, et al. Renal cell carcinoma containing fat: demonstration with CT. Radiology 1993;188(2):429–30.

34. Strotzer M, Lehner KB, Becker K. Detection of fat in a renal cell carcinoma mimicking angiomyolipoma. Radiology 1993;188(2):427–8.

35. Schuster TG, Ferguson MR, Baker DE, et al. Papillary renal cell carcinoma containing fat without calcification mimicking angiomyolipoma on CT. Am J Roentgenol 2004;183:1402–4.

36. D'Angelo PC, Gash JR, Horn AW, et al. Fat in renal cell carcinoma that lacks associated calcifications. Am J Roentgenol 2002;178:931–2.

37. Schachter LR, Bach AM, Snyder ME, et al. The impact of tumour location on the histological subtype of renal cortical tumours. BJU Int 2006;98(1):63–6.

38. Zhang J, Lefkowitz R, Ishill N, et al. Differentiation of solid renal cortical tumors by CT. Radiology 2007;244(2):494–504.

39. Jinzaki M, Tanimoto A, Mukai M, et al. Double-phase helical CT of small renal parenchymal neoplasms: correlation with pathologic findings and tumor angiogenesis. J Comput Assist Tomogr 2000;24(6):835–42.

40. Kim JK, Kim TK, Ahn HJ, et al. Differentiation of subtypes of renal cell carcinoma on helical CT scans. AJR Am J Roentgenol 2002;178(6):1499–506.

41. Sheir KZ, El-Azab M, Mosbah A, et al. Differentiation of renal cell carcinoma subtypes by multislice computerized tomography. J Urol 2005;174(2):451–5 [discussion: 455].

42. Prasad SR, Humphrey PA, Catena JR, et al. Common and uncommon histologic subtypes of renal cell carcinoma: imaging spectrum with pathologic correlation. Radiographics 2006;26:1795–806.

43. Zhang J, Lefkowitz RA, Wang L, et al. Significance of peritumoral vascularity on CT in evaluation of renal cortical tumor. J Comput Assist Tomogr 2007;31(5):717–23.

44. Kondo T, Nakazawa H, Sakai F, et al. Spoke-wheel-like enhancement as an important imaging finding of chromophobe cell renal carcinoma: a retrospective analysis on computed tomography and magnetic resonance imaging studies. Int J Urol 2004;11:817–24.

45. Prasad SR, Surabhi VR, Menias CO, et al. Benign renal neoplasms in adults: cross-sectional imaging findings. AJR Am J Roentgenol 2008;190:158–64.

46. Ambos MA, Bosniak MA, Valensi QJ, et al. Angiographic patterns in renal oncocytomas. Radiology 1978;129(3):615–22.

47. Quinn MJ, Hartman DS, Friedman AC, et al. Renal oncocytoma: new observations. Radiology 1984;153(1):49–53.

48. Kim JK, Park SY, Shon JH, et al. Angiomyolipoma with minimal fat: differentiation from renal cell carcinoma at biphasic helical CT. Radiology 2004;230(3):677–84.

49. Jinzaki M, Tanimoto A, Narimatsu Y, et al. Angiomyolipoma: imaging findings in lesions with minimal fat. Radiology 1997;205(2):497–502.

50. Silverman SG, Mortele KJ, Tuncali K, et al. Hyperattenuating renal masses: etiologies, pathogenesis, and imagin evaluation. Radiographics 2007;27:1131–43.

51. Bosniak MA. The current radiological approach to renal cysts. Radiology 1986;158(1):1–10.

52. Benjaminov O, Atri M, O'Malley MO. Enhancing component on CT to predict malignancy in cystic renal masses and interobserver agreeement of different CT features. AJR Am J Roentgenol 2006;186:665–72.

53. Siegel CL, Middleton WD, Teefey SA, et al. Angiomyolipoma and renal cell carcinoma: US differentiation. Radiology 1996;198(3):789–93.

54. Forman HP, Middleton WD, Melson GL, et al. Hyperechoic renal cell carcinomas: increase in detection at US. Radiology 1993;188(2):431–4.

55. Press GA, McClennan BL, Melson GL, et al. Papillary renal cell carcinoma: CT and sonographic evaluation. AJR Am J Roentgenol 1984;143(5):1005–9.

56. Taylor KJ, Ramos I, Carter D, et al. Correlation of Doppler US tumor signals with neovascular morphologic features. Radiology 1988;166(1 Pt 1):57–62.

57. Raj GV, Bach A, Iasonos A, et al. Utility of pre-operative color Doppler ultrasonography in predicting the histology of renal lesions. J Urology 2007;177(1):53–8.

58. Tamai H, Takiguchi Y, Oka M, et al. Contrast-enhanced ultrasonography in the diagnosis of solid renal tumors. J Ultrasound Med 2005;24(12): 1635–40.

59. Ascenti G, Mazziott S, Zimbaro G, et al. Complex cystic renal masses: characterization with contrast-enhanced US. Radiology 2007;243: 158–65.

60. Prasad SR, Saini S, Stewart S, et al. CT characterization of "indeterminate" renal masses: targeted or comprehensive scanning? J Comput Assist Tomogr 2002;26(5):725–7.

61. Pretorius ES, Wickstrom ML, Siegelman ES. MR imaging of renal neoplasms. Magn Reson Imaging Clin N Am 2000;8(4):813–36.

62. Hecht EM, Israel GM, Krinsky GA, et al. Renal masses: quantitative analysis of enhancement with signal intensity measurements versus qualitative analysis of enhancement with image subtraction for diagnosing malignancy at MR imaging. Radiology 2004;232(2):373–8.

63. Sadowski EA, Bennett LK, Chan MR, et al. Nephrogenic systemic fibrosis: risk factors and incidence estimation. Radiology 2007;243(1):148–57.

64. Broome DR, Girguis MS, Baron PW, et al. Gadodiamide-associated nephrogenic systemic fibrosis: why radiologists should be concerned. Am J Roentgenol 2007;188(2):586–92.

65. Israel GM, Hindman N, Hecht E, et al. The use of opposed-phase chemical shift MRI in the diagnosis of renal angiomyolipomas. AJR Am J Roentgenol 2005;184(6):1868–72.

66. Zhang J, Israel GM, Krinsky GA, et al. Masses and pseudomasses of the kidney: imaging spectrum on MR. J Comput Assist Tomogr 2004;28(5):588–95.

67. Semelka RC, Hricak H, Stevens SK, et al. Combined gadolinium-enhanced and fat-saturation MR imaging of renal masses. Radiology 1991;178(3): 803–9.

68. Heiss SG, Shifrin RY, Sommer FG. Contrast-enhanced three-dimensional fast spoiled gradient-echo renal MR imaging: evaluation of vascular and nonvascular disease. Radiographics 2000; 20(5):1341–52 [discussion: 1353–4].

69. Eilenberg SS, Lee JK, Brown J, et al. Renal masses: evaluation with gradient-echo Gd-DTPA-enhanced dynamic MR imaging. Radiology 1990; 176(2):333–8.

70. Semelka RC, Shoenut JP, Kroeker MA, et al. Renal lesions: controlled comparison between CT and 1.5-T MR imaging with nonenhanced and gadolinium-enhanced fat-suppressed spin-echo and breath-hold FLASH techniques. Radiology 1992; 182(2):425–30.

71. Bosniak MA, Rofsky NM. Problems in the detection and characterization of small renal masses. Radiology 1996;198(3):638–41.

72. Scialpi M, Di Maggio A, Midiri M, et al. Small renal masses: assessment of lesion characterization and vascularity on dynamic contrast-enhanced MR imaging with fat suppression. AJR Am J Roentgenol 2000;175(3):751–7.

73. Fein AB, Lee JK, Balfe DM, et al. Diagnosis and staging of renal cell carcinoma: a comparison of MR imaging and CT. AJR Am J Roentgenol 1987; 148(4):749–53.

74. John G, Semelka RC, Burdeny DA, et al. Renal cell cancer: incidence of hemorrhage on MR images in patients with chronic renal insufficiency. J Magn Reson Imaging 1997;7(1):157–60.

75. Outwater EK, Bhatia M, Siegelman ES, et al. Lipid in renal clear cell carcinoma: detection on opposed-phase gradient-echo MR images. Radiology 1997;205(1):103–7.

76. Outwater EK, Blasbalg R, Siegelman ES, et al. Detection of lipid in abdominal tissues with opposed-phase gradient-echo images at 1.5 T: techniques and diagnostic importance. Radiographics 1998;18(6):1465–80.

77. Bosniak MA. Problems in the radiologic diagnosis of renal parenchymal tumors. Urol Clin North Am 1993;20:217–30.

78. Ho VB, Allen SF, Hood MN, et al. Renal masses: quantitative assessment of enhancement with dynamic MR imaging. Radiology 2002;224(3): 695–700.

79. Rofsky NM, Bosniak MA. MR imaging in the evaluation of small (≤3.0 cm) renal masses. Magn Reson Imaging Clin N Am 1997;5:67–81.

80. Pedrosa I, Chou MT, Ngo L, et al. MR classification of renal masses with pathological correlation. Eur Radiol 2008;18(2):365–75.

81. Israel GM, Hindman N, Bosniak MA. Evaluation of cystic renal masses: comparison of CT and MR imaging by using the Bosniak classification system. Radiology 2004;231(2):365–71.

82. Gupta RK, Sinha U, Cloughesy TF, et al. Inverse correlation between choline magnetic resonance spectroscopy signal intensity and the apparent diffusion coefficient in human glioma. Magn Reson Med 1999;41:2–7.

83. Yang D, Korogi Y, Sugahara T, et al. Cerebral gliomas: prospective comparison of multivoxel 2D chemical-shift imaging proton MR spectroscopy, echoplanar perfusion and diffusion-weighted MRI. Neuroradiology 2002;44:656–66.

84. Lam WW, Poon WS, Metreweli C. Diffusion MR imaging in glioma: does it have any role in the pre-operation determination of grading of glioma? Clin Radiol 2002;57:219–25.

85. Lai PH, Ho JT, Chen WL, et al. Brain abscess and necrotic brain tumor: discrimination with proton MR spectroscopy and diffusion-weighted imaging. AJNR Am J Neuroradiol 2002;23:1369–77.

86. Murtz P, Flacke S, Traber F, et al. Abdomen: diffusion-weighted MR imaging with pulse-triggered single-shot sequences. Radiology 2002;224:258–64.

87. Yoshikawa T, Kawamitsu H, Mitchell DG, et al. ADC measurement of abdominal organs and lesions using parallel imaging technique. AJR Am J Roentgenol 2006;187:1521–30.

88. Yamada I, Aung W, Himeno Y, et al. Diffusion coefficients in abdominal organs and hepatic lesions: evaluation with intravoxel incoherent motion echo-planar MR imaging. Radiology 1999; 210:617–23.

89. Namimoto T, Yamashita Y, Sumi S, et al. Focal liver masses: characterization with diffusion-weighted echo-planar MR imaging. Radiology 1997;204: 739–44.

90. Ichikawa T, Haradome H, Hachiya J, et al. Diffusion-weighted MR imaging with a single-shot echo-planar sequence: detection and characterization of focal hepatic lesions. AJR Am J Roentgenol 1998; 170:397–402.

91. Taouli B, Vilgrain V, Dumont E, et al. Evaluation of liver diffusion isotropy and characterization of focal hepatic lesions with two single-shot echo-planar MR imaging sequences: prospective study in 66 patients. Radiology 2003;226:71–8.

92. Kim T, Murakami T, Takahashi S, et al. Diffusion-weighted single-shot echoplanar MR imaging for liver disease. AJR Am J Roentgenol 1999;173: 393–8.

93. Ichikawa T, Haradome H, Hachiya J, et al. Diffusion-weighted MR imaging with single-shot echo-planar imaging in the upper abdomen: preliminary clinical experience in 61 patients. Abdom Imaging 1999;24:456–61.

94. Namimoto T, Yamashita Y, Mitsuzaki K, et al. Measurement of the apparent diffusion coefficient in diffuse renal disease by diffusion-weighted echo-planar MR imaging. J Magn Reson Imaging 1999;9:832–7.

95. Muller MF, Prasad PV, Bimmler D, et al. Functional imaging of the kidney by means of measurement of the apparent diffusion coefficient. Radiology 1994;193:711–5.

96. Toyoshima S, Noguchi K, Seto H, et al. Functional evaluation of hydronephrosis by diffusion-weighted MR imaging. Relationship between apparent diffusion coefficient and split glomerular filtration rate. Acta Radiol 2000;41:642–6.

97. Thoeny HC, De Keyzer F, Oyen RH, et al. Diffusion-weighted MR imaging of kidneys in healthy volunteers and patients with parenchymal diseases: initial experience. Radiology 2005;235:911–7.

98. Thoeny HC, Zumstein D, Simon-Zoula S, et al. Functional evaluation of transplanted kidneys with diffusion-weighted and BOLD MR imaging: initial experience. Radiology 2006;241:812–21.

99. Cova M, Squillaci E, Stacul F, et al. Diffusion-weighted MRI in the evaluation of renal lesions: preliminary results. Br J Radiol 2004;77:851–7.

100. Chan JH, Tsui EY, Luk SH, et al. MR diffusion-weighted imaging of kidney: differentiation between hydronephrosis and pyonephrosis. Clin Imaging 2001;25:110–3.

101. Zhang J, Tehrani Y, Wang L, et al. Renal masses: characterization with diffusion-weighted MR imaging—a preliminary experience. Radiology 2008; 247(2):458–64.

102. Studer UE, Scherz S, Scheidegger J, et al. Enlargement of regional lymph nodes in renal cell carcinoma is often not due to metastases. J Urol 1990;144(2 Pt 1):243–5.

103. Hilton S. Imaging of renal cell carcinoma. Semin Oncol 2000;27(2):150–9.

104. Chae EJ, Kim JK, Kim SH, et al. Renal cell carcinoma: analysis of postoperative recurrence patterns. Radiology 2005;234(1):189–96.

Molecular Imaging of Renal Cell Carcinoma

Rodolfo Perini, MD, Daniel Pryma, MD, Chaitanya Divgi, MD*

KEYWORDS
• Molecular imaging • PET • Cancer phenotype

The recent identification of agents that have significantly influenced the therapy of clear cell renal carcinoma and the decreasing size of renal masses, usually detected serendipitously, have led to a resurgence in imaging for this condition. Although structural methods continue to be used routinely for identification of renal masses, functional and molecular techniques are showing considerable promise in their ability to characterize unique features of the renal cancer phenotype. This article discusses the evolving role of molecular imaging in the evaluation of renal cancer, including current and future applications.

IMAGING OF RENAL MASSES

The average size of detected renal masses, which now usually are detected serendipitously, has decreased considerably in the past decade.[1–3] This decrease in size has increased the need for characterization of the masses detected, because management is heavily influenced by the nature of the lesion.[3] Because most lesions are detected and then evaluated using structural imaging methodologies, particularly ultrasound, CT, and MRI, attempts have been made to use these modalities to characterize renal masses.[4–6] All these techniques seem to be useful, especially in centers with experience. All these modalities, however, including newer techniques such as dynamic contrast-enhanced MRI and measurement of tumor vascularity, are in essence structural or at best functional imaging techniques that seek to characterize renal masses based on radiodensity or blood flow.[7]

POSITRON EMISSION TOMOGRAPHY

Positron emission tomography (PET) has improved tremendously the ability to characterize the cancer phenotype. [18F]-fluorodeoxyglucose (FDG) is an excellent surrogate for glucose use, which is increased in most cancers. Renal excretion of FDG limits its usefulness in the detection of primary tumors. It is, however, an excellent agent for staging and for detection of metastases. Tumor cells constitutively use glucose (the Warburg effect)[8] and hence demonstrate greater FDG uptake than normal cells, appearing as areas of increased FDG accumulation.[9]

PET is a nuclear medicine technique that relies on the detection of energy emitted from radiotracers exogenously administered to patients. Tracers are substances that, in very low concentrations, are able to evaluate biologic functions without disturbing the milieu, a principle pioneered by Hevesy[10] in 1935.

PET images result from the detection of coincident 511-keV gamma rays originating from the annihilation of the emitted positron and a neighboring electron. These gamma rays are detected by an array of scintillation crystals, localizing the event in a linear trajectory within the patient.

PET is the most sensitive imaging tool used routinely in clinical practice, with sensitivity in the order of picomolar concentrations. Tracer uptake is indicated by the standardized uptake value, a measure of mean tissue tracer concentration relative to the mean whole body tracer concentration.[11]

PET has revolutionized the ability to study tumor biology. PET, using different radiotracers, can evaluate cellular metabolism, hypoxia, and the

Division of Nuclear Medicine and Clinical Molecular Imaging, Department of Radiology, University of Pennsylvania, 3400 Spruce Street, Philadelphia, PA 19105, USA
* Corresponding author.
E-mail address: chaitanya.divgi@uphs.upenn.edu (C. Divgi).

Urol Clin N Am 35 (2008) 605–611
doi:10.1016/j.ucl.2008.07.015

expression of cell surface markers. PET cannot distinguish between various positron-emitting radioisotopes, and therefore only one PET tracer can be studied at a given time. Most positron-emitting radioisotopes have short half-lives, however, and thus serial studies are feasible.

Because PET essentially identifies molecular features of cellular processes, it can be thought of as the pre-eminent molecular imaging modality. An overview of PET imaging of renal cancer follows.

GLUCOSE METABOLISM

FDG is the most frequently used PET radiotracer and is the only one approved by the Food and Drug Administration (FDA) for oncologic PET imaging.[12] Like glucose, FDG is transported into cells by glucose transporters and is phosphorylated by hexokinase. It is not metabolized further, however, and thus it accumulates inside cells. Tumor cells use glucose constitutively, as described by Warburg,[8] and hence demonstrate greater FDG uptake, appearing as areas of increased FDG accumulation.

FDG-PET is being used increasingly in staging and response assessment in a variety of cancers, such as lung, breast, lymphoma, melanoma, and neoplasms of the gastrointestinal tract.[12,13] Its role in renal cancer is still controversial, however.[14,15]

FDG-PET reportedly has limited use in the primary detection and staging of renal cell carcinoma. Because FDG is excreted primarily through the urine, foci of increased uptake may be mistaken as activity in the collecting system. Hydration and diuretics potentially can be used to avoid such confounding factors, as is done in bladder cancer. In addition, hybrid imaging with PET/CT scanners also has the potential to improve the sensitivity of FDG-PET in renal tumors from the levels initially reported.

Bachor and colleagues[16] initially described FDG-PET as having an overall sensitivity of 77% in detecting the primary tumor. From a group of 26 patients who had pathologically proven renal cell carcinomas, 20 were identified by FDG-PET; the diagnostic accuracy depended on the degree of tumor differentiation. Most importantly, FDG-PET proved to be a very accurate method for lymph node staging, with no false negatives in this study.

Goldberg and colleagues[17] used FDG-PET to study patients who had renal tumors and indeterminate renal cysts. The authors found that in 9 of 10 patients FDG-PET depicted solid neoplasms accurately. Except for one patient who had a renal cyst and a 4-mm papillary neoplasm, all benign lesions also were classified as such by FDG-PET.

Aide and colleagues[18] prospectively evaluated the ability of FDG-PET to characterize renal cancers and to detect distant metastasis in treatment-naïve and postnephrectomy patients. FDG-PET was less accurate than CT in imaging the primary tumors but had a greater sensitivity in detecting metastatic disease.

In a study by Kang and colleagues,[19] 66 patients who had known or suspected renal cancer were analyzed retrospectively with a total of 90 FDG-PET scans. In this study, FDG-PET was less sensitive than CT in detecting the primary tumors and metastatic disease. (One limitation of this study, however, is that the PET images were interpreted without attenuation correction; the lack of correction limits the sensitivity of any tomographic emission imaging method).

Ramdave and colleagues[20] demonstrated comparable accuracy for FDG-PET and CT in evaluating renal masses. FDG-PET was more accurate in detecting local recurrence and metastatic disease, directly affecting the treatment in 40% of the patients. **Fig. 1** shows a clear cell renal cell carcinoma.

ACETATE METABOLISM

Acetate is taken up by cells, converted into acetyl-coenzyme A in the mitochondria, and then

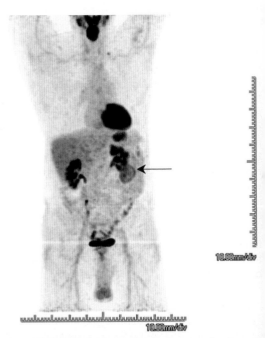

Fig. 1. FDG-PET of a patient who has renal cell carcinoma. Although the tumor can be visualized clearly (*arrow*), the intensity of uptake is much less than in the collecting system in the same kidney.

metabolized in the citric acid cycle and cleared in the form of CO_2. Acetate imaging, in the form of carbon-11 (C-11)-acetate PET, has been used mostly to evaluate myocardial oxidative metabolism.[21] C-11-acetate PET also was shown to be an accurate noninvasive technique for evaluating physiologic renal oxidative metabolism in animals, correlating with O_2 consumption and tubular sodium reabsorption.[22]

In tumor imaging, C-11-acetate has been studied most in prostate cancer, for early differentiation between benign and malignant prostate lesions and for detecting recurrence at low levels of prostate-specific antigen.[23] It has a limited role in the characterization of small renal masses. Shriki and colleagues[24] first reported C-11-acetate uptake in a patient who had renal oncocytoma. In a recent study, however, Kotzerke and colleagues[25] found no evidence of increased uptake of C-11-acetate in patients who had renal carcinoma.

OTHER METABOLIC TRACERS

Attempts have been made to characterize tumors using a variety of other tracers. Two are mentioned briefly here. Radioactive thymidine, long used to characterize cellular proliferation in vivo, has been studied with C-11 and, increasingly, with fluorine-18.[26,27] A concordance between thymidine uptake as assessed by PET and measures of cellular proliferation including Ki-67 immunohistochemistry has been demonstrated clearly.[26,27]

Radioactive choline also has been studied as a PET agent, primarily in prostate cancer.[28] One of the attractive features of using choline as a radiotracer is that elevated choline content in tumor also is detectable by proton magnetic resonance spectroscopy,[29] and thus the relationship between endogenous and exogenous choline can be studied by a combination of magnetic resonance spectroscopy and PET.

TUMOR-ASSOCIATED ANTIGENS

Antigenic features of tumors are studied in both hematologic and solid neoplasms to identify features of the cancer phenotype. In solid tumors this study usually is performed by immunohistochemistry.[30] Increasingly, the standardization of such approaches is seen as critical to their rational use in treatment decision making.[31] Immunohistochemistry is a snap-shot: it depicts the antigenic distribution in a portion of a single tumor, and only in tissue accessible to biopsy. It therefore is useful but is not always representative of the antigenic composition of all tumors in the patient.

Imaging of antigenic distribution has several advantages: it can evaluate distribution throughout the body and at various times during the course of the disease and is relatively noninvasive (especially compared with a biopsy). Such imaging has been performed using radioactive isotopes labeled to intact antibodies; the process has been termed "radioimmunodetection."[32] The limitation thus far has been the lack of suitable imaging tools. Single-photon gamma camera imaging has inherent limitations of sensitivity and specificity, and the only FDA-approved agent currently used in the evaluation of any cancer is an indium-111–labeled murine antibody that recognizes the prostate-specific membrane antigen. Imaging with this antibody is indicated for restaging patients.[33]

Antibody PET ("immunoPET") has the exquisite sensitivity of PET combined with the specificity of antibody targeting. Fluorine-18 (F-18) is the positron emitter most commonly used in PET. It has a half-life of less than 2 hours, precluding imaging at delayed time points (most antibodies accumulate slowly in solid tumors). The radiochemistry of stable conjugation of F-18 to proteins also is difficult and nonstandardized. Iodine-124 (I-124), a positron-emitting radioisotope of iodine with a half-life of 4 days,[34] addresses both limitations: iodination of proteins is standardized, and iodinated antibodies have been used successfully in humans, especially with non-internalizing proteins.[35]

IODINE-LABELED cG250

cG250 is an antibody that is being evaluated as a therapeutic agent in clear cell kidney cancer. The antibody has been studied extensively in clear cell renal cancer as a murine antibody[35,36] and as a chimeric (Fv-grafted human IgG_1) antibody.[35–37] The antibody had exquisite specificity for clear cell renal cancer, and single-photon imaging with [131I]iodine demonstrated that targeting to both primary and metastatic tumor was excellent.[35–37]

The excellent and invariable targeting of radioiodinated cG250 to clear cell renal cancer led the authors to postulate that the antibody could be used to identify clear cell renal cancer. Additionally, the availability of I-124 and the ability to attach it to cG250 raised the prospect of tumor characterization with PET.

As stated earlier,[1–3] the demographics of renal cancer have changed: an increasing proportion of patients with renal masses now are identified serendipitously, with a consequent decrease in the proportion of patients who have the clear cell

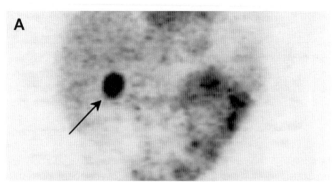

Patient with clear cell renal cancer. Uptake in the tumor is clearly evident.

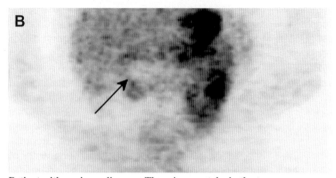

Patient with angiomyolipoma. There is no uptake in the tumor.

Fig. 2. ImmunoPET with [124I]-cG250 (*A*) in a patient who has clear cell renal cancer (uptake in the tumor is clearly evident, as indicated by the arrow) and (*B*) in a patient who has angiomyolipoma (there is no uptake in the tumor).

cancer phenotype.[38] The authors proposed a clinical trial to test the hypothesis that antibody PET with [124I]-cG250 would detect clear cell renal cancer with at least 90% accuracy. The Ludwig Institute for Cancer Research sponsored the trial, which was conducted solely at the Memorial Sloan-Kettering Cancer Center under an FDA-approved Investigational New Drug application. The demographics at the Memorial Sloan-Kettering Cancer Center[39] led the authors to anticipate a total accrual of 54 patients with an early analysis planned after 15 PET-positive patients.

Patients who had renal masses scheduled for surgical removal were entered into the study.

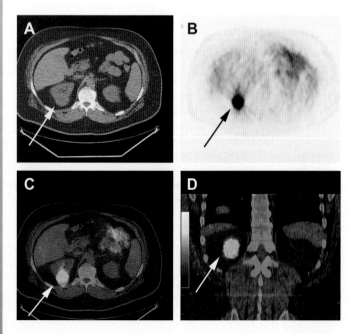

Fig. 3. ImmunoPET with [124I]-cG250. (*A*) Transaxial CT, (*B*) transaxial [124I]-cG250 PET, (*C*) transaxial fused PET-CT, and (*D*) and coronal fused PET-CT images of a 54-year-old man with right upper pole clear cell renal cancer (*arrows*). Images were acquired 5 days after intravenous infusion of 4 mCi 124I/10 mg cG250 and immediately before right upper pole partial nephrectomy.

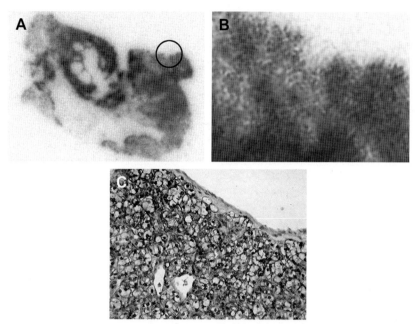

Fig. 4. (*A*) Low-power digital autoradiograph from the clear cell renal cancer seen in **Fig. 2**. The circled area in (*A*) is shown at high power as digital autoradiograph in (*B*) and as contiguous slice immunohistochemistry stained with anti-CA-9 antibody in (*C*).

Surgery was scheduled for approximately a week after antibody infusion, and PET/CT was performed before and on the day of surgery.

PET/CT using [124I]-cG250 was feasible even a week after radio-antibody infusion. All patients tolerated the infusion without acute adverse events, and none developed any side effects or an immune response to the xenogeneic protein. Fifteen of 16 patients who had clear cell renal cancer had a positive PET; the one patient who did not had necrotic tumor. All nine patients who had renal masses of a different histology had no antibody accumulation in the tumors. The positive predictive accuracy thus was 100%, and the specificity also was 100%.[40] **Figs. 2–4** show PET/CT studies using [124I]-cG250.

The results after 15 PET-positive patients were encouraging enough to lead to the initiation of a multicenter trial, sponsored and conducted by Wilex AG, in a larger group of patients. This study is adequately powered to determine the utility of [124I]-cG250 antibody PET in patients who have renal masses.

SUMMARY

Molecular imaging using PET permits in vivo characterization of metabolic and cellular characteristics of cancers. The evaluation of renal cancer using molecular imaging techniques has increased significantly because of the need to characterize the small renal masses that now are detected and because of the number of promising therapies that are becoming available for renal cancer. The metabolic characteristics of renal cancer can be studied with FDG, particularly in the evaluation of patients who have metastatic cancer. Newer methods using radiolabeled tumor-targeting moieties are being studied, and immunoPET of renal cancer with [124I]-cG250 has shown great promise in phenotypic characterization using PET. This characterization may lead to tools for stratifying patients who have cancer and thus to appropriate patient management.

REFERENCES

1. Israel GM, Bosniak MA. How I do it: evaluating renal masses. Radiology 2005;236(2):441–50.
2. Bosniak MA, Rofsky NM. Problems in the detection and characterization of small renal masses. Radiology 1996;198(3):638–41.
3. Raj GV, Thompson RH, Leibovich BC, et al. Preoperative nomogram predicting 12-year probability of metastatic renal cancer. J Urol 2008;179(6): 2146–51 [discussion 2151].
4. Raj GV, Bach AM, Iasonos A, et al. Predicting the histology of renal masses using preoperative Doppler ultrasonography. J Urol 2007;177(1):53–8.
5. Zhang J, Tehrani YM, Wang L, et al. Renal masses: characterization with diffusion-weighted MR

imaging—a preliminary experience. Radiology 2008;247(2):458–64.

6. Zhang J, Lefkowitz RA, Ishill NM, et al. Solid renal cortical tumors: differentiation with CT. Radiology 2007;244(2):494–504.

7. Prasad SR, Dalrymple NC, Surabhi VR. Cross-sectional imaging evaluation of renal masses. Radiol Clin North Am 2008;46(1):95–111, vi–vii.

8. Warburg O, Posener K, Negelein E. Ueber den Stoffwechsel der Tumoren. Biochem Z 1924;152:319–44.

9. Kim JW, Dang CV. Cancer's molecular sweet tooth and the Warburg effect. Cancer Res 2006;66(18):8927–30.

10. Hevesy G. Some applications of isotopic indicators. Les Prix Nobel en 1940–44. Stockholm (Sweden): Norstedt & Soener; 1946.

11. Weber WA, Schwaiger M, Avril N. Quantitative assessment of tumor metabolism using FDG-PET imaging. Nucl Med Biol 2000;27(7):683–7.

12. Juweid ME, Cheson BD. Positron-emission tomography and assessment of cancer therapy. N Engl J Med 2006;354(5):496–507.

13. Juweid ME, Stroobants S, Hoekstra OS, et al. Use of positron emission tomography for response assessment of lymphoma: consensus of the Imaging Subcommittee of International Harmonization Project in Lymphoma. J Clin Oncol 2007;25(5):571–8.

14. Bouchelouche K, Oehr P. Positron emission tomography and positron emission tomography/computerized tomography of urological malignancies: an update review. J Urol 2008;179(1):34–45.

15. Powles T, Murray I, Brock C, et al. Molecular positron emission tomography and PET/CT imaging in urological malignancies. Eur Urol 2007;51(6):1511–20 [discussion 1520–1].

16. Bachor R, Kotzerke J, Gottfried HW, et al. [Positron emission tomography in diagnosis of renal cell carcinoma] [German]. Der Urologe Ausg A 1996;35(2):146–50.

17. Goldberg MA, Mayo-Smith WW, Papanicolaou N, et al. FDG PET characterization of renal masses: preliminary experience. Clin Radiol 1997;52(7):510–5.

18. Aide N, Cappele O, Bottet P, et al. Efficiency of [(18)F]FDG PET in characterising renal cancer and detecting distant metastases: a comparison with CT. Eur J Nucl Med Mol Imaging 2003;30(9):1236–45.

19. Kang DE, White RL, Zuger JH, et al. Clinical use of fluorodeoxyglucose F 18 positron emission tomography for detection of renal cell carcinoma. J Urol 2004;171(5):1806–9.

20. Ramdave S, Thomas GW, Berlangieri SU, et al. Clinical role of F-18 fluorodeoxyglucose positron emission tomography for detection and management of renal cell carcinoma. J Urol 2001;166(3):825–30.

21. Choi Y, Huang SC, Hawkins RA, et al. A refined method for quantification of myocardial oxygen consumption rate using mean transit time with carbon-11-acetate and dynamic PET. J Nucl Med 1993;34(11):2038–43.

22. Juillard L, Lemoine S, Janier MF, et al. Validation of renal oxidative metabolism measurement by positron-emission tomography. Hypertension 2007;50(1):242–7.

23. Soloviev D, Fini A, Chierichetti F, et al. PET imaging with (11)C-acetate in prostate cancer: a biochemical, radiochemical and clinical perspective. Eur J Nucl Med Mol Imaging 2008;35(5):942–9.

24. Shriki J, Murthy V, Brown J. Renal oncocytoma on 1-11C acetate positron emission tomography: case report and literature review. Mol Imaging Biol 2006;8(4):208–11.

25. Kotzerke J, Linné C, Meinhardt M, et al. [1-(11)C]acetate uptake is not increased in renal cell carcinoma. Eur J Nucl Med Mol Imaging 2007;34(6):884–8.

26. Shields AF. Positron emission tomography measurement of tumor metabolism and growth: its expanding role in oncology. Mol Imaging Biol 2006;8(3):141–50.

27. Buck AK, Bommer M, Stilgenbauer S, et al. Molecular imaging of proliferation in malignant lymphoma. Cancer Res 2006;66(22):11055–61.

28. Takahashi N, Inoue T, Lee J, et al. The roles of PET and PET/CT in the diagnosis and management of prostate cancer. Oncology 2007;72(3-4):226–33.

29. Glunde K, Jacobs MA, Bhujwalla ZM. Choline metabolism in cancer: implications for diagnosis and therapy. Expert Rev Mol Diagn 2006;6(6):821–9.

30. Skinnider BF, Amin MB. An immunohistochemical approach to the differential diagnosis of renal tumors. Semin Diagn Pathol 2005;22(1):51–68.

31. Carlson RW, Moench SJ, Hammond ME, et al. HER2 testing in breast cancer: NCCN Task Force report and recommendations. J Natl Compr Canc Netw 2006;4(Suppl 3):S1–22 [quiz S23–4].

32. Lawrentschuk N, Davis ID, Bolton DM, et al. Positron emission tomography (PET), immuno-PET and radioimmunotherapy in renal cell carcinoma: a developing diagnostic and therapeutic relationship. BJU Int 2006;97(5):916–22.

33. Capromab pendetide: product approval iInformation - licensing action. Available at: http://www.fda.gov/cder/biologics/products/capcyt102896.htm. Accessed May 18, 2008.

34. Iodine-124. Available at: http://en.wikipedia.org/wiki/Iodine-124. Accessed May 18, 2008.

35. Oosterwijk E, Divgi C, Bander NH. Active and passive immunotherapy: vaccines and antibodies. BJU Int 2007;99(5 Pt B):1301–4.

36. Oosterwijk E, Divgi CR, Brouwers A, et al. Monoclonal antibody-based therapy for renal cell carcinoma. Urol Clin North Am 2003;30(3):623–31.

37. Divgi CR, O'Donoghue JA, Welt S, et al. Phase I clinical trial with fractionated radioimmunotherapy

using 131I-labeled chimeric G250 in metastatic renal cancer. J Nucl Med 2004;45(8):1412–21.

38. Huang WC, Kagiwada MA, Russo P. Surgery insight: advances in techniques for open partial nephrectomy. Nat Clin Pract Urol 2007;4(8):444–50.

39. Sorbellini M, Kattan MW, Snyder ME, et al. A postoperative prognostic nomogram predicting recurrence for patients with conventional clear cell renal cell carcinoma. J Urol 2005;173(1):48–51.

40. Divgi CR, Pandit-Taskar N, Jungbluth AA, et al. Preoperative characterisation of clear-cell renal carcinoma using iodine-124-labelled antibody chimeric G250 (124I-cG250) and PET in patients with renal masses: a phase I trial. Lancet Oncol 2007;8(4):304–10.

Prognostic Models and Algorithms in Renal Cell Carcinoma

Brian R. Lane, MD, PhD[a], Michael W. Kattan, PhD[b],*

KEYWORDS

• Renal cell carcinoma • Nomogram • Prognostic algorithms

Renal cell carcinoma (RCC) responds minimally to conventional chemotherapy and remains the most lethal of the common genitourinary cancers.[1] Cancer-specific survival correlates strongly with tumor stage, although several other factors have been shown to be independent predictive factors of disease recurrence. Long-term survival exceeds 90% in patients who have RCC that is contained within the kidney (pathologic stage T1) but is less than 5% in patients who have metastatic RCC. Although surgical treatment is curative for localized disease, 25% of patients present with locally advanced or disseminated disease, and disease recurs systemically in 20% to 30% of patients who have localized disease at presentation.[1] Only a small percentage of patients respond to interleukin-2– or interferon-based immunotherapy, and these treatments can be associated with considerable toxicity.[2] Unfortunately, the incidence of all stages of RCC continues to increase by about 2.5% per year, and RCC was responsible for more than 12,800 cancer-related deaths in the United States in 2007.[3,4] The pressing need for effective systemic therapies has led to the development of several novel treatments for metastatic RCC that are now available for clinical use. Two oral, small molecular inhibitors of the receptor for vascular endothelial growth factor (VEGF) have been approved recently by the Food and Drug Administration for the treatment of advanced RCC. Sunitinib (Sutent) and sorafenib (Nexavar) exert their anti-cancer effects primarily by blocking pathways induced by the binding of VEGF to VEGF receptor, leading to the growth of new blood vessels (angiogenesis) that supply oxygen and nutrients to the growing cancer. These agents have been shown to result in stabilization or a decrease in tumor burden in a majority of patients. They also have been shown to lengthen the time to disease progression when compared with placebo or interferon treatment.[5–8] Temsirolimus, an inhibitor of the mammalian target of rapamycin, is a third agent recently approved by the Food and Drug Administration that has been evaluated in poor-risk patients who have metastatic RCC. When administered intravenously to this patient subgroup, temsirolimus extended recurrence-free and overall survival when compared with interferon in a randomized, controlled trial.[9]

Each of the currently available treatments, as well as those currently in clinical trials, is costly and is associated with side effects. Therefore, it is important to identify patients who have the greatest likelihood of benefiting from such treatments. Determination of the risk of recurrence in patients without evidence of metastasis has been based on several predictive models that integrate known clinical risk factors for disease recurrence. More recent studies suggest that the addition of molecular markers to clinical risk factors may improve the predictive ability of RCC disease-recurrence models.[10] Prediction of disease progression or death from disease also has been investigated for use in counseling patients who have metastatic RCC and for guiding clinical decision making. This article describes the various

[a] Glickman Urological and Kidney Institute, Cleveland Clinic, 9500 Euclid Avenue, A100, Cleveland, OH 44195, USA
[b] Department of Quantitative Health Sciences, Cleveland Clinic, 9500 Euclid Avenue, Wb-4, Cleveland, OH 44195, USA
* Corresponding author.
E-mail address: kattanm@ccf.org (M.W. Kattan).

Urol Clin N Am 35 (2008) 613–625
doi:10.1016/j.ucl.2008.07.003

predictive factors and algorithms for patients who have localized and metastatic RCC.

TNM STAGING SYSTEM

Until 1990, Robson's modification of the staging system proposed by Flocks and Kadesky provided the most reliable prognostic information for clinicians caring for patients who had RCC.[11] The system most commonly used currently is the TNM staging system of the International Union Against Cancer and the American Joint Committee on Cancer. Tumor stage remains the single best prognostic indicator for RCC, although it may be viewed better as an algorithm that combines several factors, each of which provides information about outcome. Two studies have confirmed that the 2002 modification of this system has better prognostic ability than the previous 1997 staging system,[12,13] and a new staging system will become available soon. Modifications in the 2002 staging system included subclassification of pT1 tumors as pT1a (< 4 cm) and pT1b (4–7 cm), grouping extension into the renal vein and inferior vena cava below the diaphragm as T3b, and re-classifying involvement of the inferior vena cava above the diaphragm or invasion of the inferior vena cava wall as T3c. Using the 2002 staging system, cancer-specific survival at 5 years ranged from 97% for pT1a to 20% for pT4.[12] Lymph node metastases portend a poor prognosis, with cancer-specific survival rates of 5% to 30% at 5 years and 0% to 5% at 10 years.[11] Distant metastases to lung, bone, brain, or other organs are associated with survival rates of 50%, 5% to 30%, and 0% to 5% at 1, 5, and 10 years, respectively.[11]

PROGNOSTIC FACTORS

A criticism of staging systems is that they tend to provide limited prognostic ability, in part because there may be significant heterogeneity among patients in each classification, and often the systems do not take into account a number of significant predictive factors.[14] This criticism has led investigators to explore various prognostic factors, either alone or in combination with the TNM staging system and/or other factors (**Box 1**). Patients who present with either local or systemic symptoms have a worse prognosis than patients who have incidentally detected tumors.[15–18] Moreover, the presence of symptoms of cachexia, including weight loss, anorexia, or malaise, or a reduction in overall health (Karnofsky scale or Eastern Cooperative Oncology Group [ECOG] performance status)[19] at diagnosis

---

Box 1
Prognostic factors for RCC

Anatomic

Tumor size

Extension into perinephric or renal sinus fat

Adrenal involvement (direct or metastatic)

Venous involvement

Lymph node metastases

Distant metastases

Metastatic burden of disease

Clinical

Performance status (Karnofsky, ECOG)

Localized symptoms

Systemic symptoms (cachexia, > 10-pound weight loss)

Thrombocytosis

Anemia

Hypercalcemia

Elevated alkaline phosphatase

Elevated C-reactive protein

Elevated erythrocyte sedimentation rate

Histologic

Nuclear grade

Histologic subtype

Presence of sarcomatoid features

Presence of histologic necrosis

Vascular invasion

Collecting system invasion

Molecular

Hypoxia-inducible factors: CA-IX, CA-XII, CXCR3, CXCR4, HIF, IGF-1, VEGF, VEGFRs

Co-stimulatory molecules: B7-H1, B7-H3 (tumor cell/vascular), B7-H4, PD-1

Cell cycle regulators: p53, Bcl-2, PTEN, Cyclin A, p27, Skp2

Adhesion molecules: EpCAM/KSA, EMA, E-Cad, alpha-catenin, Cad-6

Other factors: Ki-67, XIAP, Survivin, EphA2, Smac/DIABLO, PCNA, Caveolin-1, AR, CD44, Annexin II, Gelsolin, Vimentin, CA-125), aberrant DNA methylation, Na-K ATPase α1 subunit, vitamin D receptor, retinoid X receptor

Data from Lane BR, Kattan MW. Predicting outcomes in renal cell carcinoma. Curr Opin Urol 2005;15: 289–97.

confers a poor prognosis in both localized and metastatic RCC.[17,18,20–24] Other prognostic factors in patients who have metastatic RCC include the number of metastases and site of metastases (**Table 1**): patients who have a solitary lung metastasis account for almost all the complete remissions observed in clinical trials.[11] Several laboratory values, including anemia (hemoglobin < 10 g/dL for females or < 12 g/dL for males), thrombocytosis, hypercalcemia, elevated alkaline phosphatase, elevated C-reactive protein, and erythrocyte sedimentation rate less than 30 mm/h, also portend poorer outcomes in patients who have RCC.[25–29]

HISTOLOGIC RENAL CELL CARCINOMA SUBTYPES

RCC is known to be a heterogeneous malignancy with several subtypes that exhibit distinct clinical and pathologic features.[30,31] Several histologic subtypes of RCC have been described, including conventional clear cell RCC (cRCC), papillary RCC, and chromophobe RCC. Papillary RCC and chromophobe RCC account for about 15% to 25% of RCC, and patients who have these subtypes generally have a better long-term disease-free survival than those who have cRCC.[30–34] Other rarer subtypes (collecting duct, medullary cell, and unclassified RCC) often display more aggressive clinical behavior. Consistent clinical behavior is not observed even within the major subtypes, however, suggesting that genetic heterogeneity exists within each subtype. The unique molecular defects that are pathogenic for each subtype are becoming defined, allowing targeted molecular approaches to be developed and tested and moving RCC to the forefront of molecular therapeutics.[35] For example, the von Hippel-Lindau (*VHL*) gene on chromosome 3p25 has been implicated in von Hippel-Lindau disease, a condition in which patients often develop multiple, bilateral cRCC. Mutations in the *VHL* gene or hypermethylation of the VHL gene promoter region have been identified in 57% to 70% of patients who have sporadic RCC.[36] A recent study, however, indicates that the presence of a detectable *VHL* mutation does not affect survival in patients who have localized cRCC.[37] Dysregulation of hypoxia-inducible factors by alterations in VHL creates a vasculogenic environment favoring tumor growth. New agents targeting several signaling pathways that derive directly or indirectly from hypoxia-inducible factors, including VEGF, platelet-derived growth factor, epidermal growth factor receptor, and mammalian target of rapamycin, have proven effective in phase II and phase III clinical trials.[5–9] Genes linked to the development of

RCC also have been identified in individuals who have hereditary papillary RCC syndrome, Birt-Hogg-Dubé syndrome, and hereditary leiomyomatosis and RCC syndrome.[35] Only 4% of patients who have RCC develop the disease within the context of these familial syndromes, however, suggesting that there are many other genes yet to be implicated in the pathogenesis of RCC. More recently, a number of molecular factors have been found to serve as independent prognostic factors for RCC.

OTHER PATHOLOGIC FACTORS

Pathologic factors, including Fuhrman nuclear grade[38,39] and the presence of sarcomatoid features,[40–42] provide prognostic information in patients who have localized RCC. Histologic tumor necrosis has been shown to be a negative prognostic indicator,[39,43–45] as has collecting system invasion in low-stage lesions.[46,47] Although the presence of multiple renal tumors may complicate surgical management, multifocality has been demonstrated to confer either a neutral or positive influence on outcomes.[48–53] In addition, although involvement of the renal vein and inferior vena cava has a negative influence on prognosis, the impact of microvascular invasion on prognosis remains controversial.[54–58]

PREOPERATIVE NOMOGRAMS FOR SUSPECTED RENAL MALIGNANCY

The authors recently have constructed a nomogram to predict the likelihood of benign or malignant pathology in patients who have a single enhancing renal neoplasm amenable to partial nephrectomy (**Fig. 1**).[59,60] Based on pathologic data obtained during 862 partial nephrectomies, 20% of suspected renal malignancies had benign histology. The predicted probability of benign disease ranged from 5% to 50% based on readily identifiable preoperative factors (tumor size, patient age and gender, symptoms at presentation, and smoking history). This information may be particularly applicable when active surveillance or tumor ablation is being considered for smaller tumors in more infirm patients. Several additional preoperative nomograms predicting recurrence-free survival have been developed,[60–62] but none performs as well as algorithms that incorporate data obtained during nephrectomy.[63] The authors believe that estimation of this end point is more useful in the postoperative setting, when this information might affect subsequent decision making (surveillance protocol, adjuvant treatment).

Table 1
Prognostic factors used in prognostic algorithms for patients who have metastatic RCC

Reference	Motzer 1999	Mekhail 2005	Motzer 2004	Boumerhi 2003	Escudier 2007	Choueiri 2007
N	670	353	137	85	300	120
Previous treatment	None	None	Immunotherapy and other therapies	Immunotherapy and other therapies	Immunotherapy	VEGF-targeted therapy
Conventional histology (%)	NA	85	92	85	93	100
Prior nephrectomy (%)	65	81	74	85	94	100
Median survival (months)	10	14.8	12.7	16.5	12.6	13.8[a]
Associated with adverse outcome?						
Less than 1 to 2 years from nephrectomy or diagnosis to metastasis	Yes	Yes	No	No	Yes	Yes
Hemoglobin below lower limit of normal	Yes	Yes	Yes	Yes	No	No
Elevated alkaline phosphatase	No	No	No	Yes	Yes	No
Abnormal corrected calcium[b]	Yes	Yes	Yes	Yes	Yes	Yes
LDH more than 1.5 × upper limit of normal	Yes	Yes	No	No	Yes	No
Reduced performance status	Yes	No	Yes	No	No	Yes
No. metastatic sites	No	Yes	No	No	Yes	No
Prior radiotherapy	No	Yes	No	No	No	No
Low platelet count	No	No	No	No	No	Yes
Low neutrophil count	No	No	No	No	No	Yes

Abbreviation: NA, not available.

Data from: Escudier B, Choueiri TK, Oudard S, et al. Prognostic factors of metastatic renal cell carcinoma after failure of immunotherapy: new paradigm from a large phase III trial with shark cartilage extract AE 941. J Urol 2007;178:1904.

[a] Progression-free survival.

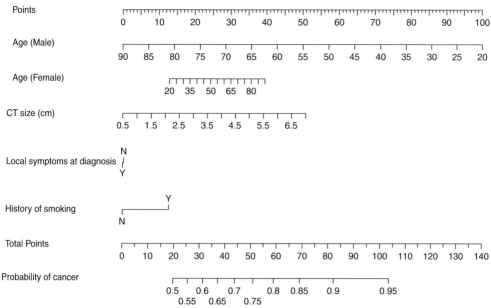

Fig. 1. Preoperative nomogram predicting the odds that an enhancing renal mass amenable to partial nephrectomy is a benign or malignant tumor. Instructions for physician: Locate the patient's age on the age axis according to gender. Draw a line upwards to the points axis to determine how many points toward cancer the patient receives for his (or her) age. Repeat this process for the other axes, each time drawing straight upward to the points axis. Sum the points achieved for each predictor, and locate this sum on the total points axis. Draw a straight line down to find the probability that cancer will be found after partial nephrectomy. Refer to this probability as P(C) and find the probability of the tumor being benign, which is 1-P(C). Inform the patient: "Mr. (or Mrs.) X, if we had 100 men (or women) exactly like you, we would expect to find a kidney cancer in P(C) of these patients after partial nephrectomy." (*From* Lane BR, Babineau D, Kattan MW, et al. A preoperative prognostic nomogram for solid enhancing renal tumors 7 cm or less amenable to partial nephrectomy. J Urol 2007;178:431; with permission.)

POSTOPERATIVE PROGNOSTIC ALGORITHMS FOR LOCALIZED RENAL CELL CARCINOMA

Several groups have developed postoperative prognostic algorithms based on clinical and pathologic features. In 2001, researchers at Memorial Sloan-Kettering Cancer Center proposed a nomogram for patients who have localized clear cell, papillary, or chromophobe RCC.[15] Prognostic factors included tumor stage, tumor size, histologic subtype, and symptoms at presentation.[15] Subsequently, the same group produced a revised nomogram for patients who had cRCC that was based on tumor stage, tumor size, nuclear grade, necrosis, vascular invasion, and symptoms at presentation (**Fig. 2**).[64] Such paper-based nomograms provide a visual aid clinicians can use during patient counseling. Software-based nomograms (www.nomograms.org) also provide accurate prognostic information and may take even less time to use during doctor–patient interactions.

Researchers at other institutions have proposed two additional postoperative prognostic systems. The University of California, Los Angeles (UCLA)

Integrated Staging System (UISS) divides patients into five groups shown to have statistically significant differences in disease-specific survival.[21] Although the UCLA group initially evaluated many potential prognostic parameters, the UISS is based solely on tumor stage, nuclear grade, and ECOG performance status.[21] In a subsequent report, the UISS was modified to identify patients who had nonmetastatic or metastatic disease at low, intermediate, or high risk of disease progression (**Table 2**).[65] This modified UISS has been validated both internally and externally in larger series of patients.[65,66] One drawback of the UISS is that it does not predict a probability of failure for an individual patient but instead places individuals into low-, intermediate-, and high-risk groups, making the information provided less meaningful for treatment decision making.

In 2002, the group at the Mayo Clinic devised the SSIGN score, in which patients who have cRCC are assigned a score based on tumor stage, tumor size, nuclear grade, and the presence of necrosis (**Table 3**).[43] The estimated cancer-specific survival for an individual patient at 1 to

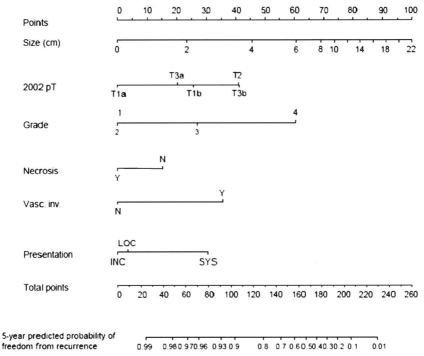

Fig. 2. Postoperative nomogram predicting recurrence of conventional RCC after nephrectomy. Instructions for physician: Locate the patient's tumor size on the size axis. Draw a line upwards to the points axis to determine how many points toward recurrence the patient receives for the tumor size. Repeat this process for the other axes, each time drawing straight upward to the points axis. Sum the points achieved for each predictor and locate this sum on the total points axis. Draw a straight line down to find the probability that the patient will remain free of recurrence for 5 years, assuming the patient does not die of another cause first. Inform the patient: "Mr. (or Mrs.) X, if we had 100 men (or women) exactly like you, we would expect (predicted percentage from nomogram) to remain free of their disease 5 years following surgery, although recurrence after 5 years is still possible." (*From* Sorbellini M, Kattan MW, Snyder ME, et al. A postoperative prognostic nomogram predicting recurrence for patients with conventional clear cell renal cell carcinoma. J Urol 2005;173:50; with permission.)

10 years then is provided based on the total of the SSIGN score (**Table 4**). The SSIGN score was based on data from more than 1800 patients but as of yet has not been validated internally or externally against additional datasets.

Many statistical methods can be used to evaluate predictive models.[14] The concordance index (c-index) is a measure of the predictive accuracy of prognostic algorithms, in which the algorithm is asked to predict which of two patients will experience clinical failure first. Comparison with the actual outcome in a large series of patient pairs determines the c-index. Perfect predictive accuracy yields the highest possible value of 1.0, whereas random chance provides a baseline value of 0.5. Although the predictive accuracy of these algorithms improves on traditional TNM staging and individual factors, such as nuclear grade and ECOG status, each of the available tools has a c-index less than 1.0, indicating room for improvement.

Comparative evaluation of prognostic algorithms should be performed with care, because c-indexes cannot be compared directly across datasets. More accurate information is obtained from head-to-head comparisons on the same validation dataset, as performed to compare the 1997 and 2002 TNM staging systems.[12,13] The discriminating ability of four prognostic algorithms was compared using an independent dataset containing more than 2400 patients.[63] Calculations of c-indexes and 95% bootstrap confidence intervals for overall survival, cancer-specific survival, and recurrence-free survival at 5 years consistently revealed the Kattan RCC nomogram to be most accurate.[63] Further studies comparing each of the prognostic models in the same datasets will help identify the most accurate nomograms. Calculation of the c-index addresses only the ranking of outcomes and does not address the absolute predictive accuracy (ie, calibration). To examine the accuracy of a particular predicted

Table 2
Modified UCLA integrated staging system

Nonmetastatic cases										
Stage	T1				T2	T3				T4
Fuhrman nuclear grade	1-2		3-4		Any	1		2-4		Any
ECOG performance status	0	≥1	0	≥1	Any	0	≥1	0	≥1	Any
Risk	Low	Intermediate								High
Metastatic cases										
Stage	N1M0	N2M0 or M1								
Fuhrman nuclear grade	Any	1		2		3		4		
ECOG performance status	Any	0	≥1	0	≥1	0	≥1	0	≥1	
Risk	Low		Intermediate	Low	Intermediate				High	

Data from Zisman A, Pantuck AJ, Wieder J, et al. Risk group assessment and clinical outcome algorithm to predict the natural history of patients with surgically resected renal cell carcinoma. J Clin Oncol 2002:20;4561.

probability, calibration usually is performed by plotting predicted versus actual probabilities. Most of the algorithms discussed in this article have been assessed for discrimination, most commonly by a bootstrapping method.

MOLECULAR FACTORS

A large number of genes that may have prognostic and therapeutic significance have been identified using high-throughput technology to investigate gene expression in RCC.[67–77] Several studies demonstrated that each histologic subtype of RCC can be differentiated by gene-expression profiling of renal tumors.[67–71,78–81] Correlation of changes in gene expression with corresponding protein expression and location can be analyzed using immunohistochemical staining of individual tissue samples. Construction of tissue microarrays can facilitate the screening of a larger number of pathologic samples, but interpretation of results accumulated in multiple datasets can be difficult.[10,82]

Many experts believe that the incorporation of both clinical and molecular factors is likely to result in the best prognostic tools. Proof-of-principle has been illustrated by the group at UCLA, who demonstrated that a clinical and molecular model (**Fig. 3**) was better than standard clinical models or a model based on molecular information alone.[10,83] The addition of expression data from five markers, including carbonic anhydrase IX (CA-IX), Ki67, gelsolin, vimentin, and p53, improved the discriminating ability of the UISS for localized RCC.[10] Other molecular factors identified as independent risk factors are B7-H1,[84,85] B7-H4,[86] PD-1,[87] EpCAM/KSA,[88] IGF-1,[89,90]

Table 3
SSIGN score algorithm

Feature	Score
T stage	
pT1	0
pT2	1
pT3 or T4	2
N stage	
pNx or N0	0
pN0 or N2	2
M stage	
pM0	0
pM1	4
Tumor size	
< 5 cm	0
≥ 5 cm	2
Furhman nuclear grade	
1 or 2	0
3	1
4	3
Necrosis	
Absent	0
Present	2

The sum of the scores is used to determine survival using **Table 4**.
Data from Frank I, Blute ML, Cheville JC, et al. An outcome prediction model for patients with clear cell renal cell carcinoma treated with radical nephrectomy based on tumor stage, size, grade and necrosis: the SSIGN score. J Urol 2002;168:2398.

Table 4
Estimated cancer-specific survival (CSS) following radical nephrectomy for cRCC according to SSIGN score

SSIGN Score	1-Year CSS (%)	5-Year CSS (%)	10-Year CSS (%)
0–1	100	99.4	97.1
2	99.1	94.8	85.3
3	97.4	87.8	77.9
4	95.4	79.1	66.2
5	91.1	65.4	50.0
6	87.0	54.0	38.8
7	80.3	41.0	28.1
8	65.1	23.6	12.7
9	60.5	19.6	14.8
10 or more	36.2	7.4	4.6

Data from Frank I, Blute ML, Cheville JC, et al. An outcome prediction model for patients with clear cell renal cell carcinoma treated with radical nephrectomy based on tumor stage, size, grade and necrosis: the SSIGN score. J Urol 2002;168:2398.

Smac/DIABLO,[91] Survivin,[85,92] PTEN,[10,93] p27,[93,94] Skp2,[94] VEGF,[95,96] VEGF receptors,[96] and EphA2.[97]

When judging a new marker, it is important to evaluate it after considering the contribution of existing markers. In other words, a new marker should improve the ability to predict outcome beyond what already can be achieved with existing markers. For example, the finding that high Ki-67 expression predicted disease recurrence was called into question by data indicating that it was simply a surrogate for histologic necrosis.[44] More recent evidence seems to indicate that each of these histologic factors has independent prognostic information.[98] To validate the cost of obtaining molecular data in current clinical practice, studies must evaluate not only the predictive ability of a new marker but also its usefulness in light of all the known clinical and pathologic risk factors. A new marker that merely replaces an existing marker is not likely to be helpful.[14]

MOLECULAR MARKER–DRIVEN THERAPIES

The two molecules that have been most rigorously evaluated at present are CA-IX, the hypoxia-induced protein product of *MN-9* gene, and the co-stimulatory molecule B7-H1. Although initial studies indicated that decreased CA-IX expression is associated independently with poor survival in patients who have advanced cRCC,[83,99] the association may not hold true in patients who have localized disease.[100] It is clear that CA-IX is expressed in the vast majority of cRCC (97%) and only rarely in other histologic subtypes, making it an attractive marker for diagnostic evaluation of renal masses.[100,101] In addition, CA-IX may serve as a marker for response to systemic therapy, making CA-IX immunostaining particularly valuable in advanced RCC. One study reported that all complete responders to immunotherapy with interleukin-2 had high CA-IX expression,[102] and a second study reported that complete response was twice as likely in this group of patients.[103] Some clinicians now are using this information to reserve high-dose interleukin-2 administration for patients who have characteristics

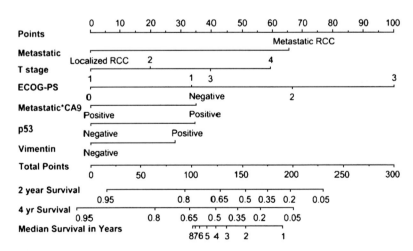

Fig. 3. Postoperative nomogram predicting disease-specific survival based on clinical variables and molecular markers (*From* Kim HL, Seligson D, Liu X, et al. Using protein expressions to predict survival in clear cell renal carcinoma. Clin Cancer Res 2004;10:5468; with permission.)

predicting the highest chance of benefit. Patients who have low CA-IX expression are not considered for interleukin-2 and are offered alternative therapies instead. One small trial, however, now indicates that CA-IX expression does not seem to predict for response to temsirolimus.[104]

B7-H1 expression in cRCC initially was found to be associated with a 4.5-fold greater risk of cancer-specific mortality,[84] This finding has been internally validated,[105] with the additional finding that high Survivin and B7-H1 expression together were associated with a 2.8-fold higher risk of cancer-specific death.[85] In addition to serving as a tumor marker for progression, B7-H1 is an attractive therapeutic target in patients who have advanced RCC. Because B7-H1 may function as an inhibitor of T-cell–mediated antitumoral immunity, blockade of its activity with a humanized neutralizing antibody has been postulated to facilitate immunotherapeutic responses in patients who have cRCC, and clinical trials are anticipated.[106]

PROGNOSTIC ALGORITHMS FOR METASTATIC RENAL CELL CARCINOMA

The group at Memorial Sloan-Kettering Cancer Center first classified patients into good-, intermediate-, and poor-risk groups according to risk factors that independently predicted overall survival in untreated patients who had metastatic RCC (see **Table 1**).[107] This model was validated externally using data from the Cleveland Clinic.[108] Mekhail and colleagues[108] found four of the five risk factors identified by Motzer and colleagues[107] to be independent predictors of overall survival. Subsequently, several analyses in previously treated patients who had metastatic RCC have been performed using similar methodology (see **Table 1**). Two papers identified risk factors predicting overall survival, largely in patients treated before the advent of molecularly-targeted therapy.[109,110] More recently, risk factors that categorize patients into good, intermediate, and poor risk for progression-free survival after treatment with agents targeting VEGF have been examined. A recent study analyzed factors predicting overall survival in 300 patients in whom disease had progressed despite immunotherapy.[111] The five independent risk factors that predicted shorter overall survival (high alkaline phosphatase, abnormal corrected calcium, lactate dehydrogenase >1.5 upper limit of normal, more than one metastatic site, and years between nephrectomy and metastasis) were incorporated into an algorithm that identified good-, intermediate-, and poor-risk groups.[111] The authors of that study concluded that these algorithms can be used to standardize patient enrollment in clinical trials better, and the authors of this article agree with this assessment. One caveat, however, is that all these studies use similar methodology, namely, the identification of risk factors with independent predictive ability in multivariable analyses and the use of these risk factors to group patients into a small number of categories. As mentioned earlier, grouping patients results in a loss of the robustness of the data and may result in the treatment of a heterogeneous group of poor-risk patients in one manner.

SUMMARY

Patients should be provided with the most accurate information about their likely individual disease course currently available to expert clinicians. A preoperative nomogram can predict the likelihood that a suspected malignancy is a cancer. Three major prognostic algorithms exist for localized RCC, each of which can assess the likelihood of disease recurrence better than the TNM staging system alone. Classification of patients who have metastatic RCC into good-, intermediate-, and poor-risk groups can define disease-specific survival better, aiding in the selection of appropriate systemic therapies or clinical trials. In each of these areas, more accurate nomograms will allow physicians to offer patients better counsel regarding their likely clinical course, will assist in the planning and tailoring of follow-up, and will identify patients who are more likely to benefit from individual treatments. Future algorithms predicting disease outcomes or response to treatment are likely to incorporate molecular factors with the potential to provide even greater information.

REFERENCES

1. Janzen NK, Kim HL, Figlin RA, et al. Surveillance after radical or partial nephrectomy for localized renal cell carcinoma and management of recurrent disease. Urol Clin North Am 2003;30:843–52.
2. Coppin C, Porzsolt F, Awa A, et al. Immunotherapy for advanced renal cell cancer. Cochrane Database Syst Rev 2005;CD001425.
3. Chow WH, Devesa SS, Warren JL, et al. Rising incidence of renal cell cancer in the United States. JAMA 1999;281:1628–31.
4. Jemal A, Siegel R, Ward E, et al. Cancer statistics, 2007. CA Cancer J Clin 2007;57:43–66.
5. Motzer RJ, Rini BI, Bukowski RM, et al. Sunitinib in patients with metastatic renal cell carcinoma. JAMA 2006;295:2516–24.
6. Motzer RJ, Hutson TE, Tomczak P, et al. Sunitinib versus interferon alfa in metastatic renal-cell carcinoma. N Engl J Med 2007;356:115–24.

7. Ratain MJ, Eisen T, Stadler WM, et al. Phase II placebo-controlled randomized discontinuation trial of sorafenib in patients with metastatic renal cell carcinoma. J Clin Oncol 2006;24:2505–12.

8. Escudier B, Eisen T, Stadler WM, et al. Sorafenib in advanced clear-cell renal-cell carcinoma. N Engl J Med 2007;356:125–34.

9. Hudes G, Carducci M, Tomczak P, et al. Temsirolimus, interferon alfa, or both for advanced renal-cell carcinoma. N Engl J Med 2007;356:2271–81.

10. Kim HL, Seligson D, Liu X, et al. Using protein expressions to predict survival in clear cell renal carcinoma. Clin Cancer Res 2004;10:5464–71.

11. Campbell SC, Novick AC, Bukowski RM. Renal tumors. In: Wein AJ, Kavoussi LR, Novick AC, et al, editors. Campbell-Walsh urology. vol. 4. 9th edition. Philadelphia: Saunders; 2007. p. 2672–731.

12. Frank I, Blute ML, Leibovich BC, et al. Independent validation of the 2002 American Joint Committee on Cancer Primary Tumor Classification for Renal Cell Carcinoma using a large, single institution cohort. J Urol 2005;173:1889–92.

13. Ficarra V, Schips L, Guille F, et al. Multiinstitutional European validation of the 2002 TNM staging system in conventional and papillary localized renal cell carcinoma. Cancer 2005;104:968–74.

14. Kattan MW. Evaluating a new marker's predictive contribution. Clin Cancer Res 2004;10:822–4.

15. Kattan MW, Reuter V, Motzer RJ, et al. A post-operative prognostic nomogram for renal cell carcinoma. J Urol 2001;166:63–7.

16. Pantuck AJ, Zisman A, Belldegrun AS. The changing natural history of renal cell carcinoma. J Urol 2001;166:1611–23.

17. Patard JJ, Dorey FJ, Cindolo L, et al. Symptoms as well as tumor size provide prognostic information on patients with localized renal tumors. J Urol 2004;172:2167–71.

18. Patard JJ, Leray E, Cindolo L, et al. Multi-institutional validation of a symptom based classification for renal cell carcinoma. J Urol 2004;172:858–62.

19. Oken MM, Creech RH, Tormey DC, et al. Toxicity and response criteria of the Eastern Cooperative Oncology Group. Am J Clin Oncol 1982;5:649–55.

20. Tsui KH, Shvarts O, Smith RB, et al. Prognostic indicators for renal cell carcinoma: a multivariate analysis of 643 patients using the revised 1997 TNM staging criteria. J Urol 2000;163:1090–5 [quiz 1295].

21. Zisman A, Pantuck AJ, Dorey F, et al. Improved prognostication of renal cell carcinoma using an integrated staging system. J Clin Oncol 2001;19:1649–57.

22. Kontak JA, Campbell SC. Prognostic factors in renal cell carcinoma. Urol Clin North Am 2003;30:467–80.

23. Kim HL, Belldegrun AS, Freitas DG, et al. Paraneoplastic signs and symptoms of renal cell carcinoma: implications for prognosis. J Urol 2003;170:1742–6.

24. Kim HL, Han KR, Zisman A, et al. Cachexia-like symptoms predict a worse prognosis in localized T1 renal cell carcinoma. J Urol 2004;171:1810–3.

25. Ljungberg B, Grankvist K, Rasmuson T. Serum acute phase reactants and prognosis in renal cell carcinoma. Cancer 1995;76:1435–9.

26. Symbas NP, Townsend MF, El-Galley R, et al. Poor prognosis associated with thrombocytosis in patients with renal cell carcinoma. BJU Int 2000;86:203–7.

27. O'Keefe SC, Marshall FF, Issa MM, et al. Thrombocytosis is associated with a significant increase in the cancer specific death rate after radical nephrectomy. J Urol 2002;168:1378–80.

28. Jacobsen J, Grankvist K, Rasmuson T, et al. Prognostic importance of serum vascular endothelial growth factor in relation to platelet and leukocyte counts in human renal cell carcinoma. Eur J Cancer Prev 2002;11:245–52.

29. Karakiewicz PI, Hutterer GC, Trinh QD, et al. C-reactive protein is an informative predictor of renal cell carcinoma-specific mortality: a European study of 313 patients. Cancer 2007;110:1241–7.

30. Cheville JC, Lohse CM, Zincke H, et al. Comparisons of outcome and prognostic features among histologic subtypes of renal cell carcinoma. Am J Surg Pathol 2003;27:612–24.

31. Lau WK, Cheville JC, Blute ML, et al. Prognostic features of pathologic stage T1 renal cell carcinoma after radical nephrectomy. Urology 2002;59:532–7.

32. Moch H, Gasser T, Amin MB, et al. Prognostic utility of the recently recommended histologic classification and revised TNM staging system of renal cell carcinoma: a Swiss experience with 588 tumors. Cancer 2000;89:604–14.

33. Amin MB, Tamboli P, Javidan J, et al. Prognostic impact of histologic subtyping of adult renal epithelial neoplasms: an experience of 405 cases. Am J Surg Pathol 2002;26:281–91.

34. Beck SD, Patel MI, Snyder ME, et al. Effect of papillary and chromophobe cell type on disease-free survival after nephrectomy for renal cell carcinoma. Ann Surg Oncol 2004;11:71–7.

35. Linehan WM, Pinto PA, Srinivasan R, et al. Identification of the genes for kidney cancer: opportunity for disease-specific targeted therapeutics. Clin Cancer Res 2007;13:671s–9s.

36. Yao M, Yoshida M, Kishida T, et al. VHL tumor suppressor gene alterations associated with good prognosis in sporadic clear-cell renal carcinoma. J Natl Cancer Inst 2002;94:1569–75.

37. Smits KM, Schouten LJ, van Dijk BA, et al. Genetic and epigenetic alterations in the von Hippel-Lindau gene: the influence on renal cancer prognosis. Clin Cancer Res 2008;14:782–7.

38. Lang H, Lindner V, de Fromont M, et al. Multicenter determination of optimal interobserver agreement using the Fuhrman grading system for renal cell carcinoma: assessment of 241 patients with > 15-year follow-up. Cancer 2005;103:625–9.

39. Lohse CM, Cheville JC. A review of prognostic pathologic features and algorithms for patients treated surgically for renal cell carcinoma. Clin Lab Med 2005;25:433–64.

40. de Peralta-Venturina M, Moch H, Amin M, et al. Sarcomatoid differentiation in renal cell carcinoma: a study of 101 cases. Am J Surg Pathol 2001;25: 275–84.

41. Mian BM, Bhadkamkar N, Slaton JW, et al. Prognostic factors and survival of patients with sarcomatoid renal cell carcinoma. J Urol 2002;167: 65–70.

42. Cheville JC, Lohse CM, Zincke H, et al. Sarcomatoid renal cell carcinoma: an examination of underlying histologic subtype and an analysis of associations with patient outcome. Am J Surg Pathol 2004;28: 435–41.

43. Frank I, Blute ML, Cheville JC, et al. An outcome prediction model for patients with clear cell renal cell carcinoma treated with radical nephrectomy based on tumor stage, size, grade and necrosis: the SSIGN score. J Urol 2002;168:2395–400.

44. Lam JS, Shvarts O, Said JW, et al. Clinicopathologic and molecular correlations of necrosis in the primary tumor of patients with renal cell carcinoma. Cancer 2005;103:2517–25.

45. Sengupta S, Lohse CM, Leibovich BC, et al. Histologic coagulative tumor necrosis as a prognostic indicator of renal cell carcinoma aggressiveness. Cancer 2005;104:511–20.

46. Uzzo RG, Cherullo EE, Myles J, et al. Renal cell carcinoma invading the urinary collecting system: implications for staging. J Urol 2002;167:2392–6.

47. Klatte T, Chung J, Leppert JT, et al. Prognostic relevance of capsular involvement and collecting system invasion in stage I and II renal cell carcinoma. BJU Int 2007;99:821–4.

48. Steinbach F, Stockle M, Griesinger A, et al. Multifocal renal cell tumors: a retrospective analysis of 56 patients treated with radical nephrectomy. J Urol 1994;152:1393–6.

49. Baltaci S, Orhan D, Soyupek S, et al. Influence of tumor stage, size, grade, vascular involvement, histological cell type and histological pattern on multifocality of renal cell carcinoma. J Urol 2000; 164:36–9.

50. Blute ML, Thibault GP, Leibovich BC, et al. Multiple ipsilateral renal tumors discovered at planned nephron sparing surgery: importance of tumor histology and risk of metachronous recurrence. J Urol 2003;170:760–3.

51. Dimarco DS, Lohse CM, Zincke H, et al. Long-term survival of patients with unilateral sporadic multifocal renal cell carcinoma according to histologic subtype compared with patients with solitary tumors after radical nephrectomy. Urology 2004; 64:462–7.

52. Lang H, Lindner V, Martin M, et al. Prognostic value of multifocality on progression and survival in localized renal cell carcinoma. Eur Urol 2004;45: 749–53.

53. Richstone L, Scherr DS, Reuter VR, et al. Multifocal renal cortical tumors: frequency, associated clinicopathological features and impact on survival. J Urol 2004;171:615–20.

54. Hatcher PA, Anderson EE, Paulson DF, et al. Surgical management and prognosis of renal cell carcinoma invading the vena cava. J Urol 1991;145:20–3 [discussion: 23–4].

55. Kim HL, Zisman A, Han KR, et al. Prognostic significance of venous thrombus in renal cell carcinoma. Are renal vein and inferior vena cava involvement different? J Urol 2004;171:588–91.

56. Ishimura T, Sakai I, Hara I, et al. Microscopic venous invasion in renal cell carcinoma as a predictor of recurrence after radical surgery. Int J Urol 2004;11: 264–8.

57. Lang H, Lindner V, Letourneux H, et al. Prognostic value of microscopic venous invasion in renal cell carcinoma: long-term follow-up. Eur Urol 2004;46: 331–5.

58. Dall'Oglio MF, Antunes AA, Sarkis AS, et al. Microvascular tumour invasion in renal cell carcinoma: the most important prognostic factor. BJU Int 2007;100:552–5.

59. Lane BR, Babineau D, Kattan MW, et al. A preoperative prognostic nomogram for solid enhancing renal tumors 7 cm or less amenable to partial nephrectomy. J Urol 2007;178:429–34.

60. Raj GV, Thompson RH, Leibovich BC, et al. Preoperative nomogram predicting 12-year probability of metastatic renal cancer. J Urol 2008;179:2146–51.

61. Yaycioglu O, Rutman MP, Balasubramaniam M, et al. Clinical and pathologic tumor size in renal cell carcinoma; difference, correlation, and analysis of the influencing factors. Urology 2002;60:33–8.

62. Cindolo L, de la Taille A, Messina G, et al. A preoperative clinical prognostic model for non-metastatic renal cell carcinoma. BJU Int 2003;92:901–5.

63. Cindolo L, Patard JJ, Chiodini P, et al. Comparison of predictive accuracy of four prognostic models for nonmetastatic renal cell carcinoma after nephrectomy. Cancer 2005;104:1362–71.

64. Sorbellini M, Kattan MW, Snyder ME, et al. A postoperative prognostic nomogram predicting

recurrence for patients with conventional clear cell renal cell carcinoma. J Urol 2005;173:48–51.

65. Zisman A, Pantuck AJ, Wieder J, et al. Risk group assessment and clinical outcome algorithm to predict the natural history of patients with surgically resected renal cell carcinoma. J Clin Oncol 2002;20: 4559–66.

66. Patard JJ, Kim HL, Lam JS, et al. Use of the University of California Los Angeles integrated staging system to predict survival in renal cell carcinoma: an international multicenter study. J Clin Oncol 2004;22:3316–22.

67. Takahashi M, Rhodes DR, Furge KA, et al. Gene expression profiling of clear cell renal cell carcinoma: gene identification and prognostic classification. Proc Natl Acad Sci U S A 2001;98:9754–9.

68. Young AN, Amin MB, Moreno CS, et al. Expression profiling of renal epithelial neoplasms: a method for tumor classification and discovery of diagnostic molecular markers. Am J Pathol 2001;158: 1639–51.

69. Higgins JP, Shinghal R, Gill H, et al. Gene expression patterns in renal cell carcinoma assessed by complementary DNA microarray. Am J Pathol 2003;162:925–32.

70. Gieseg MA, Cody T, Man MZ, et al. Expression profiling of human renal carcinomas with functional taxonomic analysis. BMC Bioinformatics 2002;3:26.

71. Boer JM, Huber WK, Sultmann H, et al. Identification and classification of differentially expressed genes in renal cell carcinoma by expression profiling on a global human 31,500-element cDNA array. Genome Res 2001;11:1861–70.

72. Moch H, Schraml P, Bubendorf L, et al. High-throughput tissue microarray analysis to evaluate genes uncovered by cDNA microarray screening in renal cell carcinoma. Am J Pathol 1999;154: 981–6.

73. Liou LS, Shi T, Duan ZH, et al. Microarray gene expression profiling and analysis in renal cell carcinoma. BMC Urol 2004;4:9.

74. Yao M, Tabuchi H, Nagashima Y, et al. Gene expression analysis of renal carcinoma: adipose differentiation-related protein as a potential diagnostic and prognostic biomarker for clear-cell renal carcinoma. J Pathol 2005;205:377–87.

75. Ami Y, Shimazui T, Akaza H, et al. Gene expression profiles correlate with the morphology and metastasis characteristics of renal cell carcinoma cells. Oncol Rep 2005;13:75–80.

76. Vasselli JR, Shih JH, Iyengar SR, et al. Predicting survival in patients with metastatic kidney cancer by gene-expression profiling in the primary tumor. Proc Natl Acad Sci U S A 2003;100:6958–63.

77. Skubitz KM, Skubitz AP. Differential gene expression in renal-cell cancer. J Lab Clin Med 2002; 140:52–64.

78. Huo L, Sugimura J, Tretiakova MS, et al. C-kit expression in renal oncocytomas and chromophobe renal cell carcinomas. Hum Pathol 2005;36:262–8.

79. Junker K, Hindermann W, von Eggeling F, et al. CD70: a new tumor specific biomarker for renal cell carcinoma. J Urol 2005;173:2150–3.

80. Tretiakova MS, Sahoo S, Takahashi M, et al. Expression of alpha-methylacyl-CoA racemase in papillary renal cell carcinoma. Am J Surg Pathol 2004; 28:69–76.

81. Yang XJ, Tan MH, Kim HL, et al. A molecular classification of papillary renal cell carcinoma. Cancer Res 2005;65:5628–37.

82. Liu X, Minin V, Huang Y, et al. Statistical methods for analyzing tissue microarray data. J Biopharm Stat 2004;14:671–85.

83. Kim HL, Seligson D, Liu X, et al. Using tumor markers to predict the survival of patients with metastatic renal cell carcinoma. J Urol 2005;173: 1496–501.

84. Thompson RH, Gillett MD, Cheville JC, et al. Costimulatory B7-H1 in renal cell carcinoma patients: indicator of tumor aggressiveness and potential therapeutic target. Proc Natl Acad Sci U S A 2004;101:17174–9.

85. Krambeck AE, Dong H, Thompson RH, et al. Survivin and b7-h1 are collaborative predictors of survival and represent potential therapeutic targets for patients with renal cell carcinoma. Clin Cancer Res 2007;13:1749–56.

86. Krambeck AE, Thompson RH, Dong H, et al. B7-H4 expression in renal cell carcinoma and tumor vasculature: associations with cancer progression and survival. Proc Natl Acad Sci U S A 2006;103: 10391–6.

87. Thompson RH, Dong H, Lohse CM, et al. PD-1 is expressed by tumor-infiltrating immune cells and is associated with poor outcome for patients with renal cell carcinoma. Clin Cancer Res 2007;13: 1757–61.

88. Seligson DB, Pantuck AJ, Liu X, et al. Epithelial cell adhesion molecule (KSA) expression: pathobiology and its role as an independent predictor of survival in renal cell carcinoma. Clin Cancer Res 2004;10: 2659–69.

89. Parker A, Cheville JC, Lohse C, et al. Expression of insulin-like growth factor I receptor and survival in patients with clear cell renal cell carcinoma. J Urol 2003;170:420–4.

90. Rasmuson T, Grankvist K, Jacobsen J, et al. Serum insulin-like growth factor-1 is an independent

predictor of prognosis in patients with renal cell carcinoma. Acta Oncol 2004;43:744–8.

91. Mizutani Y, Nakanishi H, Yamamoto K, et al. Down-regulation of Smac/DIABLO expression in renal cell carcinoma and its prognostic significance. J Clin Oncol 2005;23:448–54.

92. Byun SS, Yeo WG, Lee SE, et al. Expression of survivin in renal cell carcinomas: association with pathologic features and clinical outcome. Urology 2007;69:34–7.

93. Pantuck AJ, Seligson DB, Klatte T, et al. Prognostic relevance of the mTOR pathway in renal cell carcinoma: implications for molecular patient selection for targeted therapy. Cancer 2007;109:2257–67.

94. Langner C, von Wasielewski R, Ratschek M, et al. Biological significance of p27 and Skp2 expression in renal cell carcinoma. A systematic analysis of primary and metastatic tumour tissues using a tissue microarray technique. Virchows Arch 2004;445:631–6.

95. Jacobsen J, Rasmuson T, Grankvist K, et al. Vascular endothelial growth factor as prognostic factor in renal cell carcinoma. J Urol 2000;163:343–7.

96. Rivet J, Mourah S, Murata H, et al. VEGF and VEGFR-1 are coexpressed by epithelial and stromal cells of renal cell carcinoma. Cancer 2008;112:433–42.

97. Herrem CJ, Tatsumi T, Olson KS, et al. Expression of EphA2 is prognostic of disease-free interval and overall survival in surgically treated patients with renal cell carcinoma. Clin Cancer Res 2005; 11:226–31.

98. Tollefson MK, Thompson RH, Sheinin Y, et al. Ki-67 and coagulative tumor necrosis are independent predictors of poor outcome for patients with clear cell renal cell carcinoma and not surrogates for each other. Cancer 2007;110:783–90.

99. Bui MH, Seligson D, Han KR, et al. Carbonic anhydrase IX is an independent predictor of survival in advanced renal clear cell carcinoma: implications for prognosis and therapy. Clin Cancer Res 2003; 9:802–11.

100. Leibovich BC, Sheinin Y, Lohse CM, et al. Carbonic anhydrase IX is not an independent predictor of outcome for patients with clear cell renal cell carcinoma. J Clin Oncol 2007;25:4757–64.

101. Divgi CR, Pandit-Taskar N, Jungbluth AA, et al. Preoperative characterisation of clear-cell renal carcinoma using iodine-124-labelled antibody chimeric G250 (124I-cG250) and PET in patients with renal masses: a phase I trial. Lancet Oncol 2007;8:304–10.

102. Bui MH, Visapaa H, Seligson D, et al. Prognostic value of carbonic anhydrase IX and KI67 as predictors of survival for renal clear cell carcinoma. J Urol 2004;171:2461–6.

103. Atkins M, Regan M, McDermott D, et al. Carbonic anhydrase IX expression predicts outcome of interleukin 2 therapy for renal cancer. Clin Cancer Res 2005;11:3714–21.

104. Cho D, Signoretti S, Dabora S, et al. Potential histologic and molecular predictors of response to temsirolimus in patients with advanced renal cell carcinoma. Clin Genitourin Cancer 2007;5:379–85.

105. Thompson RH, Kuntz SM, Leibovich BC, et al. Tumor B7-H1 is associated with poor prognosis in renal cell carcinoma patients with long-term follow-up. Cancer Res 2006;66:3381–5.

106. Thompson RH, Dong H, Kwon ED. Implications of B7-H1 expression in clear cell carcinoma of the kidney for prognostication and therapy. Clin Cancer Res 2007;13:709s–15s.

107. Motzer RJ, Mazumdar M, Bacik J, et al. Survival and prognostic stratification of 670 patients with advanced renal cell carcinoma. J Clin Oncol 1999;17:2530–40.

108. Mekhail TM, Abou-Jawde RM, Boumerhi G, et al. Validation and extension of the memorial sloan-kettering prognostic factors model for survival in patients with previously untreated metastatic renal cell carcinoma. J Clin Oncol 2005;23:832–41.

109. Boumerhi G, Mekhail TM, Abou-Jawde RM, et al. Prognostic factors for survival in previously treated patients with metastatic renal cell cancer. J Clin Oncol 2003;22 [abstract 1647].

110. Motzer RJ, Bacik J, Schwartz LH, et al. Prognostic factors for survival in previously treated patients with metastatic renal cell carcinoma. J Clin Oncol 2004;22:454–63.

111. Escudier B, Choueiri TK, Oudard S, et al. Prognostic factors of metastatic renal cell carcinoma after failure of immunotherapy: new paradigm from a large phase III trial with shark cartilage extract AE 941. J Urol 2007;178:1901–5.

Renal Tumor Natural History: the Rationale and Role for Active Surveillance

Michael A.S. Jewett, MD[a],*, Alvaro Zuniga, MD[b]

KEYWORDS
- Kidney tumors • Small renal mass
- Watchful waiting • Active surveillance

Renal cell carcinoma (RCC) is the most common malignancy of the kidney and it represents 2% to 3% of newly diagnosed cancers in the United States. It is estimated that there were 51,190 new cases and 12,890 deaths from kidney cancer in 2007.[1] This incidence has been increasing in the past 20 years.[1–3] From 1983 to 2002, the overall age-adjusted incidence rate for kidney cancer rose from 7.1 to 10.8 cases per 100,000 US population, which is an increase of 52%.[4] This increase is at least in part attributable to the more frequent use of abdominal imaging.[3,5–7] All clinical stages have increased in incidence but the largest increase is in tumors smaller than 4 cm. These CT-enhancing lesions that have the characteristics of RCC have been termed small renal masses (SRMs).[8] The incidence of tumors 2 to 4 cm in size rose from 1.0 to 3.3 per 100,000.[4] Resected tumor size dropped from a maximum diameter of 7.8 cm to 5.3 cm between 1989 and 1998.[9] Diagnosis as an incidental finding increased from 7% to 13% in the early 1970s to 48% to 66% of kidney cancer currently.[5,6,10,11] Not all SRMs are RCC, and those incidentally discovered are more frequently benign. Frank and colleagues[12] reported a large series of 2770 renal tumors. Benign tumors accounted for 46.3% of those smaller than 1 cm, 22.4% of tumors 1.0 to 1.9 cm, 22.0% of tumors 2.0 to 2.9 cm, and 19.9% of tumors 3.0 to 3.9 cm and most of these incidental tumors have a lower grade than those in symptomatic patients. The greatest incidence of SRMs is in patients older than 65 years, which is an age group more likely to undergo radiological examination for other medical conditions.[1] They also have more comorbidity and are therefore at increased surgical risk. Hollingsworth and colleagues[13] in a cohort of 26,618 individuals treated surgically for localized kidney cancer, showed that the relative benefit of therapy is diminished by competing causes of mortality in older patients. Nearly one third of patients aged 70 years and older died from unrelated comorbid disease within 5 years of curative surgery.

Even though surgical morbidity is decreasing, it is still significant and has been reported in 11% to 40% of cases.[9,14–16] Despite widespread treatment at diagnosis, overall mortality rates associated with RCC have not decreased.[6] Five-year cancer-specific survival of 90% or greater with low recurrence rates is widely reported for early-stage tumors.[9,17,18] Interestingly, these results are frequently reported to be independent of margin status.[19]

These observations suggest that SRMs that are RCC may frequently be slow growing and have a reduced risk of early progression. Initial active surveillance with delayed treatment for progression for some patients should be considered.[20] This should result in an overall decrease in treatment burden and cost saving.

[a] Division of Urology, Department of Surgical Oncology, Princess Margaret Hospital and the University Health Network, University of Toronto, 610 University Avenue, 3-124, Toronto, Ontario, Canada M5G 2C4
[b] UroOncology Fellowship Program, University of Toronto, Toronto, Ontario, Canada
* Corresponding author.
E-mail address: m.jewett@utoronto.ca (M.A.S. Jewett).

Urol Clin N Am 35 (2008) 627–634
doi:10.1016/j.ucl.2008.07.004

NATURAL HISTORY

The natural history of renal tumors has not been extensively studied because the only established curative treatment for RCC has been surgery by radical or partial nephrectomy (which is done soon after diagnosis).[9,21–23]

Since 1995 there have been a number of reports that contribute to our understanding of the natural history of SRMs.[20,24–27] They all indicate that these tumors grow slowly. However, most of the clinical series are small, single institutional and retrospective.[28] Bosniak and colleagues[24] collected 40 incidentally detected renal masses < 3.5 cm in diameter with 3.25 years of follow-up. They reported a mean linear growth rate of 0.36 cm/year (0–1.1cm/year) by retrospectively reviewing available imaging obtained before surgery. Of 26 tumors removed, 22 (85%) revealed pathological RCC. Nineteen had a growth rate < 0.35 cm/year and none of the patients developed metastatic disease. These results showed that most of their reported renal masses had little or no change in size and they hypothesized that the small proportion of tumors with rapid growth rates were not curable despite early detection and treatment.[24]

We have reported our experience with prospective surveillance in 32 tumors (25 solid, 7 Bosniak III-IV) in 29 patients followed for a mean of 27.9 months (range 5.3 to 143.0). The overall average growth rate became insignificant after growing tumors were removed (nine tumors were removed after an average follow-up of 3.1 years) and growth was not associated with the initial tumor size (P = .28). For solid masses, the average growth rate was 0.11 cm^3 per year and for cystic masses it was 0.09 cm^3 per year (P = .41). Seven masses (22%) reached 4 cm in diameter after 12 to 85 months of follow-up and eight (25%) doubled their volume within 12 months. Overall, 11 (34%) fulfilled one of these two criteria of progression. Finally and importantly, four of these renal masses decreased in size (**Fig. 1**).

Kassouf and colleagues[25] reported a similar experience with SRMs. In 24 patients with 32 months of follow-up, most of the tumors had no significant growth and no metastatic disease was observed during the surveillance period. In a recently reported pooled analysis, nine single-institutional series with a total of 234 masses met the author's criteria for study.[28] Overall, the mean initial lesion size was 2.6 cm (range 1.73 to 4.08 cm) and 86% (178 of 208) were lesions smaller than 4 cm in maximal diameter at presentation. They were followed for a mean of 34 months (range 26 to 39) and the mean growth rate was 0.28 cm/year

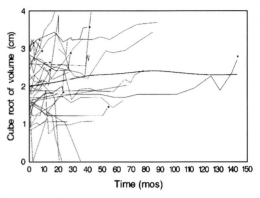

Fig. 1. Individual observed tumor volumes over time, with superimposed summary curve (*heavy line*) produced by a cubic smoothing spline routine. Growth patterns of the masses that were removed surgically are marked with asterisks. (*Reproduced from* Volpe A, Panzarella T, Rendon RA, et al. The natural history of incidentally detected small renal masses. Cancer 2004;100(4):738–45; with permission.)

(range 0.09 to 0.86 cm/year). Ninety-two percent of the lesions evaluated pathologically (42% of the tumors) were carcinoma. A comparison of size at presentation and growth rate in the 116 tumors (63 confirmed RCCs versus 53 observed without biopsy) revealed that size at presentation did not differ but that the growth rate of confirmed RCCs was greater (0.4 ± 0.36 versus 0.21 ± 0.4 cm yearly, P = .001). The difference in growth rates may have been the result of a selection bias because of treatment delay in lesions with slower growth rates.

Kouba and colleagues[29] reported a correlation between SRM growth rate and age with younger patients (60 years old or less) having more rapid growth (0.77 cm versus 0.26 cm per year). This observation supports earlier intervention in younger patients.

A lack of interval radiographic growth does not indicate benign histology. There is a wide range of growth with some lesions showing no interval growth over the short term and most of those have malignant pathology. Kunkle and colleagues[30] followed 106 enhancing renal masses for a minimum of 12 months (median 29). Pathology was available in 42 patients (40%). Overall, 33% (35/106) had no growth. The overall frequency of malignant lesions did not differ significantly between those with growth and those with zero growth (89% versus 83%, P = .56). Furthermore, they did not find any correlation between growth and patients' age, lesion size, solid/cystic appearance, or the incidental detection rate. Seventy-eight (26%) of 295 observed lesions failed to show growth. Overall, 26% to 33% of lesions under active surveillance do not grow and this characteristic does not predict for benign pathology.[30]

PROGNOSTIC FACTORS FOR TUMOR GROWTH

Clinical and pathologic stage, histologic subtype, and grade are important prognostic factors for outcome with RCC.[31] Histology and grade are less well understood factors for SRMs that are proven RCC (stage T1a).

Overall, new papillary and chromophobe RCCs appear to be smaller at presentation than clear cell carcinomas but it is not known if they have a slower growth rate.[12,32] The relationship of nuclear grade to growth is also unclear. Oda and colleagues[26] could not find a relation between growth rate and the degree of nuclear anaplasia in 16 patients. However, Kato and colleagues[33] reported that Fuhrman grade III tumors, which comprised 17% of his series of 18 incidentally detected with histologic-proven RCCs that underwent surgical resection after a median observation follow-up of 22.5 months, grew faster than Fuhrman grade I-II tumors.

Tumor size at presentation does not clearly predict growth rate. Sowery and Siemens[34] did not find a correlation in 22 patients with T1-2N0M0 tumors. Growth appeared to be slow even in those diagnosed with larger masses. Others have made the same observations that size and growth rate do not correlate.[28,35]

The presence of cystic components may be a marker of a slower growth rate but numbers reported are small and most were removed early.[36–38] Others report that the presence of cystic components does not predict slower growth.[27,36,38]

Those that are detected incidentally and are lower stage have a better survival rate (5-year cancer-specific survival 85.3% versus 62.5%).[6,7,9,11,12,18,39–41]

Molecular markers of prognosis for RCC would be very useful. Ki-67 (a nuclear antigen that is a marker of active cell proliferation), p53 protein (induces apoptosis), PTEN (a tumor suppressor gene), pAkt, nuclear akt, p27, pS6, bcl-2 (inhibits apoptosis), cyclin-D1 (a protein kinase that plays a role in cell-cycle regulation), vascular endothelial growth factor (VEGF), caveolin-1 (major structural component of caveoae that might play a role in invasion and metastatic progression), and HER-2 (an epidermal growth factor) have been studied.[33,42–49] In a recent immunohistochemistry study by Phuoc and colleagues[47] in 119 paraffin-embedded clear-cell RCCs, using univariate analyses, high Ki-67, p53, VEGF, and caveolin-1 were associated with decreased survival but high bcl-2 and cyclin-D1 were associated with increased survival. On multivariate analysis, expression of p53 or bcl-2 was an independent predictor of disease-specific survival. In addition, low PTEN expression was associated with decreased survival. Kim and colleagues[44] developed a multivariate clinical prognostic model based on the UCLA Integrated Staging System. CA9, CA12 (cell surface transmembrane carbonic anhydrases that are normally up-regulated by hypoxia-inducible factor in a low oxygen environment), PTEN, vimentin (epithelial cell adhesion molecule expressed on cell surface of carcinomas), p53, T stage, and performance status were significant predictors of survival.

Most of these studies included renal masses larger than 3 cm. However, Kato and colleagues[33] investigated the natural history of incidentally discovered SRMs and evaluated several features including cell proliferation and apoptosis. The cell activity was measured by immunostaining using Ki-67 and TUNEL (tranferase-mediated dUTP-biotin nick). They found that tumor growth rate is not associated with Ki-67 immunostaining and apoptosis was related to growth rate. However, Oda and colleagues[45] failed to establish a correlation between cell proliferation, apoptosis, and angiogenesis (measured with CD34 immunoanalysis) and tumor growth. Fujimoto and colleagues,[43] in a study of 18 patients with incidental renal tumors, reported that the argyrophilic nucleolar organizer regions (AgNORs) and proliferating cell nuclear antigen (PCNA) activity immunohistochemically correlated with the tumor doubling time (DT). DT was inversely and significantly correlated with AgNORs and PCNA. At this time, molecular markers of progression by tumor growth or metastatic potential have not been established as clinically useful triggers for therapy when active surveillance is being conducted or being considered.

There has been considerable effort to establish genomic markers of progression and response to treatment in RCC, as has been reported in retinoblastoma for example.[50,51] Genomic features of RCC have been studied using microarrays.[52–59] Higgins and colleagues[52] characterized different types of RCC. Takahashi and colleagues[57] used 21,632 element arrays to prognostically stratify 29 clear-cell carcinoma patients. They found two groups of patients and identified 40 genes that predict patients' prognosis, which are related to matrix metalloproteinase and angiogenesis activity. One group had a 100% 5-year survival with 88% of these without clinical evidence of metastatic disease. The remainder had an average survival time of 25.4 months with a 0% 5-year survival rate. This stratification by gene expression was superior to stage but similar to grade.

Zhao and colleagues[59] studied 177 clear-cell carcinomas and identified different types by distinct gene expression patterns with differing prognosis. They developed a set of 259 genes that predicted survival. By multivariate analysis, the gene expression pattern was a strong predictor of survival independent of tumor stage, grade, and performance status. Vasselli and colleagues[58] studied 58 archived tumors from patients with sporadic, stage IV RCC and 8 matched grossly normal-appearing kidney samples. They identified two patterns of gene expression, which correlated with a significant difference in overall survival. Although several reports using microarray data have been published in the past decade, variations among studies and lack of consistency between different platforms exist. At present, expression array data have limited clinical utility.

RISK OF PROGRESSION TO METASTATIC DISEASE

Progression to metastases as opposed to progression in tumor stage in patients under observation therapy is rare and poorly documented. In the recent pooled analysis, only 3 patients progressed to metastatic disease, representing 1% (3 in 286) of the total lesions.[28,34,35,60] It is important to point out that all of these patients were symptomatic at the time of disease progression. They reported the lesion size at presentation, the growth rate and follow-up in two patients. One patient presented with an 8.8-cm lesion and was followed for 111 months with a growth rate of 0.2 cm per year. The other developed metastatic disease after 54 months of follow-up, with a 2.0-cm lesion at the presentation and a growth rate of 1.3 cm per year.[60]

BIOPSY OF RENAL MASSES

The role of percutaneous biopsy remains controversial but is increasingly being discussed because of the rising incidental discovery of SRMs.[61,62] Tissue diagnosis may be useful to direct therapy and to avoid unnecessary nephrectomies. However, biopsy of indeterminate renal masses is not standard practice in the urology community.[63] In a recent survey, 43% of the consultant urologists never use biopsy, whereas 34% always employ it for the diagnosis and 23% of urologists use biopsy in selected cases. These results probably reflect perceptions of the complication rate and accuracy of early reports.[64] However, several new studies have shown that biopsy with fine needle aspiration (FNA) and/or

core is a safe procedure with a good accuracy.[65–67] The largest recent series with core and FNA biopsy reported a low incidence of complication.[68–74] There are only six cases of tumor seeding in the clinical literature, so the overall estimated risk is less than 0.01%.[75–81] There are no recent reports of implantation; probably owing to better technique including the use of guiding cannulas.[65–67] Other complications such as infection, arteriovenous fistula, and pneumothorax are extremely unlikely. Smith reported in 16,000 fine needle biopsies an overall mortality rate of 0.031%.[82] Maturen and colleagues[66] studied the accuracy of imaging-guided percutaneous renal mass biopsy and its impact on clinical management. They performed 152 biopsies in 125 patients with 97% malignancy sensitivity and 100% of specificity. These results are supported by several others reports showing a sensitivity and specificity of 70% to 100% and 100%, respectively, but the average sensitivity of FNA for cancer diagnosis is lower (76% to 97%) than needle cores.[64,83–85] However, some report false-negative rates of up to 24%.[64] False-negative biopsies result from sampling necrotic zones or missing the tumor entirely (which is easy to do, yielding normal kidney or blood for example). These biopsies should be classified as insufficient or unsatisfactory to make a diagnosis to establish the incidence of false-negative biopsies.

Lesion size is important. Rybicki and colleagues[86] cautioned that negative results in percutaneous biopsies should be interpreted with caution in masses smaller than 3 cm and larger than 6 cm (10% of false-negative rates). Also, Lechevailler and colleagues[71] showed that the rate of biopsy failures increase in smaller lesions. Renal masses smaller than 3 cm had a higher incidence of biopsy failure compared with lesions larger than 3 cm (37% versus 9%). Technical changes by the same group improved results.[72]

A good biopsy can establish tumor subtype and grade, which may be helpful. Renshaw and colleagues[87] studied 38 renal FNA specimens. Seventy-four percent of the primary renal lesions and all oncocytomas and the two chromophobe tumors were correctly classified. With regard to tumor grade, Lechevallier and colleagues[71] reported a 74% concordance between surgical tissue and percutaneous biopsy, with a 69% concordance in lesions under 4 cm. However, other studies have shown better correlation between pathological grade and the preoperative FNA (89% and 92% interobserver and intraobserver, variability).[88]

The use of percutaneous biopsies can have a remarkable effect on decision making and cost. Wood and colleagues[89] reported a 44% change in treatment plan in patients because of the biopsy result. In 152 masses biopsied, Maturen and colleagues[66] showed that patient management changed in 60.5%. Others report similar change.[72] There are limited data regarding the health care cost saving attributable to biopsy.[90] In our institution, we recommend CT-guided biopsy of all SRMs before treatment to confirm malignancy, to classify the histologic subtype, and establish grade with a reported 84% diagnostic accuracy and 100% concordance with the final pathology (Jewett and colleagues, unpublished data, July 2008).

ROLE FOR ACTIVE SURVEILLANCE IN THE MANAGEMENT OF SMALL RENAL MASSES

The treatment paradigm for enhancing renal masses that are consistent with RCC has been immediate removal or more recently probe ablation in selected cases. The rationale has been that early treatment will improve survival. However, as we treat more and smaller tumors (usually detected incidentally) without metastases or symptoms, kidney cancer mortality continues to rise.[4] The natural history evidence that many of these small tumors have a low malignant potential to progress has been presented. Therefore, a period of initial active surveillance delaying treatment for evidence of progression is attractive, particularly in the elderly and infirm.

The evidence to support biopsy followed by a period of surveillance includes the following:

1. A significant proportion of SRMs turn out to be benign when biopsied or removed. We should not assume that enhancing masses are all RCC.
2. Even with histologic confirmation of RCC, most SRMs appear to have a slow growth rate and a very low potential to metastasize, at least in the first few years. This may be in part because of the larger proportion that are papillary or chromophobe RCC and that have a low grade.
3. Many SRMs are detected in elderly patients with comorbidities. The risk of perioperative mortality and morbidity is higher and often appears to exceed the risk of progression.
4. If progression in tumor stage is detected early, and treatment delivered, survival may not be compromised, although this remains to be firmly established. There does not appear to be increased surgical morbidity attributable to treatment of larger tumors in this setting.

We do not yet recommend this approach for fit and young patients until the safety is established or until we have more accurate prognostic factors.

We do however recommend an attempt to biopsy all SRMs before treatment to establish that they are indeed malignant.

The trigger point for progression to treatment is not well defined. An upper limit of 3 to 4 cm for the maximum tumor diameter is commonly used to identify renal masses that are at very low risk of metastasizing.[91–93] We are currently testing the hypothesis that masses that reach 4 cm in maximum dimension, or volume doubling in less than 12 months, are at risk of further progression and should be treated. Surveillance is conducted by imaging, usually every 6 months, or annually if the tumor appears benign on biopsy. As we reported previously, 34% of our patients appear to progress.[27] No patients progressed to metastatic disease and two patients died of unrelated causes. In our Canadian prospective trial we have observed metastatic progression in 2% of patients, which is the reason we are very cautious about recommending this approach in younger patients.[94] We believe that risk stratification of patients by age, potential morbidity of therapy, and biopsy result is appropriate before treatment of enhancing SRMs.

REFERENCES

1. Ries LAG, Melbert D, Krapcho M, et al, editors. SEER cancer statistics review, 1975–2004. Bethesda (MD): National Cancer Institute; 2007.
2. Karumanchi SA, Merchan J, Sukhatme VP. Renal cancer: molecular mechanisms and newer therapeutic options. Curr Opin Nephrol Hypertens 2002; 11:37–42.
3. Pantuck AJ, Zisman A, Belldegrun AS. The changing natural history of renal cell carcinoma. J Urol 2001; 166:1611–23.
4. Hollingsworth JM, Miller DC, Daignault S, et al. Rising incidence of small renal masses: a need to reassess treatment effect. J Natl Cancer Inst 2006;98: 1331–4.
5. Chow WH, Devesa SS, Warren JL, et al. Rising incidence of renal cell cancer in the United States. JAMA 1999;281:1628–31.
6. Hock LM, Lynch J, Balaji KC. Increasing incidence of all stages of kidney cancer in the last 2 decades in the United States: an analysis of surveillance, epidemiology and end results program data. J Urol 2002;167:57–60.
7. Tsui KH, Shvarts O, Smith RB, et al. Renal cell carcinoma: prognostic significance of incidentally detected tumors. J Urol 2000;163:426–30.
8. Rendon RA, Stanietzky N, Panzarella T, et al. The natural history of small renal masses. J Urol 2000; 164:1143–7.

9. Lee CT, Katz J, Shi W, et al. Surgical management of renal tumors 4 cm or less in a contemporary cohort. J Urol 2000;163:730–6.

10. Jayson M, Sanders H. Increased incidence of serendipitously discovered renal cell carcinoma. Urology 1998;51:203–5.

11. Luciani LG, Cestari R, Tallarigo C. Incidental renal cell carcinoma—age and stage characterization and clinical implications: study of 1092 patients (1982–1997). Urology 2000;56:58–62.

12. Frank I, Blute ML, Cheville JC, et al. Solid renal tumors: an analysis of pathological features related to tumor size. J Urol 2003;170:2217–20.

13. Hollingsworth JM, Miller DC, Daignault S, et al. Five-year survival after surgical treatment for kidney cancer: a population-based competing risk analysis. Cancer 2007;109:1763–8.

14. Mejean A, Vogt B, Quazza JE, et al. Mortality and morbidity after nephrectomy for renal cell carcinoma using a transperitoneal anterior subcostal incision. Eur Urol 1999;36:298–302.

15. Stephenson AJ, Hakimi AA, Snyder ME, et al. Complications of radical and partial nephrectomy in a large contemporary cohort. J Urol 2004;171:130–4.

16. Uzzo RG, Novick AC. Nephron sparing surgery for renal tumors: indications, techniques and outcomes. J Urol 2001;166:6–18.

17. Kattan MW, Reuter V, Motzer RJ, et al. A postoperative prognostic nomogram for renal cell carcinoma. J Urol 2001;166:63–7.

18. Licht MR, Novick AC, Goormastic M. Nephron sparing surgery in incidental versus suspected renal cell carcinoma. J Urol 1994;152:39–42.

19. Sutherland SE, Resnick MI, Maclennan GT, et al. Does the size of the surgical margin in partial nephrectomy for renal cell cancer really matter? J Urol 2002;167:61–4.

20. Wehle MJ, Thiel DD, Petrou SP, et al. Conservative management of incidental contrast-enhancing renal masses as safe alternative to invasive therapy. Urology 2004;64:49–52.

21. Fergany AF, Hafez KS, Novick AC. Long-term results of nephron sparing surgery for localized renal cell carcinoma: 10-year followup. J Urol 2000;163:442–5.

22. Morgan WR, Zincke H. Progression and survival after renal-conserving surgery for renal cell carcinoma: experience in 104 patients and extended follow-up. J Urol 1990;144:852–8.

23. Novick AC. Nephron-sparing surgery for renal cell carcinoma. Br J Urol 1998;82:321–4.

24. Bosniak MA, Birnbaum BA, Krinsky GA, et al. Small renal parenchymal neoplasms: further observations on growth. Radiology 1995;197:589–97.

25. Kassouf W, Aprikian AG, Laplante M, et al. Natural history of renal masses followed expectantly. J Urol 2004;171:111–3.

26. Oda T, Miyao N, Takahashi A, et al. Growth rates of primary and metastatic lesions of renal cell carcinoma. Int J Urol 2001;8:473–7.

27. Volpe A, Panzarella T, Rendon RA, et al. The natural history of incidentally detected small renal masses. Cancer 2004;100:738–45.

28. Chawla SN, Crispen PL, Hanlon AL, et al. The natural history of observed enhancing renal masses: meta-analysis and review of the world literature. J Urol 2006;175:425–31.

29. Kouba E, Smith A, McRackan D, et al. Watchful waiting for solid renal masses: insight into the natural history and results of delayed intervention. J Urol 2007;177:466–70.

30. Kunkle DA, Crispen PL, Chen DY, et al. Enhancing renal masses with zero net growth during active surveillance. J Urol 2007;177:849–53.

31. Girgin C, Tarhan H, Hekimgil M, et al. P53 mutations and other prognostic factors of renal cell carcinoma. Urol Int 2001;66:78–83.

32. Cheville JC, Lohse CM, Zincke H, et al. Comparisons of outcome and prognostic features among histologic subtypes of renal cell carcinoma. Am J Surg Pathol 2003;27:612–24.

33. Kato M, Suzuki T, Suzuki Y, et al. Natural history of small renal cell carcinoma: evaluation of growth rate, histological grade, cell proliferation and apoptosis. J Urol 2004;172:863–6.

34. Sowery RD, Siemens DR. Growth characteristics of renal cortical tumors in patients managed by watchful waiting. Can J Urol 2004;11:2407–10.

35. Lamb GW, Bromwich EJ, Vasey P, et al. Management of renal masses in patients medically unsuitable for nephrectomy—natural history, complications, and outcome. Urology 2004;64:909–13.

36. Corica FA, Iczkowski KA, Cheng L, et al. Cystic renal cell carcinoma is cured by resection: a study of 24 cases with long-term followup. J Urol 1999;161:408–11.

37. Koga S, Nishikido M, Hayashi T, et al. Outcome of surgery in cystic renal cell carcinoma. Urology 2000;56:67–70.

38. Nassir A, Jollimore J, Gupta R, et al. Multilocular cystic renal cell carcinoma: a series of 12 cases and review of the literature. Urology 2002;60:421–7.

39. Bretheau D, Lechevallier E, Eghazarian C, et al. Prognostic significance of incidental renal cell carcinoma. Eur Urol 1995;27:319–23.

40. Sweeney JP, Thornhill JA, Graiger R, et al. Incidentally detected renal cell carcinoma: pathological features, survival trends and implications for treatment. Br J Urol 1996;78:351–3.

41. Thompson IM, Peek M. Improvement in survival of patients with renal cell carcinoma—the role of the serendipitously detected tumor. J Urol 1988;140:487–90.

42. Delahunt B, Bethwaite PB, Thornton A, et al. Proliferation of renal cell carcinoma assessed by fixation-resistant polyclonal Ki-67 antibody labeling. Correlation with clinical outcome. Cancer 1995;75:2714–9.

43. Fujimoto N, Sugita A, Terasawa Y, et al. Observations on the growth rate of renal cell carcinoma. Int J Urol 1995;2:71–6.

44. Kim HL, Seligson D, Liu X, et al. Using tumor markers to predict the survival of patients with metastatic renal cell carcinoma. J Urol 2005;173:1496–501.

45. Oda T, Takahashi A, Miyao N, et al. Cell proliferation, apoptosis, angiogenesis and growth rate of incidentally found renal cell carcinoma. Int J Urol 2003;10:13–8.

46. Pantuck AJ, Seligson DB, Klatte T, et al. Prognostic relevance of the mTOR pathway in renal cell carcinoma: implications for molecular patient selection for targeted therapy. Cancer 2007;109:2257–67.

47. Phuoc NB, Ehara H, Gotoh T, et al. Immunohistochemical analysis with multiple antibodies in search of prognostic markers for clear cell renal cell carcinoma. Urology 2007;69:843–8.

48. Shin Lee J, Seok Kim H, Bok Kim Y, et al. Expression of PTEN in renal cell carcinoma and its relation to tumor behavior and growth. J Surg Oncol 2003;84:166–72.

49. Zhang X, Takenaka I. Cell proliferation and apoptosis with BCL-2 expression in renal cell carcinoma. Urology 2000;56:510–5.

50. Dimaras H, Gallie BL. The p75 NTR neurotrophin receptor is a tumor suppressor in human and murine retinoblastoma development. Int J Cancer 2008;122:2023–9.

51. Dimaras H, Khetan V, Halliday W, et al. Loss of RB1 induces non-proliferative retinoma; increasing genomic instability correlates with progression to retinoblastoma. Hum Mol Genet 2008;10:1363–72.

52. Higgins JP, Shinghal R, Gill H, et al. Gene expression patterns in renal cell carcinoma assessed by complementary DNA microarray. Am J Pathol 2003;162:925–32.

53. Hirata H, Hinoda Y, Matsuyama H, et al. Polymorphisms of DNA repair genes are associated with renal cell carcinoma. Biochem Biophys Res Commun 2006;342:1058–62.

54. Jones J, Otu H, Spentzos D, et al. Gene signatures of progression and metastasis in renal cell cancer. Clin Cancer Res 2005;11:5730–9.

55. Kosari F, Parker AS, Kube DM, et al. Clear cell renal cell carcinoma: gene expression analyses identify a potential signature for tumor aggressiveness. Clin Cancer Res 2005;11:5128–39.

56. Sultmann H, von Heydebreck A, Huber W, et al. Gene expression in kidney cancer is associated with cytogenetic abnormalities, metastasis formation, and patient survival. Clin Cancer Res 2005;11:646–55.

57. Takahashi M, Rhodes DR, Furge KA, et al. Gene expression profiling of clear cell renal cell carcinoma: gene identification and prognostic classification. Proc Natl Acad Sci U S A 2001;98:9754–9.

58. Vasselli JR, Shih JH, Iyengar SR, et al. Predicting survival in patients with metastatic kidney cancer by gene-expression profiling in the primary tumor. Proc Natl Acad Sci U S A 2003;100:6958–63.

59. Zhao H, Ljungberg B, Grankvist K, et al. Gene expression profiling predicts survival in conventional renal cell carcinoma. PLoS Med 2006;3:e13.

60. Crispen PL, Uzzo RG. The natural history of untreated renal masses. BJU Int 2007;99:1203–7.

61. Lane BR, Samplaski MK, Herts BR, et al. Renal mass biopsy—a renaissance? J Urol 2008;179:20–7.

62. Volpe A, Kachura JR, Geddie WR, et al. Techniques, safety and accuracy of sampling of renal tumors by fine needle aspiration and core biopsy. J Urol 2007;178:379–86.

63. Khan AA, Shergill IS, Quereshi S, et al. Percutaneous needle biopsy for indeterminate renal masses: a national survey of UK consultant urologists. BMC Urol 2007;7:10.

64. Campbell SC, Novick AC, Herts B, et al. Prospective evaluation of fine needle aspiration of small, solid renal masses: accuracy and morbidity. Urology 1997;50:25–9.

65. Beland MD, Mayo-Smith WW, Dupuy DE, et al. Diagnostic yield of 58 consecutive imaging-guided biopsies of solid renal masses: should we biopsy all that are indeterminate? AJR Am J Roentgenol 2007;188:792–7.

66. Maturen KE, Nghiem HV, Caoili EM, et al. Renal mass core biopsy: accuracy and impact on clinical management. AJR Am J Roentgenol 2007;188:563–70.

67. Wunderlich H, Hindermann W, Al Mustafa AM, et al. The accuracy of 250 fine needle biopsies of renal tumors. J Urol 2005;174:44–6.

68. Brierly RD, Thomas PJ, Harrison NW, et al. Evaluation of fine-needle aspiration cytology for renal masses. BJU Int 2000;85:14–8.

69. Eshed I, Elias S, Sidi AA. Diagnostic value of CT-guided biopsy of indeterminate renal masses. Clin Radiol 2004;59:262–7.

70. Hara I, Miyake H, Hara S, et al. Role of percutaneous image-guided biopsy in the evaluation of renal masses. Urol Int 2001;67:199–202.

71. Lechevallier E, Andre M, Barriol D, et al. Fine-needle percutaneous biopsy of renal masses with helical CT guidance. Radiology 2000;216:506–10.

72. Neuzillet Y, Lechevallier E, Andre M, et al. Accuracy and clinical role of fine needle percutaneous biopsy with computerized tomography guidance of small (less than 4.0 cm) renal masses. J Urol 2004;171: 1802–5.

73. Richter F, Kasabian NG, Irwin RJ Jr, et al. Accuracy of diagnosis by guided biopsy of renal mass lesions classified indeterminate by imaging studies. Urology 2000;55:348–52.

74. Vasudevan A, Davies RJ, Shannon BA, et al. Incidental renal tumours: the frequency of benign lesions and the role of preoperative core biopsy. BJU Int 2006;97:946–9.

75. Abe M, Saitoh M. Selective renal tumour biopsy under ultrasonic guidance. Br J Urol 1992;70:7–11.

76. Auvert J, Abbou CC, Lavarenne V. Needle tract seeding following puncture of renal oncocytoma. Prog Clin Biol Res 1982;100:597–8.

77. Gibbons RP, Bush WH Jr, Burnett LL. Needle tract seeding following aspiration of renal cell carcinoma. J Urol 1977;118:865–7.

78. Herts BR, Baker ME. The current role of percutaneous biopsy in the evaluation of renal masses. Semin Urol Oncol 1995;13:254–61.

79. Kiser GC, Totonchy M, Barry JM. Needle tract seeding after percutaneous renal adenocarcinoma aspiration. J Urol 1986;136:1292–3.

80. Shenoy PD, Lakhkar BN, Ghosh MK, et al. Cutaneous seeding of renal carcinoma by Chiba needle aspiration biopsy. Case report. Acta Radiol 1991;32:50–2.

81. Wehle MJ, Grabstald H. Contraindications to needle aspiration of a solid renal mass: tumor dissemination by renal needle aspiration. J Urol 1986;136:446–8.

82. Smith EH. Complications of percutaneous abdominal fine-needle biopsy. Radiology 1991;178:253–8 [review].

83. Cristallini EG, Paganelli C, Bolis GB. Role of fine-needle aspiration biopsy in the assessment of renal masses. Diagn Cytopathol 1991;7:32–5.

84. Juul N, Torp-Pedersen S, Gronvall S, et al. Ultrasonically guided fine needle aspiration biopsy of renal masses. J Urol 1985;133:579–81.

85. Niceforo J, Coughlin BF. Diagnosis of renal cell carcinoma: value of fine-needle aspiration cytology in patients with metastases or contraindications to nephrectomy. AJR Am J Roentgenol 1993;161:1303–5.

86. Rybicki FJ, Shu KM, Cibas ES, et al. Percutaneous biopsy of renal masses: sensitivity and negative predictive value stratified by clinical setting and size of masses. AJR Am J Roentgenol 2003;180:1281–7.

87. Renshaw AA, Lee KR, Madge R, et al. Accuracy of fine needle aspiration in distinguishing subtypes of renal cell carcinoma. Acta Cytol 1997;41:987–94.

88. Cajulis RS, Katz RL, Dekmezian R, et al. Fine needle aspiration biopsy of renal cell carcinoma. Cytologic parameters and their concordance with histology and flow cytometric data. Acta Cytol 1993;37:367–72.

89. Wood BJ, Khan MA, McGovern F, et al. Imaging guided biopsy of renal masses: indications, accuracy and impact on clinical management. J Urol 1999;161:1470–4.

90. Silverman SG, Deuson TE, Kane N, et al. Percutaneous abdominal biopsy: cost-identification analysis. Radiology 1998;206:429–35.

91. Frank I, Blute ML, Cheville JC, et al. An outcome prediction model for patients with clear cell renal cell carcinoma treated with radical nephrectomy based on tumor stage, size, grade and necrosis: the SSIGN score. J Urol 2002;168:2395–400.

92. Walther MM, Choyke PL, Glenn G, et al. Renal cancer in families with hereditary renal cancer: prospective analysis of a tumor size threshold for renal parenchymal sparing surgery. J Urol 1999; 161:1475–9.

93. Zisman A, Pantuck AJ, Chao D, et al. Reevaluation of the 1997 TNM classification for renal cell carcinoma: T1 and T2 cutoff point at 4.5 rather than 7 cm better correlates with clinical outcome. J Urol 2001;166:54–8.

94. Mattar K, Basiuk J, Finelli A, et al. Active surveillance of small renal masses: a prospective multi-centre Canadian trial. Presented at the Annual EAU Congress, Milan, Italy. March 26–29, 2008.

The Medical and Oncological Rationale for Partial Nephrectomy for the Treatment of T1 Renal Cortical Tumors

Paul Russo, MD, FACS[a],*, William Huang, MD[b]

KEYWORDS

- Renal cancer • Partial nephrectomy
- Chronic kidney disease

The medical and oncologic rationale for partial nephrectomy has evolved over the last 10 years and is based on the following factors: an enhanced understanding of renal tumor histology, the proven oncological equivalency of partial and radical nephrectomy for T1 renal cancers, and new concerns regarding chronic kidney disease (CKD) and its potential adverse impact on cardiovascular health and overall survival. Historically, partial nephrectomy was reserved for patients with tumor in a solitary kidney, bilateral renal tumors, or tumor in a patient with underlying medical diseases of the kidney or renal insufficiency. For the last 15 years, the concept of partial nephrectomy for patients with a renal tumor and a normal contralateral kidney (kidney sparing or nephron sparing), has generated increasing acceptance both in the United States and abroad, and, over the last 5 years, has crystallized as the treatment of choice for small renal masses. In this article we discuss the oncological and medical rationale for partial nephrectomy as the treatment of choice whenever possible for T1 (<7 cm) renal tumors.

RENAL CORTICAL TUMORS: A DIVERSITY OF TUMORS AND POTENTIAL THREATS

Renal cortical tumors (RCTs) are members of a complex family with unique histologies, cytogenetic defects, and variable metastatic potentials ranging from the benign oncocytoma, to the indolent papillary and chromophobe carcinomas, to the more malignant conventional clear carcinoma.[1] At our center, Memorial Sloan Kettering Cancer Center (MSKCC), the conventional clear cell tumor accounts for 90% of all metastatic RCTs but only 54% of the renal tumors undergoing resection. Two groups of patients with RCTs currently exist. The first group consists of patients with symptomatic, large, locally advanced tumors often presenting with regional adenopathy, adrenal invasion, and extension into the renal vein or inferior vena cava. Despite radical nephrectomy in conjunction with regional lymphadenectomy and adrenalectomy, progression to distant metastasis and death from disease occurs in approximately 30% of these patients. For patients presenting with isolated metastatic disease, metastasectomy in carefully selected patients has been associated with long-term survival.[2] For patients with diffuse metastatic disease and an acceptable performance status, cytoreductive nephrectomy, compared to cytokine therapy alone, may add several additional months of survival.[3] Cytoreductive nephrectomy also prepares patients for integrated treatment, now in neoadjuvant and adjuvant

a Department of Surgery, Urology Service, Weill Cornell College of Medicine, Memorial Sloan Kettering Cancer Center, 1275 York Avenue, New York, NY 10021, USA
b Department of Urology, New York University School of Medicine, 150 East 32nd Street, Suite 200, New York, NY 10016, USA
* Corresponding author.
E-mail address: russop@MSKCC.org (P. Russo).

Urol Clin N Am 35 (2008) 635–643
doi:10.1016/j.ucl.2008.07.008

clinic trials, with the new multitargeted tyrosine kinase inhibitors (sunitinib, sorafenib) and mammalian target of rapamycin inhibitors (temsirolimus, RAD001).

The second group of RCTs consists of small renal tumors (median tumor size <4 cm, T1a) often incidentally discovered in asymptomatic patients during imaging for nonspecific abdominal or musculoskeletal complaints or during unrelated cancer care. A greater than 90% survival rate, depending on the tumor histology,[4] is expected following partial or radical nephrectomy. Despite vast improvements in modern CT, ultrasound, and MRI imaging of the kidney, these studies are nonspecific and between 16.4% and 23% of patients undergoing tumor resection are ultimately found to have a benign lesion, including angiomyolipoma, oncocytoma, metanephric adenoma, or hemorrhagic cyst.[5,6] Although CT-guided percutanous renal biopsy can easily be performed, the differentiation between a benign and malignant tumor and the determination of tumor histologic subtypes by current radiological and biopsy techniques alone or in combination is only 70% accurate.[7] Active research to determine if immunohistochemical and cytogenetic techniques can substantially improve the accuracy of RCT percutaneous biopsy is ongoing. An alternative strategy to image the more malignant clear cell carcinoma with a specific radio-labeled antibody that reacts to carbonic anhydrase 9 124I-cG250 is under active investigation and has shown a high sensitivity and specificity in preliminary studies. This immuno–positron emission tomographic scan may play an important role in the future for planning surgeries, selecting for active surveillance, determining the response to novel local and systemic therapies, and evaluating extent of disease.[8]

PARTIAL NEPHRECTOMY IS AS EFFECTIVE AS RADICAL NEPHRECTOMY FOR T1 TUMORS

Contemporary surgical oncology (eg, for breast cancer, soft tissue sarcoma) now favors surgical approaches that preserve organs and limbs whenever possible, and is often used in conjunction with adjuvant therapies, with resulting local tumor control and long-term survival equivalent to their more radical counterparts. Partial nephrectomy, once used only for the essential indications, is now considered a preferred alternative to radical nephrectomy for patients with T1 tumors, normal renal function, and two intact kidneys.[9] Studies from the United States and abroad have shown that partial nephrectomy for tumors of 4 cm or less provides equivalent tumor control compared with radical nephrectomy.[10,11] Previous deterrents to

partial nephrectomy, including proximity to collecting system or major segmental vessels, endophytic tumor location, concern for tumor multifocality, and the desire for a 1-cm surgical margin, are now routinely managed effectively in the operating room. Tumor localization using intraoperative ultrasound for endophytic and multifocal tumors,[12] suture repair of the collecting system and blood vessels, and closed suction retroperitoneal drainage, has made open partial nephrectomy a highly effective operation. Complication rates are less than 10% and mostly relate to prolonged urinary fistula with only the rare need for reoperation or endoscopic interventions.[13] Renoprotective measures of ice slush and mannitol seem effective in limiting damage to the kidney with normalization of renal function by 12 months postoperatively. Prolonged ischemia time, increasing blood loss, and partial nephrectomy in a solitary kidney, all indicators of a more challenging operation, are associated with early declines in glomerular filtration rate (GFR) but not long-term damage.[14] It is our practice to perform partial nephrectomy with no ischemia (no renal artery cross-clamping) whenever possible to limit potential glomerular damage, which may not be detectable by serum markers or formulas that estimate kidney function. If renal artery clamping is required to limit blood loss during the resection of a large tumor or an endophytic tumor, mannitol (12.5 gm/250 mL of saline) and ice slush are routinely used with every attempt to limit cold ischemia to less than 30 minutes. In addition, careful visual inspection of the kidney and the use of intraoperative ultrasound address the small likelihood (<5%) of a previously unrecognized tumor satellite, which can also be excised at the same operation.[15]

Recent studies have demonstrated that gross resection of all tumors, as assessed by the operating surgeon, even in the presence of only microscopically negative surgical margins, provides excellent local tumor control without an increased risk of local tumor recurrence and without the need for a 1-cm margin of surrounding renal parenchyma. One-centimeter margins are easily achievable goal for an exophytic tumor, but often not technically feasible for a renal sinus tumor, a juxtahilar tumor, or an intraparenchymal tumor. Complete resection of RCTs in these less-accessible locations increases the percentage of patients eligible for kidney-sparing operations and renders an excellent prognosis with a high likelihood (>90%) of freedom from local, regional, and metastatic recurrence,[16] particularly because a significant percentage of patients with central tumors have indolent or benign histology (30.2%).[17] In the event of a positive microscopic surgical margin on final pathology, previous recommendations for a "completion" radical nephrectomy appear unnecessary. In recently published study of 1344 partial nephrectomies from MSKCC and the Mayo Clinic, 77 patients (5.5%) were found to have positive surgical margins on final pathology. This was more likely to occur during the resection of a tumor in a solitary kidney or one in a technically challenging location. Although the surgeon should make every effort to achieve a complete resection at the time of a partial nephrectomy, a final pathologic positive surgical margin was not associated with an increased likelihood of local tumor recurrence or metastatic disease.[18]

Partial nephrectomy has been safely extended to tumors of 7 cm or less, when technically feasible, with disease-free intervals equivalent to those in similar patients treated with radical nephrectomy across all histologic subtypes.[9,11] MSKCC investigators compared the results of 45 patients undergoing partial nephrectomy to 151 patients undergoing radical nephrectomy (22 of whom were originally slated to have a partial nephrectomy but were converted to radical nephrectomy) for T1b (4–7 cm) conventional clear cell carcinomas. Disease-free survival between the groups were no different, but the serum creatinine levels, a relatively crude indicator of overall renal function, were substantially better in patients undergoing partial nephrectomy at 3, 6, and 12 months.[19]

Clinical local recurrence in the partial nephrectomy bed is a rare event (<1%) and is often associated with a grossly positive surgical margin at the time of the initial resection, which is more likely to occur in patients with multifocal tumors or a large tumor in a solitary kidney. A recent publication from Pahernik and colleagues[20] from Mainz, Germany, confirmed the oncological efficacy of partial nephrectomy in tumors larger than 4 cm. New tumor formation in the operated kidney is an uncommon event, occurring at a lifetime risk, in the absence of familial or hereditary syndromes, in less than 5% of patients.[14] Following either partial nephrectomy or radical nephrectomy, the contralateral kidney also retains a lifetime risk of approximately 5% for the development of new tumor formation necessitating lifelong surveillance.[21] At some finite point, likely measured in years, the risk of a new ipsilateral or contralateral tumor formation exceeds the risk of metastatic disease development from the index tumor. In any case, long-term surveillance with a yearly renal imaging study (CT, ultrasonography, or MRI) and chest radiograph (for clear cell, chromophobe, papillary renal cancer, but not benign oncocytoma or metanephric adenoma) to assess local or systemic recurrence is recommended. With this approach, disease-free survival rates of greater than 90% are achieved using partial nephrectomy for T1 RCTs across all histologic subtypes.[22]

KIDNEY TUMOR PATIENTS AND UNRECOGNIZED MEDICAL RENAL DISEASE

A historical misconception is that radical nephrectomy, although likely to cause a detectable and permanent rise in serum creatinine because of the sacrifice of normal renal parenchyma not involved by tumor, will not cause serious long-term side effects as long as the patient has a normal contralateral kidney. The renal transplant literature is often cited as the clinical evidence to support this view since patients undergoing donor nephrectomy have not been reported to have higher rates of kidney failure requiring dialysis or resulting in death.[23] However, distinct differences between renal donors and renal tumor patients exist. Donors tend to be carefully selected, screened for medical comorbidities, and are generally young (age 40 or less).[24,25] In contrast, renal tumor patients are not screened, are older (mean age 61 years), and often have significant comorbidities that can affect kidney function, including metabolic syndrome, hypertension, obesity, vascular disease, and diabetes, alone or in combination. As patients age, particularly beyond the age of 60, nephrons atrophy and GFRs progressively decreases.[26]

A recent clinical and pathologic study from the Harvard Medical School examined the non–tumor-bearing kidney of patients undergoing resection of RCTs and demonstrated a far greater degree of unsuspected underlying renal disease in kidney tumor patients than previously appreciated.[27] The nonneoplastic renal tissue in 110 nephrectomy specimens, including 67 clear cell carcinomas of which 39 were less than 5 cm, were correlated to the patient's clinical history. Only 10% of patients had completely normal adjacent renal tissue and 28% were found to have vascular sclerotic changes. In the remaining 62% of cases, evidence of significant intrinsic renal abnormalities, including diabetic nephropathy, glomerular hypertrophy, mesangial expansion, and diffuse glomerulosclerosis, was noted. In this study, 91 patients (83%) underwent radical nephrectomy for the treatment of their tumors. This study indicates that the loss of functional nephrons during radical nephrectomy, coupled with pre-existing renal diseases, which may or may not be clinically apparent but is present at the pathologic level in the vast majority of patients, causes the worsening of overall renal function.

CHRONIC KIDNEY DISEASE IS AN INDEPENDENT RISK FACTOR FOR CARDIOVASCULAR DISEASE

CKD is increasingly viewed as a major public health problem in the United States. Currently it is estimated that there are 19 million adults in the United States in the early stages of CKD and that by the year 2030, 2 million will be in need of chronic dialysis or renal transplantation.[28] CKD is defined as a GFR of less than 60 mL/min/1.73m². Traditional risk factors for CKD include age greater than 60, hypertension, diabetes, cardiovascular disease, and family history of renal disease. The prevalence and incidence of kidney failure requiring either dialysis or renal transplantation have increased from 1988 to 2004. Also, a significant trend has been a 10% increase in the prevalance of earlier stages of CKD, as indicated by decreased GFR, increased proteinuria, or both. These findings were determined by the National Health and Nutrition Examination Surveys, which compared 15,488 adults from 1988 to 1994 to 13,233 adults from 1999 to 2004. A higher rate of diabetes and hypertension during a later time frame in the United States is thought to be responsible for the increase in earlier stages of CKD.

Recommendations for assessing patients at increased risk for CKD include measurement of urine albumin and estimation of GFR using equations based on the level of serum creatinine.[29] In 2003, the National Kidney Foundation; the American Heart Association; and the Seventh Joint National Committee on Prevention, Detection, Evaluation, and Treatment of High Blood Pressure classified CKD as an independent cardiovascular risk factor.[30–34] Certain serum factors, including elevated inflammatory and prothrombotic factors (C-reactive protein, fibrinogen, IL-6, and IL-8) and decreased hemoglobin levels and lipoprotein A may mechanistically contribute to the elevated cardiovascular risk. Therefore, medical interventions designed to modify well-known traditional risk factors, such as systolic blood pressure greater than 140 mm Hg, diabetes, cigarette smoking, high-density lipoprotein less than 40, low-density lipoprotein more than 130, body mass index over 30, physical inactivity, and left ventricular hypertrophy, may be effective in reducing the cardiovascular mortality risk in CKD.

Two widely used formulas, the Modification in Diet and Renal Disease (MDRD) equation and the Cockcroft-Gault equation, are superior to serum creatinine alone in estimating the GFR.[29] These formulas have been extensively evaluated in populations of patients, including blacks, whites, and Asians; people with and without diabetes or kidney disease; and transplant donors. Both equations are more accurate in evaluating kidney function in patients with CKD, as opposed to younger patients, those with type 1 diabetes without microalbuminuria, or healthy potential kidney donors.[35]

An estimated GFR of less than 60 mL/min/1.73 m², stage 3 CKD, is associated with a graded increase in the risk of progression to end-stage kidney disease and premature death caused by cardiovascular disease. A clinician can quickly calculate the estimated GFR using a Web site that only requires patient age, sex, race, and serum creatinine (http://www.nephron.com/MDRD_GFR.cgi). In our practice, the routine use of the MDRD equation to estimate GFR has become an essential part of the initial evaluation of the renal tumor patient and is critical for surgical planning and counseling.[36]

The adverse clinical impact of a decline in estimated GFR was reported by investigators at Kaiser Permanente in California who estimated the longitudinal GFR in 1,120,295 patients between 1996 and 2000 who had not undergone dialysis or kidney transplantation. The investigators examined the multivariable association between estimated GFR and the risks of death, cardiovascular events, and hospitalization. The median patient age was 52 years, 55% of the patients were women, and median follow-up was 2.84 years. The risk of death increased as the estimated GFR decreased below 60 mL/min/1.73 m² with the adjusted hazard ratios of 1.2 (GFR 45–59 mL/min/1.73 m²), 1.8 (GFR 30–44 mL/min/1.73 m²), 3.2 (GFR 15–29 mL/min/1.73 m²), and 5.9 (GFR <15 mL/min/1.73 m²) respectively. The adjusted risk of hospitalization followed a similar pattern.[37] The link between CKD and cardiovascular risk factors was also reported by Foley and colleagues,[38] who analyzed data from 15,837 noninstitutionalized adults from 1988 to 1994 in the Third National Health and Nutrition Examination Survey. Data were gathered on nine cardiovascular risk factors (smoking, obesity, hypertension, high total cholesterol, C-reactive protein, glycosylated hemoglobin, homocysteine levels, low hemoglobin, high urinary albumin to creatinine ratio) and estimated GFR. Estimated GFR was greater than 60 mL/min/1.73 m² in 93.3% of patients, between 30 and 59 mL/min/1.73 m² (stage 3 CKD) in 6.2%, and less than 30 mL/min/1.73 m² (stage 4 and 5 CKD) in 0.5%. As kidney function deteriorated, the percentage of subjects with two associated cardiovascular risk factors increased from 34.7% (stage 1 and 2 CKD), to 83.6% (for stage 3), to 100% for stage 4 and 5 subjects. Patients with CKD were far more likely to require medical interventions to treat cardiovascular disease than those with normal renal function. The low prevalence of patients with stage 4 or 5 CKD is attributable to their 5-year survival rates of only 30%.[38]

PARTIAL NEPHRECTOMY PRESERVES RENAL FUNCTION

Data comparing late renal functional and oncological results in over 450 patients undergoing partial nephrectomy or radical nephrectomy for tumors measuring less than 4 cm were first reported from the Mayo Clinic in 2000 and from MSKCC in 2002. The Mayo Clinic study showed that patients undergoing radical nephrectomy were more likely to have serum creatinine levels elevated to more than 2.0 ng/mL and proteinuria.[39] The MSKCC study resulted in similar findings even when study patients were carefully matched for associated risk factors, including diabetes, smoking history, preoperative serum creatinine, and American Society of Anesthesiologists score.[40] In both studies, oncological outcomes were highly favorable (>90% survival rates) whether partial nephrectomy or radical nephrectomy was done. Investigators from MSKCC later created a postoperative prognostic nomogram for renal insufficiency that used percent changes in kidney volume as calculated from CT scans, preoperative serum creatinine, American Society of Anesthesiologists score, patient age, and sex. In this study, serum creatinine of greater than 2 was described as renal insufficiency. The investigators studied 161 patients undergoing partial nephrectomy and 857 patients undergoing radical nephrectomy. A total of 111 patients (10.9%), of which 105 underwent radical nephrectomy (95%), experienced renal insufficiency at a median of 14.4 months following surgery. Using a multivariate analysis, patient age, sex, preoperative creatinine, and percent change in kidney volume were all significant factors associated with freedom from renal insufficiency with preoperative serum creatinine greater than 1.0 contributing nearly 70 points to the nomogram.[41] Skeptics pointed out that these studies failed to demonstrate an increased risk of dialysis in the radical nephrectomy patients but their comments failed to mention the cardiovascular morbidity and mortality associated with CKD for patients not yet requiring dialysis.

MSKCC investigators recently analyzed their partial nephrectomy and radical nephrectomy experience using the MDRD abbreviated formula to estimate GFR in a retrospective cohort study of 662 patients with a normal serum creatinine and two healthy kidneys that underwent either elective partial nephrectomy or radical nephrectomy for an RCT 4 cm or less in diameter. Data was analyzed using two threshold definitions of CKD: a GFR less than 60 mL/min/1.73 m^2 or a GFR less than 45 mL/min/1.73 m^2. To the surprise of the investigators, 171 patients (26%) had pre-existing CKD (GFR <60) before operation despite two intact, normal-appearing kidneys and a serum creatinine within normal limits. After surgery, the 3-year probability of freedom from new onset of GFR less than 60 was 80% after partial nephrectomy but only 35% after radical nephrectomy. Corresponding values for 3-year probability of GFR less than 45, a more severe level of CKD, was 95% for partial nephrectomy and 64% for radical nephrectomy. Multivariable analysis indicated that radical nephrectomy remained an independent risk factor for the development of new-onset CKD.[42] Also, a detectable decline in renal function also occurred in the patients undergoing partial nephrectomy. A recent study from the Mayo Clinic queried their nephrectomy registry between 1989 and 2003 and identified 648 patients treated with radical nephrectomy or partial nephrectomy for a solitary renal tumor less than or equal to 4 cm (excluding perinephric fat, nodal, and distant metastases patients) and a normal contralateral kidney. Overall survival was calculated in 327 patients younger than 65 at the time of operation and it was found that radical nephrectomy was significantly associated with an increased risk of death, which persisted after adjusting for year of surgery, diabetes at presentation, Charlson-Romano index, and tumor histology.[43] These studies, when taken together, raise serious concerns regarding the long-term effects of radical nephrectomy, particularly when used in a population of patients with small RCTs at low risk for the development of metastatic disease and a long anticipated survival who remain at risk for the common aforementioned medical diseases.

Currently, active investigation, using both institutional databases and national databases, is underway to confirm these initial reports regarding increased cardiovascular events and decreased overall survival when radical nephrectomy rather than partial nephrectomy is used in the treatment of small, favorable-prognostic renal masses. This important data strongly suggest that routine radical nephrectomy for small renal tumors is unjustified on oncological grounds and has potential adverse consequences on the long-term cardiovascular and renal health of the patient. Short-term end points stressed by some investigators in the recent laparoscopic literature regarding length of hospital stay, analgesic requirements postoperatively, and cosmetic elements while advocating laparoscopic radical nephrectomy must now be tempered with the new concerns that radical nephrectomy for the treatment of small renal tumors, by either open or laparoscopic techniques, may worsen or cause CKD and decrease overall patient survival.

PARTIAL NEPHRECTOMY IS UNDERUSED

In 2008, more than 54,390 patients will develop RCTs in the United States, according to estimates,[44] and approximately 70% of those will be incidentally detected at 4 cm or less, a size considered amenable to partial nephrectomy. At many academic centers, partial nephrectomy comprises 60% to 70% of the operations for RCTs. Yet, when investigators took a cross-sectional view of clinical practice using the Nationwide Inpatient Sample, they reported that only 7.5% of kidney tumor operations in the United States from 1988 to 2002 were partial nephrectomies.[45] Using the Surveillance Epidemiology and End Results database, investigators from the University of Michigan reported that from 2001, only 20% of all RCTs between 2 and 4 cm were treated by partial nephrectomy despite an already well-established literature supporting partial nephrectomy.[46] In England, a similar underuse of partial nephrectomy was reported in 2002 with only 108 (4%) partial nephrectomies out of 2671 nephrectomies performed.[47]

Many factors likely account for this reluctance to integrate partial nephrectomies into widespread clinic practice, despite mounting evidence of the virtues of partial nephrectomies both for local tumor control and preservation of long-term renal function. Open kidney surgery as a common element of training programs has been markedly reduced since the introduction of percutaneous, ureteroscopic, and extracorporeal approaches for the treatment of kidney stones over the last 20 years. Many of the surgical techniques employed in partial nephrectomy for tumors, including vascular isolation, ice slush, and suture repair of the collecting system, emanated from operations initially designed to treat complex kidney (staghorn) stones. Possibly, because of demographics of RCTs and regional referral patterns, only certain centers have had the numbers of extensive open renal tumor operations sufficient enough for training residents and staff.

The development of minimally invasive laparoscopic renal tumor surgery and tumor ablative techniques, such as radiofrequency and cryoablation, has been ongoing for 17 years by committed investigators in the United States and abroad. The advantages of cosmetic incisions, decreased perioperative analgesic requirements, and more rapid return to normal activity were emphasized in early publications and short-term oncologic end points seemed equivalent to those of their open-surgical counterparts. However, at centers with expertise in both open and minimally invasive surgery approaches for RCT, published experiences revealed inconsistencies in the management of small renal tumors. Open surgeons were more likely to perform partial nephrectomy, and laparoscopic surgeons were more likely to perform radical nephrectomy. These reports suggested that skills related to minimally invasive surgery were being acquired through surgery involving small renal tumors (<4 cm), despite the above-described clinical data that this was surgical overkill and deleterious to the patients' overall renal function.[48] Unique issues relative to minimally invasive surgery, such as the problem of tumor-bearing kidney retrieval (ie, morcellation vs. an open extraction incision for removal) were debated in the literature. The case load required to extend the surgical limits for minimally invasive surgery was not known and the decision to perform an open kidney procedure rather than a minimally invasive kidney procedure often depended upon the relative surgical expertise of the individual surgeon rather than more clearly defined guidelines relating to tumor size and concerns about future renal function.

By 2000, because of the well-described benefits of partial nephrectomy, several minimally invasive surgery groups began concerted efforts to develop laparoscopic partial nephrectomy techniques that would closely simulate the open procedure, initially with smaller, exophytic renal tumors and, with time and increasing experience, with more complex centrally located or cystic renal tumors. Valiant attempts to duplicate the renal protective effects of cold ischemia, readily obtained in open partial nephrectomy, were reported and included cold renal arterial and ureteral perfusions and, recently, laparoscopic ice slush placement. Nonetheless, the majority of laparoscopic partial nephrectomies (many of which are complex) continue to be performed under warm ischemic conditions with the hope that rapid completion of the operation will limit any ischemic effects on the kidney. Even for these expert surgeons, laparoscopic partial nephrectomy is currently described as a "complex" or "advanced" operation with published complication rates that are three to four times higher than those for their open counterparts.[49,50] Interestingly, laparoscopic partial nephrectomy teams report similar rates of benign lesions resected (20%–30%) and similar beneficial effects on overall renal function as described above in the open partial nephrectomy experience.

Recently, investigators from the Mayo Clinic, Cleveland Clinic, and Johns Hopkins pooled their data on 1800 partial nephrectomies, of which 771 were performed laparoscopically and 1028 were performed open for T1 tumors between 1998 and 2005. Even though the surgeons at these centers were experts in their respective laparoscopic and open operations, careful case selection was apparent. Open partial nephrectomy patients had larger tumors that were more likely centrally located and malignant; were at higher risk of perioperative complications as defined by their older age, increased comorbidities, and decreased performance status; and had decreased renal function at the time of operation, all of which may have contributed to longer hospital stays for open partial nephrectomy (5.8 days) versus laparoscopic partial nephrectomy (3.3 days). Patients in the laparoscopic partial nephrectomy group were more likely to have elective indications than imperative or absolute indications for partial nephrectomy yet laparoscopic partial nephrectomy was associated with longer ischemic time; more postoperative complications, particularly urologic; and increased number of subsequent procedures to treat complications. This comprehensive study leaves little doubt that the laparoscopic partial nephrectomy is a technically challenging operation, even in the hands of such experts, where careful case selection may decrease the chance of surgical and urological complications.[51]

As the virtues of partial nephrectomy, by any technique, are apparent, an open alternative to laparoscopy is a miniflank supra–11th rib incision, which can be in the range of 8 to 10 cm. This approach leaves an incision only 1 to 2 cm larger than the extraction incisions for laparoscopic radical nephrectomy or the hand-assist ports for hand-assisted laparoscopic surgery, avoids the painful rib resection, and is associated with a low rate of incidence of flank bulge and hernias (<5%) compared with more traditional open flank operations (30%–40%). This approach may allow urologists trained in open surgery to perform partial nephrectomy with lesser patient morbidity and without the more elaborate training and learning curve associated with laparoscopic partial nephrectomy.[52] For patients with small renal tumors, the long-lasting value of renal preservation by partial nephrectomy, whether performed by laparoscopic or open techniques, now far supersedes the rapid recovery offered by laparoscopic radical nephrectomy.

Also under active investigation are the renal tumor ablative modalities of percutaneous radiofrequency ablation and percutaneous and laparoscopic cryoablation.[53] These are offered often to patients who are old or comorbidly ill. With short overall follow-up and lack of pathologic resection to confirm the completeness of the ablation, it is not known whether ablation is as effective as surgical resection and whether or not the radiological images postablation represent complete or partial tumor destruction or simply a renal tumor, partially treated, not in active growth. In a recent report from the Cleveland Clinic, which has substantial experience in both radiofrequency ablation and cryoablation, documented recurrence rates for cryoablation were 13 of 175 cases (7.4%) and 26 of 104 cases (25%) for radiofrequency ablation whose mean preablation tumor sizes were 3.0 and 2.8 cm respectively. Repeat ablations were performed in 26 patients but 12 patients were not candidates for repeat ablation because of large tumor size, disease progression, or repeat ablation failure. Of these, 10 patients underwent attempted resection with only 2 patients being eligible for partial nephrectomy (open) and 7 patients requiring radical nephrectomy. One operation was aborted. From this data, it appears that a failed ablative procedure in a patient originally eligible for a partial nephrectomy, likely translates into a radical nephrectomy as salvage procedure because of extensive postablation scarring.[54] Carefully designed "ablate and resect" clinical protocols need to be done, much like those done in the 1990s with cryotherapy and localized prostate cancer, to determine the true effectiveness of these approaches. For this same population of elderly patients or comorbidly ill patients with small renal tumors, active surveillance is increasingly being suggested as an alternative to invasive treatments.[55,56]

SUMMARY

The value of partial nephrectomy in the management of small renal cortical tumors is gaining wider recognition thanks to (1) enhanced understanding of the biology of renal cortical tumors; (2) better knowledge about tumor size and stage migration to small tumors at the time of presentation; (3) studies indicating the oncologic efficacy of kidney-sparing surgery, whether performed by open or laparoscopic techniques, and (4) increasing awareness of the wide prevalence of CKD and its associated cardiovascular morbidity and mortality. The argument by many minimally invasive surgeons for laparoscopic radical nephrectomy and its associated rapid convalescence and cosmesis is not sufficiently compelling when iatrogenic initiation or worsening of CKD is the result. The overzealous use of radical nephrectomy for small renal tumors, whether by open or laparoscopic techniques, must now be considered detrimental to the long-term health and safety of the patient with a small RCT. Widespread training in partial nephrectomy and enhanced use, whether by open or laparoscopic approaches, is clearly indicated in the United States and abroad.

REFERENCES

1. Linehan WM, Walther MM, Zbar B. The genetic basis of cancer of the kidney. J Urol 2003;170:2163–72.
2. Russo P, Snyder M, Vickers A, et al. Cytoreductive nephrectomy and nephrectomy/complete metastasectomy for renal cancer. The Scientific World Urology 2007;2:42–52.
3. Flanigan RC, Salmon SE, Blumenstein BA, et al. Nephrectomy followed by interferon alfa-2b compared with interferon alfa-2b alone for metastatic renal-cell cancer. N Engl J Med 2001;345:1655–9.
4. Russo P. Renal cell carcinoma: presentation, staging, and surgical treatment. Semin Oncol 2000;27:160–76.
5. McKiernan JM, Yossepowitch O, Kattan MW, et al. Partial nephrectomy for renal cortical tumors: pathological findings and impact on outcome. Urology 2002;60:1003–9.
6. Snyder ME, Bach A, Kattan MW, et al. Incidence of benign lesions for clinically localized renal masses <7cm in radiological diameter: influence of gender. J Urol 2006;176:2391–6.
7. Dechet CB, Zincke H, Sebo TJ, et al. Prospective analysis of computerized tomography and needle biopsy with permanent sectioning to determine the nature of solid renal masses in adults. J Urol 2003;169:71–4.
8. Divgi C, Pandit-Taskar N, Jungbluth AA, et al. Preoperative characterization of clear cell renal carcinoma using iodine-124 labeled antibody chimeric G250 (124I–cG250) and positron emission tomography (PET): phase 1 surgical validation in patients with renal masses. Lancet Oncol 2007;4:304–10.
9. Russo P, Goetzl M, Simmons R, et al. Partial nephrectomy: the rationale for expanding the indications. Ann Surg Oncol 2002;9:680–7.
10. Lee CT, Katz J, Shi WW, et al. Surgical management of renal tumors of 4 cm or less in a contemporary cohort. J Urol 2000;163:730–6.
11. Leibovich BC, Blute ML, Cheville JC, et al. Nephron sparing surgery for appropriately selected renal cell carcinoma between 4 and 7 cm resulting in outcome similar to radical nephrectomy. J Urol 2004;171:1066–70.
12. Gilbert BR, Russo P, Zirinsky K, et al. Intraoperative sonography. Application in renal cell carcinoma. J Urol 1988;139:582–4.
13. Stephanson A, Hakimian A, Snyder ME, et al. Complications of radical and partial nephrectomy in a large contemporary cohort. J Urol 2004;171:130–4.
14. Yossepowitch O, Eggener SE, Serio A, et al. Temporary renal ischemia during nephron-sparing surgery is associated with short-term but not long-term impairment of renal function. J Urol 2006;176(4 Pt 1):1339–43.
15. Richstone L, Scherr DS, Reuter VR, et al. Multifocal renal cortical tumors: frequency, associated clinicopathological features, and impact on survival. J Urol 2004;171:615–20.
16. Tismit MO, Razin JP, Thionunn N, et al. Prospective study of the safety margins in partial nephrectomy: intraoperative assessment and contribution of frozen section analysis. Urology 2006;67:923–6.
17. Schachter LR, Bach AM, Snyder ME, et al. The impact of tumor location on histological subtype of renal cortical tumors. BJU Int 2006;98(1):63–6.
18. Yossepowitch O, Thompson RH, Leibovitch BC, et al. Predictors and oncological outcomes following positive surgical margins at partial nephrectomy. J Urol 2008;179(6):2158–63.
19. Dash A, Vickers AJ, Schachter LR, et al. Comparison of outcomes in elective partial vs. radical nephrectomy for clear cell renal cell carcinoma of 4–7 cm. BJU Int 2006;97:939–45.
20. Pahernik S, Roos F, Rohrig B, et al. Elective nephron sparing surgery for renal cell carcinoma larger than 4 cm. J Urol 2008;179:71–4.
21. Patel MI, Simmons R, Kattan MW, et al. Long term follow up of bilateral sporadic renal tumors. Urology 2003;61:921–5.
22. Kattan MW, Reuter V, Motzer RJ, et al. A postoperative prognostic nomogram for renal cell. J Urol 2001;166:63–7.
23. Najaraian JS, Chavers BM, McHugh LE, et al. 20 years or more of follow-up of living kidney donors. Lancet 1992;340:807–10.
24. Fehrman-Ekholm I, Duner F, Brink B, et al. No evidence of loss of kidney function in living kidney donors from cross sectional follow up. Transplantation 2001;72:444–9.
25. Goldfarb DA, Matin SF, Braun WE, et al. Renal outcome 25 years after donor nephrectomy. J Urol 2001;166:2043–7.
26. Kaplan C, Pasternack B, Shah H, et al. Age-related incidence of sclerotic glomeruli in human kidneys. Am J Pathol 1975;80:227–34.
27. Bijol V, Mendez GP, Hurwitz S, et al. Evaluation of the nonneoplastic pathology in tumor nephrectomy specimens: predicting the risk of progressive renal failure. Am J Surg Pathol 2006;30:575–84.
28. Coresh J, Selvin E, Stevens LA, et al. Prevalence of chronic kidney disease in the United States. JAMA 2007;298:2038–47.
29. Stevens LA, Coresh J, Green T, et al. Assessing kidney function—measured and estimated glomerular filtration rate. N Engl J Med 2006;354:2473–83.

30. Sarnak M, Leavey AS, Schoolwerth AC, et al. Kidney disease as a risk factor for the development of cardiovascular disease: a statement from the American Heart Association Council on Kidney in Cardiovascular Disease. High blood pressure research, clinical cardiology, and epidemiology and prevention. Circulation 2003;108:2154–69.

31. Chobanian AV, Bakris GL, Black HR, et al. The seventh report of the Joint National Committee on TN Prevention, Detection, Evaluation, and Treatment of High Blood Pressure: the JNC 7 report. JAMA 2003;289:2560–72.

32. Kidney Disease Outcome Quality Imitative. K/DOQI clinical guideline for chronic kidney disease evaluation, classification, stratification. 51:5246. Am J Kidney Dis 2002;39(Suppl 2):39–47.

33. Ritz E, McClellan WW. Overview: increased cardiovascular risk in patients with minor renal dysfunction: an emerging issue with far-reaching consequences. J Am Soc Nephrol 2004;15:513–6.

34. Shlipak MG, Fried LF, Cushman M, et al. Cardiovascular mortality risk in chronic kidney disease. JAMA 2005;293:1737–45.

35. Poggio ED, Wang X, Greene T, et al. Performance of the modification of diet in renal disease and Cockcroft-Gault equations in the estimation of GFR in health and in chronic kidney disease. J Am Soc Nephrol 2005;16:459–66.

36. Levey AS, Coresh J, Greene T, et al. Chronic Kidney Disease Epidemiology Collaboration. Using standardized serum creatinine values in the modification of diet in renal disease study equation for estimating glomerular filtration rate. Ann Intern Med 2006; 145(4):247–54.

37. Go AS, Chertow GM, Fan D, et al. Chronic kidney disease and the risks of death, cardiovascular events, and hospitalization. N Engl J Med 2004;351:1296–305.

38. Foley RN, Wang C, Collins AJ. Cardiovascular risk factor profiles and kidney function stage in the US general population: the NHANES 3 study. Mayo Clin Proc 2005;80:1270–7.

39. Lau WK, Blute ML, Weaver AL, et al. Matched comparison of radical nephrectomy vs. nephron-sparing surgery in patients with unilateral renal cell carcinoma and a normal contra lateral kidney. Mayo Clin Proc 2000;75:1236–42.

40. McKiernan J, Simmons R, Katz J, et al. Natural history of chronic renal insufficiency after partial and radical nephrectomy. Urology 2002;59:816–20.

41. Sorbellini M, Kattan MW, Snyder ME, et al. Prognostic nomogram for renal insufficiency after radical or partial nephrectomy. J Urol 2006;176:472–6.

42. Huang WC, Levey AS, Serio AM, et al. Chronic kidney disease after nephrectomy in patients with renal cortical tumors: a retrospective cohort study. Lancet Oncol 2006;7:735–40.

43. Thompson HR, Boorjian SA, Lohse CM, et al. Radical nephrectomy for pT1a renal masses may be associated with decreased overall survival compared to partial nephrectomy. J Urol 2008;179:468–73.

44. Jemal A, Siegel R, Ward E, et al. Cancer statistics, 2008. CA Cancer J Clin 2008;58:71–96.

45. Hollenback BK, Tash DA, Miller DC, et al. National utilization trends of partial nephrectomy for renal cell carcinoma: a case of underutilization? Urology 2006;67:254–9.

46. Miller DC, Hollingsworth JM, Hafez KS, et al. Partial nephrectomy for small renal masses. An emerging quality of care concern? J Urol 2006;175:853–7.

47. Nuttail M, Cathcart P, van der Meulen J, et al. A description of radical nephrectomy practice and outcomes in England. 1995–2002. BJU Int 2005;96:58–61.

48. Scherr DS, Ng C, Munver R, et al. Practice patterns among urologic surgeons treating localized renal cell carcinoma in the laparoscopic age: technology vs. oncology. Urology 2003;62:1007–11.

49. Ramani AP, Desai MM, Steinberg AP, et al. Complications of laparoscopic partial nephrectomy in 200 cases. J Urol 2005;173:42–7.

50. Kim FJ, Rha KH, Hernandez F, et al. Laparoscopic radical versus partial nephrectomy: assessment of complications. J Urol 2003;170:408–11.

51. Gill IS, Kavoussi LR, Lane BR, et al. Comparison of 1800 laparoscopic and open partial nephrectomies for single renal tumors. J Urol 2007;178:41–6.

52. Diblasio CJ, Snyder ME, Russo P. Mini flank supra-eleventh incision for open partial or radical nephrectomy. BJU Int 2006;97(1):149–56.

53. Gill IS, Remer EM, Hasan WA, et al. Renal cryoablation: outcome at 3 years. J Urol 2005;173:1903–7.

54. Nguyen CT, Lane BR, Kaouk JH, et al. Surgical salvage of renal cell carcinoma recurrence after thermal ablative therapy. J Urol 2008;180:104–9.

55. Wehle MJ, Thiel DD, Petrou SP, et al. Conservative management of incidental contrast-enhancing renal masses as safe alternative to invasive therapy. Urology 2004;64:49.

56. Volpe A, Jewett MA. The role of surveillance for small renal masses. Nat Clin Pract Urol 2007;4:2–3.

Choice of Operation for Clinically Localized Renal Tumor

Carvell T. Nguyen, MD, PhD[a], Steven C. Campbell, MD, PhD[b], Andrew C. Novick, MD[a],*

KEYWORDS
- Renal cell carcinoma • Radical nephrectomy
- Partial nephrectomy • Laparoscopy • Thermal ablation

EVOLUTION OF THE SURGICAL MANAGEMENT OF LOCALIZED RENAL CELL CARCINOMA

Intensive study of the biology of renal cell carcinoma (RCC) has advanced the understanding of its pathogenesis and led to novel adjuvant therapies, such as tyrosine kinase inhibitors. Even in this era of molecular targeted therapy, however, surgical excision remains the primary curative treatment for RCC. Historically, radical nephrectomy (RN), with or without ipsilateral adrenalectomy and regional lymphadenectomy, has been the reference standard for curative treatment of localized RCC. With prevailing data showing excellent oncologic efficacy, RN long has been the treatment of choice in patients who have localized unilateral RCC and a normally functioning contralateral kidney.[1]

With the advent of laparoscopy, minimally invasive techniques have been applied to RN resulting in an appealing alternative to open surgery that is associated with decreased morbidity and quicker convalescence. Generally used in the management of localized RCC without invasive features or substantial venous or nodal involvement, these techniques have had survival outcomes comparable with those of the open approach, and laparoscopic RN now is firmly established as one of the standards in this field.[2–5]

Despite its long history and proven efficacy in treating kidney cancer, changes in the epidemiology of RCC and recent data clarifying a link between RN and chronic kidney disease have called into question the status of RN as the treatment of choice in patients who have a normal contralateral kidney. During the last decade, there has been stage and size migration in RCC because of the increased incidental detection of small (< 4 cm) renal masses, which now account for the majority of cases that present for surgical management.[6] Moreover, there now is evidence demonstrating that renal preservation is critical even in patients who have normal contralateral renal function because there is a higher risk of subsequent chronic kidney disease following RN for RCC.[7–9]

As a result, surgical options for localized RCC have expanded in the past 2 decades to include nephron-sparing surgery (NSS), which encompasses open and laparoscopic partial nephrectomy (OPN and LPN, respectively) as well as newer modalities based on thermal ablation. Partial nephrectomy (PN) has demonstrated curative potential equal to RN in the treatment of localized RCC according to comparison studies. For example, Lau and colleagues[7] performed a matched comparison of 164 patients treated with either RN or PN and reported no significant differences between the two treatment groups in overall and cancer-specific survival, complication rate, and development of metastatic disease. Patients who underwent PN, however, demonstrated

[a] Glickman Urological & Kidney Institute, Cleveland Clinic Foundation, 9500 Euclid Avenue A100, Cleveland, OH 44195, USA

[b] Section of Urological Oncology, Glickman Urological and Kidney Institute, Cleveland Clinic Foundation, 9500 Euclid Avenue A100, Cleveland, OH 44195, USA

* Corresponding author.

E-mail address: novicka@ccf.org (A.C. Novick).

Urol Clin N Am 35 (2008) 645–655
doi:10.1016/j.ucl.2008.07.002

a decreased incidence of chronic kidney disease (defined by a serum creatinine > 2 mg/dL) as well as a decreased rate of proteinuria at a follow-up of 10 years. Other groups have demonstrated similar findings, and the increased incidence of renal insufficiency following RN persists even after controlling for potential confounding factors such as diabetes or hypertension.[10,11]

The primary concern from these studies is that RN can have deleterious effects on a patient's long-term renal function and overall health, because population-based studies have shown a correlation between chronic kidney disease and increased risks of morbid cardiac events, hospitalization for any reason, and death. Another concern with indiscriminate application of RN is the possibility of late recurrence of RCC in the contralateral kidney; options for salvage treatment become more limited in the context of a solitary kidney. Overall, the current evidence supports a judicious use of RN in the treatment of localized renal masses that otherwise may be amenable to NSS, and this principle now is an overriding consideration in the management of patients who have small renal masses. Undoubtedly, RN remains a viable option when the primary tumor is prohibitively large (ie, > 7 cm), replaces too much renal parenchyma, is in a location not amenable to NSS, or in some older patients who desire surgical excision but for whom the risks associated with a complex PN may not be acceptable.

THE ASCENDANCY OF ELECTIVE PARTIAL NEPHRECTOMY

PN involves the complete resection of a localized renal mass with adequate surgical margins while preserving as much normal renal parenchyma as possible. Historically, PN has been used in patients who have imperative indications for renal preservation to avoid the need for renal replacement therapy. Such patients include individuals who have a solitary kidney (functional or anatomic), those who have bilateral tumors, or those affected by local or systemic conditions that may place them at high risk for subsequent renal failure (eg, diabetes, hypertension, or renovascular disease).[12–14]

The indications for NSS have expanded during the past 2 decades, and elective PN now is established as a standard of care for small (< 4 cm) renal tumors in patients who have a normal opposite kidney (**Table 1**). Elective PN is concordant with the current mandate to optimize renal function on a long-term basis but also offers a variety of other important advantages. It avoids overtreatment of benign renal histologies that represent

approximately 20% of all small, enhancing renal tumors,[10,15–17] its cost effectiveness is equivalent to that of RN,[8,18–20] and some studies also demonstrate better quality of life after PN than after RN.[21,22] With careful patient selection and adequate expertise, PN also can provide a perioperative morbidity profile similar to that of RN.

Although preservation of renal function and prevention of chronic kidney disease are important considerations, local cancer control is still the primary goal of any cancer surgery, and equivalent oncologic efficacy must be demonstrated before PN can be accepted as a viable alternative to RN in an elective setting. In fact, the technical success rate of PN for RCC is excellent, and the prevailing data indicate extended cancer-specific survival rates on par with those observed after RN.[14,23] The largest reported study of PN for localized RCC is from the Cleveland Clinic and reviewed the results of 485 patients who had sporadic RCC, demonstrating overall and cancer-specific 5-year survival rates of 81% and 92%, respectively.[24] Long-term results of PN for localized RCC have confirmed its enduring oncologic efficacy. Fergany and colleagues[25] demonstrated a 10-year cancer-specific survival rate of 73% as well as preservation of renal function in 93% of patients treated for localized sporadic RCC. Likewise, Herr[26] reported overall and metastasis-free survival rates of 93% and 97%, respectively, at a median follow-up of 10 years in a cohort of patients who had unilateral renal tumors and a normal opposite kidney. Furthermore, studies from institutions with extensive experience with PN have found no significant differences in survival between patients who had low-stage, localized RCC treated with either PN or RN. Butler and colleagues[27] noted 5-year cancer-specific survival rates of 97% and 100% for patients treated with RN and PN, respectively, and investigators from the Mayo Clinic noted similar rates of 96% and 92%.[28]

Careful patient selection, which probably contributed to the favorable outcomes demonstrated in these reports, can help determine which patients will benefit from elective PN versus RN. This precaution will ensure that PN is used safely and appropriately, thereby optimizing outcomes and reducing the incidence of tumor recurrence. Preoperative patient characteristics that may predict postoperative renal insufficiency after RN include elevated preoperative serum creatinine level, proteinuria, and hypertension,[29] and a nomogram to predict postnephrectomy renal insufficiency incorporating some of these variables has been developed by investigators at the Memorial Sloan-Kettering Cancer Center.[30] In addition, a number

Table 1
Outcomes after elective partial nephrectomy for unilateral renal tumor and normal opposite kidney

Series	No. of Patients	Disease-Specific Survival (%)	Local Recurrence (%)	Mean Tumor Size (cm)
Bazeed et al (1986)	23	100	0	3.3
Carini et al (1988)	10	90	0	3.5
Morgan and Zincke (1990)	20	100	0	3.1
Selli et al (1991)	20	90	0	< 3.5
Provet et al (1991)	19	100	0	2.6
Steinbach et al (1992)	72	94.4	2.7 (2 cases)	N/A
Moll et al (1993)	98	100	1 (1 cases)	4
Thrasher et al (1994)	6	—	0	4.3
Lerner et al (1996)	54	92	5.6 (3 cases)	< 4
D'Armiento et al (1997)	19	96	0	3.34
van Poppel et al (1998)	51	98	0	3
Herr (1999)	70	97.5	1.5 (2 cases)	3
Hefez et al (1999)	45	100	0	< 4
Barbalias et al (1999)	41	97.5	7.3 (3 cases)	3.5
Belldegrun et al (1999)	63	100	3.2 (2 cases)	< 4
Filipas et al (2000)	180	98	1.6 (3 cases)	3.3
Delakas et al (2002)	118	97.3	3.9 (cases)	3.4
Total	909	90–100	0–7.3	2–4.3 cm

Abbreviation: N/A, not available.
Data from Campbell SC, Novick AC, Bukow ski RM (2007) Renal tumors. In: Wein AJ, Kavoussi LR, Novick AC, et al, editors. Campbell-Walsh urology. Philadelphia: Saunders Elsevier; 2007. p. 1614.

of clinical criteria related to low tumor burden seem to be associated with improved patient outcomes following PN, including small tumor size (eg, < 4 cm), low tumor stage, and a solitary lesion. In another study from the Cleveland Clinic, PN performed in patients fitting these criteria resulted in a 5-year cancer-specific survival of 100% with no cases of postoperative tumor recurrence.[13]

A significant concern with the use of PN in RCC is indeed the risk of local recurrence in the ipsilateral kidney. Fortunately, overall rates of local recurrence following NSS in the literature range from 0% to 10%, and when considering tumors smaller than 4 cm (ie, the types of tumors commonly treated with elective PN), the incidence is approximately 1% to 3%.[14] Taken together, these data justify the growing confidence in PN as an oncologically equivalent alternative to RN in patients who have a solitary, unilateral tumor smaller than 4 cm and normal contralateral renal function.

UPPER LIMITS OF TUMOR SIZE FOR ELECTIVE PARTIAL NEPHRECTOMY

Initial studies assessing the impact of tumor size on treatment outcomes following NSS for localized

RCC demonstrated a significantly lower rate of recurrence and improved survival for tumors smaller than 4 cm.[24] Such data provided the rationale for using a 4-cm cutoff as the upper limit for elective PN and a revision of the American Joint Committee on Cancer staging system for confined RCC in 2002. During the last decade, PN has indeed become a standard of care for the treatment of T1a tumors. With the excellent oncologic efficacy displayed by PN and the importance of renal preservation, some institutions now are expanding the indications for elective PN to include T1b tumors (4–7 cm) (**Fig. 1**).

Several studies have suggested that elective PN in carefully selected patients can achieve oncologic efficacy equivalent to RN in the treatment of stage T1b renal masses.[31–33] For example, a large multi-institutional study demonstrated no significant difference in the rates of distant or local recurrence or cancer-specific mortality between patients undergoing PN and those undergoing RN for T1b tumors.[31] Similarly, Leibovich and colleagues[32] found comparable cancer-specific and distant metastases-free survival rates for patients treated with either PN or RN for pT1b tumors after controlling for pathologic features such as stage,

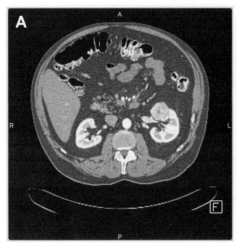
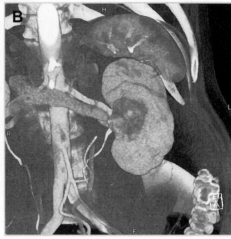

Fig. 1. A 50-year-old man who had no significant past medical history presented with microscopic hematuria and was found to have a 4.8-cm left renal mass abutting the renal vein and branches of the renal artery (*A*), The contralateral kidney was normal. Despite the precarious hilar location, three-dimensional reconstructed images (*B*) revealed a potential plane of dissection between the mass and the hilar vessels. OPN was performed, resulting in complete excision of the tumor with negative margins while preserving 75% of the left kidney. Final pathology was grade 3, pT2 clear cell RCC. At 2-year follow-up, the patient is without evidence of recurrence and has normal renal function (serum creatinine, 1.0 mg/dL).

grade, and histologic subtype. Although such data are encouraging, patient selection almost certainly contributed to the favorable outcomes in these series; patients who underwent PN tended to be younger, and their tumors tended to be smaller as well as of lower stage and grade.[33] Peripheral tumor location also was more common in these series. Elective PN for T1b tumors in a broader patient population remains controversial.[34]

OPEN VERSUS LAPAROSCOPIC PARTIAL NEPHRECTOMY

Significant advances in the field have allowed current laparoscopic techniques to duplicate the essential surgical principles of OPN, including clamping of the renal vasculature to provide a bloodless field when necessary, careful resection of the mass with a rim of normal parenchyma, and intracorporeal suturing to close the collecting system and repair the capsular defect.[35,36] Nevertheless, LPN can be technically demanding, and certain obstacles remain, including longer warm ischemia times and hemostatic concerns. As such, the decision to perform LPN versus OPN currently may depend more on the experience and comfort level of the surgeon than on oncologic guidelines. Not surprisingly, the practice of LPN has been limited largely to specialized tertiary care centers.

A recent multicenter study comparing OPN and LPN for single renal masses addressed the questions of oncologic efficacy, impact on renal function, and postoperative morbidity and provides useful information about the relative merits of these approaches.[37] This study comprised 1800 patients including 771 undergoing LPN and 1029 undergoing OPN for a single renal tumor smaller than 7 cm. Similar cancer-specific survival (99.3% versus 99.2% at 3 years) and postoperative renal function (97.9% versus 99.6% functioning renal units at 3 months) was demonstrated. Compared with OPN, LPN was associated with decreased operative time, blood loss, and hospital stay but demonstrated longer warm ischemia times and more postoperative complications requiring additional interventions (**Table 2**).[37] In particular, urologic complications (primarily urine leak and hemorrhage) were more common after LPN (9.2% versus 5.0%, *P* = .0006), and postoperative hemorrhage was almost threefold more common after LPN (4.2% versus 1.6%, *P* = .0002). It should be noted that patients treated with OPN were a higher-risk group than the LPN cohort: a greater percentage of patients in the OPN group demonstrated decreased performance status, impaired renal function, and symptomatic presentation. Furthermore, tumors in the OPN cohort more often were malignant, were larger on average, and more were centrally located or involved a solitary kidney (see **Table 2**). These observations suggest that in this study patient selection and tumor biology were substantially different in the two groups, with all comparisons reflecting a higher-risk population for OPN.

Table 2
Comparison of patient characteristics, perioperative parameters, and outcome in OPN and LPN

	OPN	LPN
No. patients	1029	771
ECOG performance status $\geq$ 1 (%)	14.7	1.4
Mean preoperative serum creatinine (mg/dL)	1.25	1.01
% Symptomatic at presentation	33.5	8.8
Mean tumor size (cm)	3.5	2.7
% central tumors	53.3	34.4
% solitary kidney	21.6	4.2
Mean operative time (min)[a]	266	201
Mean warm ischemia time (min)	20.1	30.7
Mean blood loss (cm^3)[a]	376	300
% with RCC on final pathology[a]	83	72
Mean hospital stay (days)[a]	5.8	3.3
% intraoperative complications	1	1.8
% postoperative urologic complications[a]	5	9.2
% postoperative hemorrhage[a]	1.6	4.2
% postoperative urine leak	2.3	3.1
% patients requiring subsequent procedure[a]	3.5	6.9

Abbreviation: ECOG, Eastern Cooperative Oncology Group.
[a] Statistically significant.
Data from Gill IS, Kavoussi LR, Lane BR, et al. Comparison of 1,800 laparoscopic and open partial nephrectomies for single renal tumors. J Urol 2007;178:41–6.

Long-term oncologic outcomes following LPN have become available recently and seem to be comparable with those observed after OPN. A recent long-term study from the Cleveland Clinic including 56 patients, each of whom had completed a minimum of 5 years of follow-up after LPN, demonstrated overall and cancer-specific survival rates of 86% and 100%, respectively, at a median follow-up of 6 years.[38] There was one case of local recurrence, and no patients developed metastatic disease. Likewise, in a retrospective comparison of LPN and OPN, Permpongkosol and colleagues[39] demonstrated 5-year disease-free survival rates of 91.4% and 97.6% and actuarial survival rates of 93.8% and 95.8%, respectively. Rates of local and distant recurrence after OPN and LPN also were comparable.

Encouragingly, despite longer warm ischemic times, LPN, like its open counterpart, has been shown to have protective effects on long-term renal function when compared with RN.[40,41] Finally, although financial concerns should not be the primary determinant of treatment method, there are data showing that LPN is less costly than OPN, primarily because of reduced length of stay.[42]

Although OPN remains the standard mode of NSS in patients who have localized RCC, the overall data suggest that LPN, in the hands of an experienced laparoscopic surgeon, can be an effective treatment option in select patients, with equivalent early cancer control, minimal impact on postoperative renal function, reduced blood loss, and more rapid convalescence. The increased warm ischemic times and postoperative urologic complications (eg, hemorrhage) are concerning, however, and mandate careful patient selection. Complex scenarios for PN such as centrally located tumor, tumor in a solitary kidney, predominantly cystic tumor, and multifocal disease probably are managed best with an open technique. All these challenging situations have been addressed successfully by experienced laparoscopic surgeons, however, and these conditions are best considered relative rather than absolute contraindications to LPN.[35,43–45]

THERMAL ABLATION FOR LOCALIZED RENAL MASSES

Conventional surgical excision may not be suitable for all patients, particularly those of advanced age or those who have multiple medical comorbidities. For such high-risk surgical candidates, thermal ablation represents a less invasive way to manage small renal masses proactively and seems to be associated with reduced morbidity and improved quality of life.[46–48] Established ablative techniques include cryoablation and radiofrequency ablation (RFA), both of which can be performed laparoscopically or percutaneously. The laparoscopic approach is preferred when mobilization away from adjacent organs is required. The percutaneous approach is even less invasive and is particularly suited to posteriorly located tumors.[49]

Because of the relatively recent application of thermal ablation to renal tumors, the long-term oncologic efficacy of these techniques has not been established to the same degree as surgical excision. There currently is greater experience with cryoablation, and there now are some studies with at least 5 years of follow-up data that suggest durable cancer control. Hegarty and colleagues[50] reported on 66 patients, all of whom had at least 5 years of follow-up after laparoscopic renal cryoablation, and demonstrated 5-year overall and cancer-specific survival rates of 81% and 98%, respectively. Another series of 48 patients with minimum and median follow-ups of 3 years and 64 months, respectively, demonstrated a cancer-specific survival of 100%.[51] RFA is less established than cryoablation, and its technology is still evolving; a number of different RFA generators and probes are commercially available.[52] A review of the literature indicates that RFA can be effective in treating small renal masses, providing cancer-specific survival ranging from 83% to 100% at a mean follow-up of 20 months.[53] Long-term data ($\geq$ 5 years) are required to establish the true oncologic efficacy of RFA and the optimal method for delivering radiofrequency energy.

Because it is less invasive, thermal ablation has gained considerable traction in the field recently. This technology comes with several potential limitations that must be considered carefully during patient counseling and clinical decision making, however. The current literature suggests that local cancer control with thermal ablation is inferior to that achieved with PN. Recent meta-analyses reported higher local recurrence rates with cryoablation and RFA than with surgical excision: 4.6%, 7.9%, and 2.7%, respectively, in the study by Weld and Landman[54] and relative rates of 7.45, 18.23, and 1.0, respectively, in the study by Kunkle and colleagues.[55] Furthermore, the validity of the radiographic definition of postablative success has been called into question, with recent data demonstrating that a small percentage of patients are found to have viable cancer on biopsy of an ablated tumor despite lack of enhancement on MRI.[56] Such data suggest that recurrence may be more common after thermal ablation,

particularly after RFA, than previously appreciated. Another disadvantage of thermal ablation is the lack of a pathologic diagnosis following treatment and an inability to confirm complete tumor kill.

Most local recurrences after thermal ablation can be managed successfully with repeat ablation, but indiscriminate use of thermal ablation in patients who otherwise may tolerate conventional surgery may hinder subsequent salvage attempts. A recent study from the Cleveland Clinic demonstrated that salvage surgery after previous ablation can be challenging, and in many cases partial nephrectomy or laparoscopic surgery were not possible.[57] A final limitation of thermal ablation relates to tumor size: success rates fall substantially for tumor diameters of 3.5 cm or greater. When all these potential limitations are considered, thermal ablation currently cannot be recommended as definitive therapy for the general patient population and may be best suited for high-risk surgical candidates who have small, exophytic renal masses.

SURGICAL APPROACH TO BILATERAL RENAL TUMORS

Because preservation of renal parenchyma is paramount in patients who have bilateral synchronous masses, NSS should be performed whenever possible, generally in a bilateral staged fashion. Unilateral RN may be required if conditions such as local extension, unfavorable location, or extremely large tumor size preclude PN. At the Cleveland Clinic the general strategy is to operate first on the kidney with the less-complicated tumor (eg, based on size and location), with the intent of preserving as much renal parenchyma as possible and establishing baseline function of the remnant ipsilateral kidney. This approach provides increased flexibility when planning the contralateral operation, and the flexibility can be very helpful in complex situations. This strategy also abrogates the need for temporary dialysis in the postoperative period because the contralateral kidney can protect against acute ischemic renal failure. Others have described simultaneous management of both kidneys with favorable results, and this approach is particularly appealing if one side requires either minimal or no hilar clamping.[58] Thermal ablation also can be considered as a nephron-sparing strategy in carefully selected patients.

SURGICAL APPROACH TO HEREDITARY RENAL CELL CARCINOMA

The presentation and natural history of hereditary RCC, represented by von Hippel-Lindau disease, familial papillary RCC, hereditary leiomyomatosis and RCC syndrome, and the Birt-Hogg-Dube syndrome, differ from sporadic RCC and mandate adjustments in surgical management. Although each of these syndromes is characterized by distinct genetic anomalies and histologic correlates, they all tend to present at a younger age and demonstrate a higher tumor burden, often displaying bilateral and multifocal disease. Kidneys of patients who have hereditary RCC also often harbor several hundred microscopic tumors, and local recurrences are common after PN as these occult lesions mature.[59,60]

Management options in hereditary RCC include NSS, RN, or active surveillance. Because of the high tumor burden associated with hereditary RCC, PN typically is the first-line treatment, allowing pathologic confirmation of the diagnosis as well as addressing all grossly evident lesions. Despite high rates of local recurrence, cancer-specific survival rates for patients who had von Hippel-Lindau disease and localized RCC range from 70% to 100% at 5 years with a minority of patients (23%) developing end-stage renal disease and requiring renal replacement therapy.[61,62] These data suggest that PN is an effective treatment option in patients who have hereditary RCC, allowing prolonged survival, preservation of renal function, and avoidance or delay of renal replacement therapy. Active surveillance is a viable option for patients who have recurrent disease whose dominant tumors are smaller than 3 cm, given that tumors below this size cutoff rarely metastasize.[63,64] This "3-cm rule" can be applied to all the familial forms of RCC except hereditary leiomyomatosis, which tends to be a more aggressive phenotype. Surgical intervention can be delayed until this size threshold is surpassed, limiting the morbidity and financial burden of repeated operations and optimizing renal function on a long-term basis.

RN effectively eliminates the possibility of local tumor recurrence but may represent overtreatment in most patients and hasten the development of end-stage renal failure. RN, however, may be indicated in patients who have hereditary leiomyomatosis, which is associated with renal tumors that are aggressive at presentation and represent a significant cause of mortality in these patients.[65,66] Some patients who have hereditary RCC may even require bilateral nephrectomy if the primary tumor is extensive bilaterally, although these patients should be in the minority. Some of these patients may be considered for subsequent renal transplantation, and this approach has been substantiated in the von Hippel-Lindau population.[67]

PN remains the preferred management for locally recurrent disease, but thermal ablation represents an attractive option for certain patients, particularly those who have a history of previous ipsilateral surgery, impaired renal function that may be compromised further by hilar clamping, or significant multifocal disease.[68,69] Along these lines, some have described a combined approach using PN for dominant lesions and thermal ablation to manage remaining evident lesions, with the goal of minimizing warm ischemic times while rendering the kidney grossly free of disease.

SURGICAL APPROACH TO A TUMOR IN A SOLITARY KIDNEY

Another absolute indication for NSS is the presence of a tumor involving a functional solitary kidney. When contemplating PN for such patients, it is critical to realize that at least 20% of a normal kidney must be spared to avoid end-stage renal failure and dialysis.[70,71] Even if this amount of residual renal parenchyma is spared successfully after partial nephrectomy, a minority of patients still may require dialysis in the postoperative period on a temporary (8% of cases) or permanent basis (4%).[72] When considering LPN versus OPN in this scenario, it is important to consider the adverse effect of prolonged ischemia time on postoperative renal function of solitary kidneys. Thompson and colleagues[73] reported on a multicenter study assessing the functional effects of vascular clamping in patients who had solitary kidneys and found that both warm and cold ischemia were associated with a significantly increased risk of acute and chronic renal failure and with need for temporary dialysis. In particular, a warm ischemia time longer than 20 minutes resulted in a greater incidence of chronic renal insufficiency and permanent dialysis.

These data emphasize the importance of selecting the nephron-sparing approach that allows adequate control of the renal hilum while limiting ischemia time. A study from the Cleveland Clinic compared 169 open and 30 laparoscopic PN performed for stage T1 tumors in a solitary kidney.[74] Despite equivalent postoperative renal function at 3 months, LPN, compared with OPN, was associated with a longer warm ischemia time (mean difference of 9 minutes, $P < .0001$), a 2.51-fold higher chance of postoperative complications ($P < .05$), and a higher rate of postoperative dialysis (10% versus 0.6%, respectively; $P = .01$). As such, OPN may represent the better treatment approach in patients who have localized RCC involving a solitary kidney who are at high risk for chronic kidney disease. Thermal ablation also can be a viable option for NSS in select patients. It must be emphasized, however, that most tumors in a solitary kidney can be managed safely and effectively with PN, which is still the standard of care for this patient population, assuming the patient is a reasonable surgical candidate.

SURGICAL APPROACH TO CENTRALLY LOCATED RENAL TUMORS

In the past, certain high-risk tumor characteristics, such as central location or proximity to the hilar vessels, were contraindications to PN, committing patients to RN instead. The risk of local recurrence for such precariously placed tumors was believed to be higher because of the difficulty in achieving the traditional 1- to 2-cm margin of normal parenchyma. Recent studies, however, have demonstrated that margin size has no effect on the risk of subsequent local recurrence as long as the final parenchymal margins are negative for tumor involvement.[75–77] Furthermore, tumor location itself does not affect treatment outcomes. Analyzing a cohort of patients who had solitary, unilateral tumors smaller than 4 cm who were treated with either PN or RN, Hafez and colleagues[78] found that there were no significant differences between central and peripheral tumors with respect to stage and grade distribution, survival, tumor recurrence, or postoperative renal function. Although PN was more technically challenging for central tumors than for peripheral tumors, as evidenced by longer ischemia times and more frequent violation of the collecting system, treatment with PN or RN was equally effective in this patient cohort regardless of tumor location.[78]

The initial experience with LPN for central tumors has confirmed its technical feasibility in this patient population, although the degree of technical difficulty is increased.[44] A retrospective comparison of LPN for central versus peripheral tumors demonstrated longer warm ischemia time, operative time, and hospital stay for central tumors, but the rate of perioperative complications and the median blood loss were similar.[45] Given individual surgeon expertise and experience, indications for LPN can be expanded to include central tumors, but OPN is still the better approach in most patients. RN remains a viable option when PN cannot achieve negative margins, reconstruction of the remnant kidney is not feasible, or in centers where expertise with PN is not available.

SUMMARY

The surgical treatment of localized RCC has undergone much change during the past decade.

Driven by the substantial evidence that preservation of renal function is a relevant clinical consideration for all patients, increasing efforts have been made to employ nephron-sparing approaches whenever possible. Efforts that once focused on avoiding dialysis now should be directed toward optimizing renal function. The prevailing data indicate that PN provides effective curative treatment for localized renal tumors on par with RN and should be the first-line treatment option for most patients, given requisite surgeon expertise. OPN is particularly suited to complex situations such as tumor in a solitary kidney or a central or hilar tumor, because this approach is more versatile and because the current database suggests that perioperative morbidity is lower than with LPN. Currently, the use of LPN for a given clinical scenario will depend primarily on patient selection and individual surgeon experience, but its growing importance in the armamentarium of cancer operations cannot be denied. Thermal ablation is a novel modality with great potential, particularly in high-risk surgical candidates, but its role as either a means of definitive therapy or as a supplement to current surgical approaches remains to be determined.

REFERENCES

1. Lam JS, Shvarts O, Pantuck AJ. Changing concepts in the surgical management of renal cell carcinoma. Eur Urol 2004;45:692–705.
2. Cadeddu JA, Ono Y, Clayman RV, et al. Laparoscopic nephrectomy for renal cell cancer: evaluation of efficacy and safety: a multicenter experience. Urology 1998;52:773–7.
3. Chan DY, Cadeddu JA, Jarrett TW, et al. Laparoscopic radical nephrectomy: cancer control for renal cell carcinoma. J Urol 2001;166:2095–9.
4. Gill IS, Meraney AM, Schweizer DK, et al. Laparoscopic radical nephrectomy in 100 patients: a single center experience from the United States. Cancer 2001;92:1843–55.
5. Permpongkosol S, Chan DY, Link RE, et al. Laparoscopic radical nephrectomy: long-term outcomes. J Endourol 2005;19:628–33.
6. Russo P. Open partial nephrectomy: an essential operation with an expanding role. Curr Opin Urol 2007;17:309–15.
7. Lau WK, Blute ML, Weaver AL, et al. Matched comparison of radical nephrectomy vs nephron-sparing surgery in patients with unilateral renal cell carcinoma and a normal contralateral kidney. Mayo Clin Proc 2000;75:1236–42.
8. McKiernan J, Simmons R, Katz J, et al. Natural history of chronic renal insufficiency after partial and radical nephrectomy. Urology 2002;59:816–20.

9. Huang WC, Levey AS, Serio AM, et al. Chronic kidney disease after nephrectomy in patients with renal cortical tumours: a retrospective cohort study. Lancet Oncol 2006;7:735–40.

10. McKiernan J, Yossepowitch O, Kattan MW, et al. Partial nephrectomy for renal cortical tumors: pathologic findings and impact on outcome. Urology 2002;60:1003–9.

11. Matin SF, Gill IS, Worley S, et al. Outcome of laparoscopic radical and open partial nephrectomy for the sporadic 4 cm. or less renal tumor with a normal contralateral kidney. J Urol 2002;168:1356–9.

12. Ghavamian R, Zincke H. Nephron-sparing surgery. Curr Urol Rep 2001;2:34–9.

13. Licht MR, Novick AC, Goormastic M. Nephron sparing surgery in incidental versus suspected renal cell carcinoma. J Urol 1994;152:39–42.

14. Uzzo RG, Novick AC. Nephron sparing surgery for renal tumors: indications, techniques and outcomes. J Urol 2001;166:6–18.

15. Glassman D, Chawla SN, Waldman I, et al. Correlation of pathology with tumor size of renal masses. Can J Urol 2007;14:3616–20.

16. Silver DA, Morash C, Brenner P, et al. Pathologic findings at the time of nephrectomy for renal mass. Ann Surg Oncol 1997;4:570–4.

17. Snyder ME, Bach A, Kattan MW, et al. Incidence of benign lesions for clinically localized renal masses smaller than 7 cm in radiological diameter: influence of sex. J Urol 2006;176:2391–5.

18. Shekarriz B, Upadhyay J, Shekarriz H, et al. Comparison of costs and complications of radical and partial nephrectomy for treatment of localized renal cell carcinoma. Urology 2002;59:211–5.

19. Stephenson AJ, Hakimi AA, Snyder ME, et al. Complications of radical and partial nephrectomy in a large contemporary cohort. J Urol 2004;171:130–4.

20. Uzzo RG, Wei JT, Hafez K, et al. Comparison of direct hospital costs and length of stay for radical nephrectomy versus nephron-sparing surgery in the management of localized renal cell carcinoma. Urology 1999;54:994–8.

21. Clark PE, Schover LR, Uzzo RG, et al. Quality of life and psychological adaptation after surgical treatment for localized renal cell carcinoma: impact of the amount of remaining renal tissue. Urology 2001;57:252–6.

22. Lesage K, Joniau S, Fransis K, et al. Comparison between open partial and radical nephrectomy for renal tumours: perioperative outcome and health-related quality of life. Eur Urol 2007;51:614–20.

23. Campbell SC, Novick AC. Surgical technique and morbidity of elective partial nephrectomy. Semin Urol Oncol 1995;13:281–7.

24. Hafez KS, Fergany AF, Novick AC. Nephron sparing surgery for localized renal cell carcinoma: impact of tumor size on patient survival, tumor recurrence and TNM staging. J Urol 1999;162:1930–3.

25. Fergany AF, Hafez KS, Novick AC. Long-term results of nephron sparing surgery for localized renal cell carcinoma: 10-year followup. J Urol 2000;63:442–5.

26. Herr HW. Partial nephrectomy for unilateral renal carcinoma and a normal contralateral kidney: 10-year followup. J Urol 1999;161:33–4.

27. Butler BP, Novick AC, Miller DP, et al. Management of small unilateral renal cell carcinomas: radical versus nephron-sparing surgery. Urology 1995;45:34–40.

28. Lerner SE, Hawkins CA, Blute ML, et al. Disease outcome in patients with low stage renal cell carcinoma treated with nephron sparing or radical surgery. J Urol 1996;155:1868–73.

29. Ito K, Nakashima J, Hanawa Y, et al. The prediction of renal function 6 years after unilateral nephrectomy using preoperative risk factors. J Urol 2004;171:120–5.

30. Sorbellini M, Kattan MW, Snyder ME, et al. Prognostic nomogram for renal insufficiency after radical or partial nephrectomy. J Urol 2006;176:472–6.

31. Patard JJ, Shvarts O, Lam JS, et al. Safety and efficacy of partial nephrectomy for all T1 tumors based on an international multicenter experience. J Urol 2004;171:2181–5.

32. Leibovich BC, Blute ML, Cheville JC, et al. Nephron sparing surgery for appropriately selected renal cell carcinoma between 4 and 7 cm results in outcome similar to radical nephrectomy. J Urol 2004;171:1066–70.

33. Dash A, Vickers AJ, Schachter LR, et al. Comparison of outcomes in elective partial vs radical nephrectomy for clear cell renal cell carcinoma of 4-7 cm. BJU Int 2006;97:939–45.

34. Campbell SC, Novick AC. Expanding the indications for elective partial nephrectomy: is this advisable? Eur Urol 2006;49:952–4.

35. Gill IS, Desai MM, Kaouk JH, et al. Laparoscopic partial nephrectomy for renal tumor: duplicating open surgical techniques. J Urol 2002;167:469–76.

36. Desai MM, Gill IS, Kaouk JH, et al. Laparoscopic partial nephrectomy with suture repair of the pelvicaliceal system. Urology 2003;61:99–104.

37. Gill IS, Kavoussi LR, Lane BR, et al. Comparison of 1,800 laparoscopic and open partial nephrectomies for single renal tumors. J Urol 2007;178:41–6.

38. Lane BR, Gill IS. 5-Year outcomes of laparoscopic partial nephrectomy. J Urol 2007;177:70–4.

39. Permpongkosol S, Bagga HS, Romero FR, et al. Laparoscopic versus open partial nephrectomy for the treatment of pathological T1N0M0 renal cell carcinoma: a 5-year survival rate. J Urol 2006;176:1984–8.

40. Kim FJ, Rha KH, Hernandez F, et al. Laparoscopic radical versus partial nephrectomy: assessment of complications. J Urol 2003;170:408–11.

41. Zorn KC, Gong EM, Orvieto MA, et al. Comparison of laparoscopic radical and partial nephrectomy: effects on long-term serum creatinine. Urology 2007;69: 1035–40.

42. Link RE, Permpongkosol S, Gupta A, et al. Cost analysis of open, laparoscopic, and percutaneous treatment options for nephron-sparing surgery. J Endourol 2006;20:782–9.

43. Gill IS, Colombo JR Jr, Moinzadeh A, et al. Laparoscopic partial nephrectomy in solitary kidney. J Urol 2006;175:454–8.

44. Gill IS, Colombo JR Jr, Frank I, et al. Laparoscopic partial nephrectomy for hilar tumors. J Urol 2005;174: 850–3.

45. Frank I, Colombo JR Jr, Rubinstein M, et al. Laparoscopic partial nephrectomy for centrally located renal tumors. J Urol 2006;175:849–52.

46. Hinshaw JL, Lee FT Jr. Image-guided ablation of renal cell carcinoma. Magn Reson Imaging Clin N Am 2004;12:429–47.

47. Lowry PS, Nakada SY. Renal cryotherapy: 2003 clinical status. Curr Opin Urol 2003;13:193–7.

48. Murphy DP, Gill IS. Energy-based renal tumor ablation: a review. Semin Urol Oncol 2001;19:133–40.

49. Hafron J, Kaouk JH. Ablative techniques for the management of kidney cancer. Nat Clin Pract Urol 2007;4:261–9.

50. Hegarty NJ, Gill IS, Kaouk JH, et al. Renal cryoablation: 5 year outcomes. [abstract 1091]. J Urol 2006; 175(Suppl):351.

51. Davol PE, Fulmer BR, Rukstalis DB. Long-term results of cryoablation for renal cancer and complex renal masses. Urology 2006;68(1 Suppl): S2–6.

52. Mulier S, Miao Y, Mulier P, et al. Electrodes and multiple electrode systems for radiofrequency ablation: a proposal for updated terminology. Eur Radiol 2005;15:798–808.

53. Park S, Cadeddu JA. Outcomes of radiofrequency ablation for kidney cancer. Cancer Control 2007;14: 205–10.

54. Weld KJ, Landman J. Comparison of cryoablation, radiofrequency ablation and high-intensity focused ultrasound for treating small renal tumours. BJU Int 2005;96:1224–9.

55. Kunkle DA, Egleson BL, Uzzo RG. Excise, ablate, or observe: the small renal mass dilemma–a meta-analysis and review. J Urol 2008;179:1227–33.

56. Hegarty NJ, Kaouk J, Remer EM, et al. Lack of enhancement on 6-month MRI does not guarantee complete cancer cell kill following radiofrequency ablation of small renal tumors. [abstract 1718]. J Urol 2006;175(4 Suppl):552.

57. Nguyen CT, Lane BR, Kaouk J, et al. Surgical salvage of renal cell carcinoma recurrence after thermal ablative therapy. J Urol 2008;180: 104–9.

58. Blute ML, Amling CL, Bryant SC, et al. Management and extended outcome of patients with synchronous bilateral solid renal neoplasms in the absence of von Hippel-Lindau disease. Mayo Clin Proc 2000;75: 1020–6.

59. Novick AC, Streem SB. Long-term followup after nephron sparing surgery for renal cell carcinoma in von Hippel-Lindau disease. J Urol 1992;147: 1488–90.

60. Roupret M, Hopirtean V, Mejean A, et al. Nephron sparing surgery for renal cell carcinoma and von Hippel-Lindau's disease: a single center experience. J Urol 2003;170:1752–5.

61. Lund GO, Fallon B, Curtis MA, et al. Conservative surgical therapy of localized renal cell carcinoma in von Hippel-Lindau disease. Cancer 1994;74: 2541–5.

62. Steinbach F, Novick AC, Zincke H, et al. Treatment of renal cell carcinoma in von Hippel-Lindau disease: a multicenter study. J Urol 1995;153:1812–6.

63. Duffey BG, Choyke PL, Glenn G, et al. The relationship between renal tumor size and metastases in patients with von Hippel-Lindau disease. J Urol 2004;172:63–5.

64. Walther MM, Choyke PL, Glenn G, et al. Renal cancer in families with hereditary renal cancer: prospective analysis of a tumor size threshold for renal parenchymal sparing surgery. J Urol 1999; 161:1475–9.

65. Launonen V, Vierimaa O, Kiuru M, et al. Inherited susceptibility to uterine leiomyomas and renal cell cancer. Proc Natl Acad Sci U S A 2001;98:3387–92.

66. Tomlinson IP, Alam NA, Rowan AJ, et al. Germline mutations in FH predispose to dominantly inherited uterine fibroids, skin leiomyomata and papillary renal cell cancer. Nat Genet 2002;30:406–10.

67. Goldfarb DA, Neumann HP, Penn I, et al. Results of renal transplantation in patients with renal cell carcinoma and von Hippel-Lindau disease. Transplantation 1997;64:1726–9.

68. Shingleton WB, Sewell PE Jr. Percutaneous renal cryoablation of renal tumors in patients with von Hippel-Lindau disease. J Urol 2002;167:1268–70.

69. Mabjeesh NJ, Avidor Y, Matzkin H. Emerging nephron sparing treatments for kidney tumors: a continuum of modalities from energy ablation to laparoscopic partial nephrectomy. J Urol 2004;171:553–60.

70. Novick AC, Gephardt G, Guz B, et al. Long-term follow-up after partial removal of a solitary kidney. N Engl J Med 1991;325:1058–62.

71. Campbell SC, Novick AC, Bukowski RM. Renal tumors. In: Wein AJ, Kavoussi LR, Novick AC, editors. Campbell-Walsh urology, vol. 2. Philadelphia: Saunders Elsevier; 2007. p. 1616–9.

72. Campbell SC, Novick AC, Streem SB, et al. Complications of nephron sparing surgery for renal tumors. J Urol 1994;151:1177–80.

73. Thompson RH, Frank I, Lohse CM, et al. The impact of ischemia time during open nephron sparing surgery on solitary kidneys: a multi-institutional study. J Urol 2007;177:471–6.

74. Lane BR, Novick AC, Babineau D, et al. Comparison of laparoscopic and open partial nephrectomy for tumor in a solitary kidney. J Urol 2008;179: 847–51.

75. Timsit MO, Bazin JP, Thiounn N, et al. Prospective study of safety margins in partial nephrectomy: intraoperative assessment and contribution of frozen section analysis. Urology 2006;67:923–6.

76. Castilla EA, Liou LS, Abrahams NA, et al. Prognostic importance of resection margin width after nephron-sparing surgery for renal cell carcinoma. Urology 2002;60:993–7.

77. Sutherland SE, Resnick MI, Maclennan GT, et al. Does the size of the surgical margin in partial nephrectomy for renal cell cancer really matter? J Urol 2002;167:61–4.

78. Hafez KS, Novick AC, Butler BP. Management of small solitary unilateral renal cell carcinomas: impact of central versus peripheral tumor location. J Urol 1998;159:1156–60.

Resection of Renal Tumors Invading the Vena Cava

Chad Wotkowicz, MD*, Matthew F. Wszolek, MD,
John A. Libertino, MD

KEYWORDS

- Renal cell carcinoma • Inferior vena cava
- Surgical management

Renal cell carcinoma (RCC) has been called the "internists' tumor" for many years because of the myriad of vague symptoms associated with this malignancy. Patients historically presented with metastatic disease at the time of their initial diagnosis. At the present time, approximately 70% of the patients who have RCC are diagnosed as a result of enhanced imaging capabilities. This early diagnosis has produced a stage migration because many RCCs are discovered incidentally. Kidney cancer is the third most common urologic malignancy in the United States, representing 3.5% of the newly diagnosed cancers in the United States, and accounts for 2.3% of cancer-related deaths.[1] During the past 20 years, the incidence of RCC has been increasing worldwide at a rate of 2.5% every year. This increased incidence is a result of increased abdominal imaging and an aging population.[2–4] In addition, RCC is a highly vascular malignancy with a tendency to invade the venous system and create a tumor thrombus either in the renal vein or the inferior vena cava (IVC). An estimated 4% to 10% of RCCs have a tumor thrombus present in the venous circulation, specifically the renal vein and IVC, and a subpopulation of 1% has extension into the right atrium.[5] Despite advances in radiation, chemotherapy, and immunotherapy the reference standard for RCC with tumor thrombus remains surgical resection. Several contemporary series have demonstrated 5-year survival rates of up to 60% in the absence of metastatic disease in patients who have venous tumor thrombus treated with radical nephrectomy and tumor thrombectomy.[5–11]

CLINICAL PRESENTATION

The advent of cross-sectional imaging for the work-up of abdominal pain has resulted in an increase of RCC prevalence. A number of patients who have venous tumor thrombus can be asymptomatic depending on the level of the tumor thrombus and the extent of occlusion of the IVC. Significant venous congestion as a result of caval intrusion can present with varying symptoms, including significant lower extremity edema, varicocele formation, proteinuria, caput medusae, and even pulmonary emboli. If the tumor extends above the level of the hepatic veins, Budd-Chiari syndrome may result from obstruction of the major hepatic veins, resulting in a triad of hepatomegaly, abdominal fullness/pain, and ascites. The resulting varices produce massive collaterals with associated impaired hepatic function and portal hypertension. Additional symptoms of RCC include flank discomfort, hematuria, and constitutional changes (fever, weight loss, fatigue). These constitutional symptoms usually indicate the presence of metastatic disease with an overall poor prognosis.

DIAGNOSTIC IMAGING AND PREOPERATIVE EVALUATION

All patients who have renal masses must have imaging studies, including chest radiographs and bone scans when appropriate, to rule out metastatic disease. In patients who have venous extension, additional studies are necessary to define the extent of the tumor thrombus. For this subset of

Department of Urology, Lahey Clinic, Burlington, MA, USA
* Corresponding author.
E-mail address: Chad.wotkowicz@lahey.org (C. Wotkowicz).

Urol Clin N Am 35 (2008) 657–671
doi:10.1016/j.ucl.2008.07.013

patients the authors' preferred imaging modality is MRI, specifically magnetic resonance venography, in combination with CT studies and three-dimensional reformatted images (**Fig. 1**). Tumor at or above the level of the diaphragm requires transesophageal echocardiography and may necessitate angiography to delineate the extent of the tumor thrombus. At the present time positron emission tomography (PET) scans have a limited diagnostic role; however, this modality is being evaluated at the Lahey Clinic as part of the preoperative evaluation and postoperative follow-up. The authors have noted that PET CT has demonstrated lesions in the liver that have not been detected on ordinary CT or MRI (**Fig. 2**).

A report from Zini and colleagues[12] suggests that preoperative measurements of the renal vein and IVC diameter with associated tumor thrombus correlate with the rate of renal ostial wall invasion and may serve as another prognostic indicator.

The importance of preoperative imaging for surgical planning cannot be overemphasized. Tumor thrombus extending to the level of the hepatic veins or higher may require cardiopulmonary bypass and circulatory arrest to provide insurance against excessive blood loss. Patients slated for cardiopulmonary bypass and circulatory arrest should have a cardiac evaluation, which may include stress testing or a coronary angiogram. If significant coronary artery disease is discovered, it may be treated with either a stent or bypass grafting. In five of the authors' patients bypass grafting was performed concomitantly with the radical nephrectomy and IVC thrombectomy.[13]

Bland thrombus often can be distinguished from tumor thrombus during the preoperative evaluation, and anticoagulation therapy or placement of an IVC filter should be considered to limit further propagation and the possibility of a pulmonary embolus. Transesophageal echocardiography identifies the presence of tumor thrombus in the right atrium and is an important adjunctive intraoperative diagnostic modality.[14]

RENAL ANGIOINFARCTION

Although only one prospective trial of preoperative angioinfarction is available to validate its use, the authors find that preoperative renal artery embolization is an important adjunctive tool in the treatment for advanced RCC, including patients who have venous tumor involvement.[15] Preoperative renal angioinfarction facilitates the dissection of the renal tumor as a result of local tissue edema from hypoxia and tissue necrosis. In addition, it potentially may decrease the extent of the tumor thrombus while minimizing intraoperative blood loss associated with extensive venous collaterals. Renal angioinfarction also allows the surgeon to ligate or transect the renal vein before controlling or occluding the renal artery. Clinicians must be aware of the postinfarction syndrome caused by innate and humoral immune responses to the infracted kidney.[16] This syndrome is characterized by chills, fevers, flank pain, malaise, hematuria, transient hypertension, and hyponatremia, all of which are self limiting.[17]

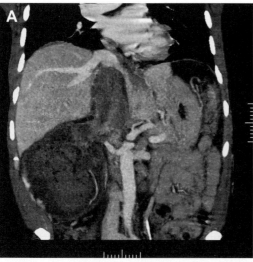 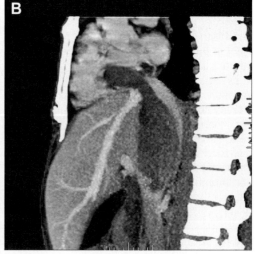

Fig. 1. (*A*) Coronal scan demonstrates the extent of tumor thrombus to the level of the major hepatic veins. (*B*) Lateral reconstructions indicate thrombus above the diaphragm. Cardiopulmonary bypass was required to resect this tumor.

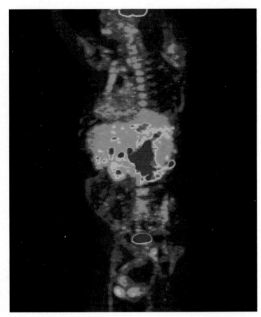

Fig. 2. PET scan obtained during preoperative evaluation for planned radical nephrectomy demonstrates increased uptake in multiple sites of the liver.

CLINICAL STAGING AND PROGNOSTICS FACTORS

There have been numerous proposals for staging RCCs and venous invasion. The current TNM staging system (**Box 1**) designates tumor thrombus in the renal vein up to the diaphragm as T3b. Numerous retrospective studies at the Lahey Clinic and elsewhere advocate revision based on difference in survival when only the renal vein is involved.[18,19] Literature, however, supports the current classification scheme, leaving the debate open for further discussion.[20] In addition to the level of the tumor thrombus, a variety of centers are exploring additional prognostic factors for a revision of the current staging. The UCLA Integrated Staging System incorporates TNM stage, Fuhrman tumor grade, and the Eastern Cooperative Oncology Group performance status.[21] Kattan and colleagues[22] have developed a nomogram based on the TNM stage, patient symptoms, tumor size, grade, and vascular invasion or tumor necrosis. The SSIGN (stage, size, grade necrosis) model from the Mayo Clinic also has been evaluated in more than 1800 patients.[23]

SURGICAL TREATMENT STRATEGIES

This discussion of surgical planning covers the following levels of tumor thrombus: renal vein, infrahepatic, retrohepatic, suprahepatic, supradiaphragmatic, and intra-atrial. Aggressive surgical management (radical nephrectomy, IVC

Box 1
American Joint Committee on Cancer 2002 TNM staging system for renal cell carcinoma

T: Primary tumor

Tx: Primary tumor cannot be assessed

T0: No evidence of primary tumor

T1: Tumor <7 cm in diameter, limited to kidney

T1a: Tumor 0–4 cm in greatest diameter, confined to kidney

T1b: Tumor 4–7 cm in greatest diameter, confined to kidney

T2: Tumor > 7 cm in greatest diameter, confined to kidney

T3: Tumor extends into major veins or invades adrenal gland or perinephric tissues but not beyond Gerota's fascia

T3a: Tumor directly invades adrenal gland or perirenal and/or renal sinus fat but not beyond Gerota's fascia

T3b: Tumor grossly extends into the renal vein or its segmental (ie, muscle-containing) branches or into the vena cava below the diaphragm

T3c: Tumor grossly extends into the vena cava above the diaphragm or invades the wall of the vena cava

T4: Tumor invades beyond Gerota's fascia

N: Regional lymph nodes

NX: Regional lymph nodes cannot be assessed

N0: No regional lymph node metastasis

N1: Metastasis in a single regional lymph node

N2: Metastasis in more than one regional lymph node

M: Distant metastases

MX: Metastases cannot be assessed

M0: No distant metastases

M1: Distant metastases

---

thrombectomy, lymph node dissection, and potential metastectomy) remains the primary treatment modality, with the level of the tumor thrombus dictating the surgical approach. Tumors involving the caval venous system represent one of the most technically challenging and rewarding procedures for urologists because the 5-year survival rates, even in the face of intra-atrial tumor thrombus, are comparable to those for lesions confined to the kidney. A stepwise approach is discussed for each level of vein involvement focusing on techniques the authors have found successful in treating more 243 patients over a 30-year period (**Fig. 3**).[24] Additional techniques used by other urologic surgeons also are discussed in conjunction with specific scenarios.

RENAL VEIN INVOLVEMENT

The invasion of the tumor thrombus at the level of the renal vein often can be approached using the principles of traditional radical nephrectomy first described by Robson and colleagues[25] in 1969. The kidney and the great vessels can be exposed, mobilized, and controlled using a thoracoabdominal incision (**Fig. 4**). In general a ninth or tenth intercostal incision is preferred. Significant venous collaterals can develop in the setting of venous tumor thrombus, particularly the lumbar drainage system. After ligation of the renal artery, the tumor thrombus is palpated gently to ensure that no further extension into the vena cava is present. A Satinsky clamp then is placed at the level of the renal vein ostium, sparing any lumbar tributaries. A circumferential incision is made at the level of the renal vein ostium. The caval defect is closed with running 4-0 polypropylene sutures, with caution taken to avoid constricting the diameter of the vena cava. With the venous system and arterial system ligated, a standard nephrectomy is performed with or without a lymph node dissection for staging purposes. In rare instances it is possible to spare the adrenal gland in lower pole tumors.

SUPRARENAL (INFRAHEPATIC TUMOR THROMBUS)

The authors categorize the presence of tumor thrombus below the level of the liver edge as infrahepatic. It often is possible to resect these lesions without bypass, because caval wall resection is rarely necessary, and bleeding can be controlled. The initial portion of this operation is to control

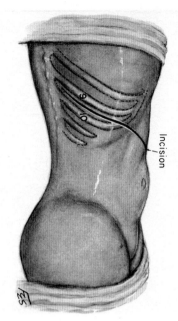

Fig. 4. Thoracoabdominal incision landmarks.

the IVC with limited manipulation to prevent tumor embolus. The vena cava is dissected anteriorly and mobilized so that a Rummel tourniquet can be placed above and below the tumor thrombus and around each renal vein. Transesophageal echocardiography is performed to rule out propagation of the tumor thrombus. A chevron incision is made from the tip of the eleventh rib to the tip of the contralateral eleventh rib. The aorta and vena cava are exposed, and dissection is continued to allow placement of the Rummel tourniquets. As mentioned previously, large upper pole tumors also can be approached via a thoracoabdominal incision. The renal artery, associated lumbar and minor hepatic veins, and the contralateral renal vein are isolated and are dissected circumferentially. In many instances renal angioinfarction may produce an inflammatory response that precludes arterial mobilization; in this instance the authors defer ligation of the renal artery until the tumor thrombectomy has been completed. After the Rummel tourniquets are applied as described previously, a longitudinal cavatomy is made, and the thrombus is freed from the caval wall to the level of the renal vein ostium (**Fig. 5**) The IVC then is gently flushed with heparinized saline and is evaluated for residual fragments. The cavotomy is closed with continuous 4-0 polypropylene sutures. The infrarenal clamp is released initially to purge the system and to limit the chance of embolus. Radical nephrectomy and/or lymph node dissection is performed after closure of the vena cava has been completed.

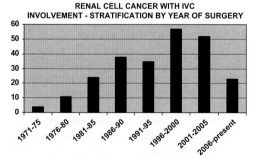

Fig. 3. Surgical stratification of renal cell cancer with tumor thrombus at the Lahey Clinic.

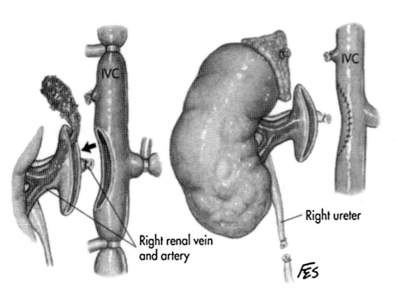

Fig. 5. Removal of larger right-sided infrahepatic tumor without cardiopulmonary bypass.

IVC

Right ureter

Right renal vein and artery

SUPRARENAL THROMBUS (RETROHEPATIC AND SUPRADIAPHRAGMATIC)

Surgical removal of RCC with suprarenal retrohepatic tumor thrombus can be accomplished with a variety of surgical techniques with equivalent oncologic outcomes. The authors' experience with hypothermic circulatory arrest and cardiopulmonary bypass is one of the largest series published to date with outcomes comparable to those of contemporary colleagues.[26] The authors have described techniques of vascular and liver mobilization that have provided excellent exposure to the retrohepatic portion of the IVC (**Fig. 6**). After a chevron incision is made and the absence of metastatic disease is confirmed, the anterior surface of the IVC is identified and is palpated gently to confirm the cephalad extent of the tumor

thrombus. In some cases the thrombus can be gently milked caudally for clamp placement. This procedure must be performed with caution to prevent embolization of the thrombus. Traditionally the duodenum is kocherized, and the Langenbuch maneuver is used to mobilize the liver cephalad and to the left, thus exposing the retrohepatic portion of the IVC (**Fig. 7**). The kidney is mobilized completely with the exception of the renal vein and associated tumor thrombus (**Fig. 8**). The IVC then is mobilized completely from the renal vein to the cephalad extent of the tumor thrombus, ensuring retroperitoneal hemostasis before heparinization and cardiopulmonary bypass. The right subclavian artery and superior vena cava are cannulated, and cardiopulmonary bypass is initiated (**Fig. 9**). Thiopental and methylprednisolone are given as the core temperature is cooled to 18° to

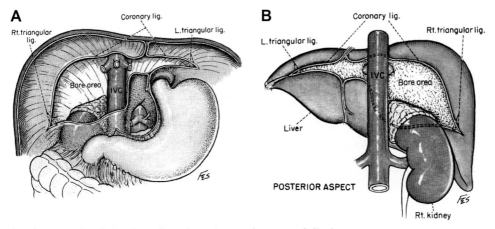

Fig. 6. (*A, B*) Anatomic relationship of IVC, hepatic vasculature, and diaphragm.

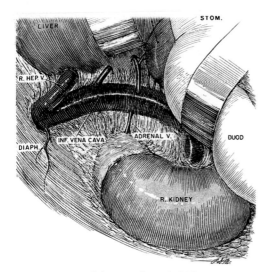

Fig. 7. Exposure of the retrohepatic IVC.

20°C and the patient is exsanguinated. Patients can withstand up to 40 minutes of circulatory arrest time without neurologic insult and may be exposed to extended periods with the use of retrograde cerebral perfusion.[27] A right atriotomy provides distal control of the tumor thrombus, minimizing the risk of embolization (**Fig. 10**). An anterior cavotomy is made from the level of the renal vein to the level of the hepatic veins, and the thrombus is extracted with the patient in Trendelenberg's position and using positive-pressure respiration (**Fig. 11**). In some situations a Fogarty catheter is passed into the atrium and/or hepatic veins to retrieve portions of the tumor thrombus. The authors use venacavascopy with a flexible cystoscope to ensure that tumor thrombus removal is complete. Efforts should be made to

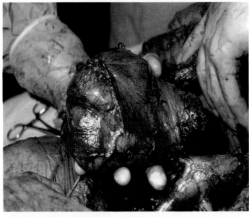

Fig. 8. Intraoperative photograph demonstrating the complete mobilization of the kidney except for the renal vein and associated tumor thrombus.

remove the kidney and thrombus as one specimen (**Fig. 12**). The advantage of bypass is an essentially bloodless operative field, but the authors recognize and accept the complications of bypass, including coagulopathy and the potential for neurologic complications.

MINIMALLY INVASIVE CARDIOPULMONARY BYPASS

Cardiopulmonary bypass has been done at the Lahey Clinic using a minimally invasive approach since 1998.[28] It was developed initially for aortic valve replacements but suited the authors' need to carry out cardiopulmonary bypass and circulatory arrest in patients who have tumor thrombus extending beyond the hepatic veins or into the atrium.[29] Unlike the traditional approach, the kidney is not mobilized during the initial exposure; rather, a chevron incision is made, and surveillance for intra-abdominal metastatic disease is performed. The anterior vena cava and renal vein are identified using a "no-touch" technique, minimizing the possibility of a pulmonary embolus. (The initiative for this approach stemmed from a lethal pulmonary embolism during the removal of a large left-sided adrenal tumor with associated retrohepatic tumor thrombus.)

Next, the right subclavian artery is mobilized via a small infraclavicular incision. Then a small (2-inch) right parasternal incision is made at the heads of the third and fourth ribs. This incision allows resection of the rib cartilage and ligation of the right internal thoracic artery. Periosteum muscles and pleura are preserved for closure, and the right pericardium is opened exposing the superior vena cava and right atrium. Systemic heparinization is initiated as an 8-mm synthetic graft is sewn to the right subclavian artery for arterial return while a two-stage venous cannula is positioned into the right atrium for venous outflow (**Fig. 13**). Cardiopulmonary bypass then is initiated, and the patient is cooled in a fashion similar to that used for patients undergoing traditional bypass procedures. A formal right atriotomy is made, and the distal components of the thrombus are identified while the urologic surgeon opens the IVC. Tumor thrombus is removed from the cava, and a sponge stick or laparotomy pad is passed up to the cardiothoracic team to be certain that all residual thrombus has been removed (**Fig. 14**). Flexible cystoscopy may be performed to confirm the presence or absence of clot or venous wall invasion. Fogarty balloons may be used to address thrombus in the hepatic veins. Radical nephrectomy is performed while the

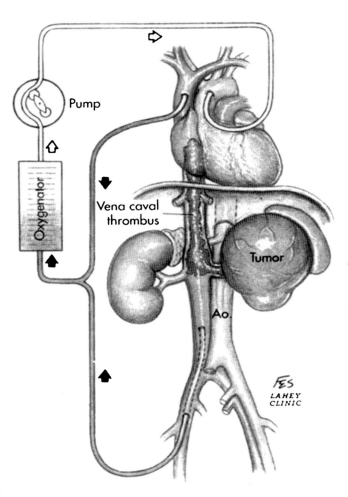

Fig. 9. Traditional cardiopulmonary bypass requiring median sternotomy.

patient is being rewarmed and is coming off bypass. Then protamine sulfate is given to offset the effect of heparin; fresh frozen plasma, platelets, and desmopressin can be to given to address any coagulopathy. Unlike traditional bypass, coronary revascularization cannot be done.

The authors have performed more than 50 caval thrombectomies using cardiopulmonary bypass and circulatory arrest. They have performed minimal-access bypass procedures in more than 30 patients to date with results demonstrating shorter operative and hospital times and decreased rates of transfusion and of mechanical ventilatory support (**Table 1**).[26] Eliminating the median sternotomy reduces the dose of postoperative analgesics required and also avoids reoperative sternotomy in patients who have had a prior coronary artery bypass procedure. Close monitoring for hematologic and neurologic complications must be observed in the immediate postoperative period.[30] Thus far these authors have had no serious neurologic sequelae from cardiopulmonary

bypass and circulatory arrest in their experience of more than 50 patients.

VENOVENOUS BYPASS

Patients who have minimal extension of thrombus above the level of the diaphragm can be managed with venovenous bypass via a caval-atrial shunt.[31,32] With this approach the vena cava needs to be controlled at the infrarenal level, at the level of both renal veins, and at its intrapericardial portion. Once control is established, the cannulas can be placed in the right atrium or axillary vein and the femoral veins, and bypass can be initiated before cavotomy. Bleeding from the hepatic venous system can be managed by cross-clamping the hepatic veins or by the Pringle maneuver. The Pringle maneuver can be used for up to 45 minutes before liver metabolism is affected significantly. Although this technique avoids cardiopulmonary bypass and circulatory arrest, the incidence of hepatic venous bleeding can be significant.

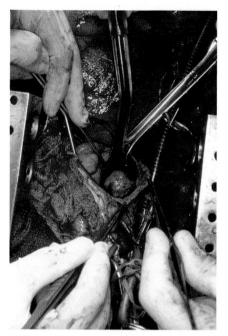

Fig. 10. Right atriotomy exposing tumor thrombus after circulatory arrest has been achieved.

LIVER TRANSPLANTATION MOBILIZATION

Mobilization of the liver has been used successfully to treat similar tumors except in cases with significant intra-atrial tumor thrombus burden. Liver mobilization avoids the use of bypass, as described by the authors' group and by Ciancio and colleagues.[33–35] The liver is mobilized to the left after the division of the ligamentum teres, falciform ligament, triangular ligament, and superior coronary ligament of the liver. The porta hepatis is accessed via the foramen of Winslow, and the Pringle maneuver is employed. This technique provides excellent access to the retrohepatic portion of the vena cava and allows mobilization of the liver from the vena cava, leaving only the major hepatic veins in continuity. After liver mobilization the surgeon can palpate and milk the tumor thrombus caudally below the confluence of the hepatics veins to limit hepatic venous congestion associated with hepatic clamping. All cases are performed with the use of transesophageal echo monitoring.

SUPRADIAPHRAGMATIC AND ATRIAL TUMOR RESECTION WITHOUT BYPASS

A case report from D'Ancona and colleagues[36] describes the removal of a suprarenal tumor thrombus using extracorporeal circulation and deep hypothermic arrest without violation of the thoracic cavity. After exposure of the vena cava, the liver is retracted inferiorly to expose the pericardium at the level of the diaphragmatic insertion. Retraction again is facilitated via division of multiple perihepatic ligamentous structures, as described previously. A pericardial window permits cardiac defibrillation. Extracorporeal

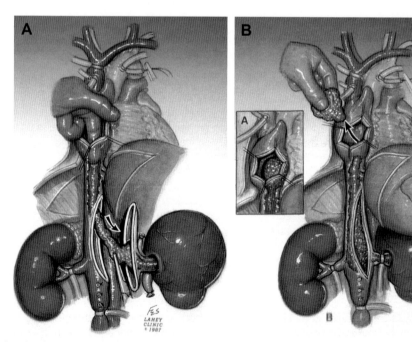

Fig. 11. (*A, B*) Schematic demonstrating the removal of atrial tumor thrombus. When tumor burden is too large, the atrial component may be fractured and removed first.

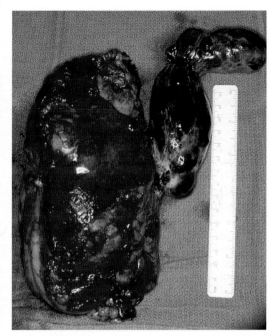

Fig. 12. Radical nephrectomy specimen and associated tumor thrombus.

circulation is established via the right femoral artery and the right femoral and subclavian veins, and core hypothermia to 20°C achieved before circulatory arrest commences. Infrahepatic and suprahepatic longitudinal incisions provide access for thrombus removal. In contrast to other reports, a nephrectomy is performed while gaining access to the femoral circulation and before extracorporeal circulation is established. Chowdhury and colleagues[37] discuss another alternative for intra-atrial tumor thrombus using cardiopulmonary bypass, mild hypothermia, and an intermittent cross-clamping of the supraceliac aorta to avoid the risks associated with circulatory arrest.

ENDOLUMINAL OCCLUSION AND CAVAL THROMBUS

The authors have used Fogarty balloon catheters in efforts to eliminate thrombus from the vena cava or, in some instances, thrombus that has extended into the hepatic veins, into the contralateral renal veins, or caudally toward the common iliac bifurcation. Zini and colleagues[38] describe an alternative technique of transesophageal echocardiography–guided endoluminal occlusion cranial to tumor thrombus, eliminating the need for extensive caval mobilization. Although the inherent risk of emboli during catheter placement seems high, their series of 13 procedures (6 retrohepatic and 7 suprahepatic) included only one event, which was asymptomatic. The authors claim that extensive caval mobilization used with liver transplant techniques carries an even higher risk of emboli. This technique should be approached with caution when the thrombus seems to invade caval wall, as evidenced by resistance to the catheter placement.

LAPAROSCOPIC MANAGEMENT IN RENAL CELL TUMOR THROMBUS

Laparoscopy has been used in the successful resection of renal carcinomas with renal vein thrombus via pure and hand-assisted approaches. Intraoperative ultrasound can help establish the extent of thrombus and guide the placement of distal clamps.[39] Hand-assisted approaches using a subcostal incision also have been reported for

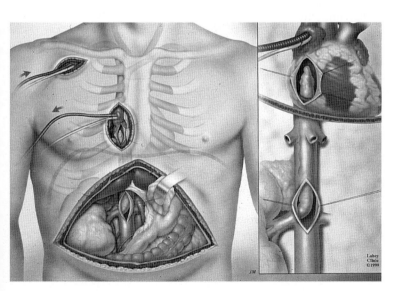

Fig. 13. Minimal access cardiopulmonary bypass using a parasternal incision.

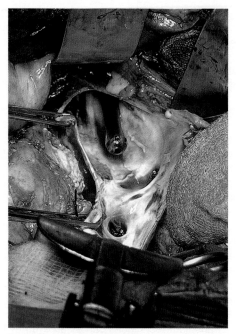

Fig. 14. Yankeur suction passed from the thoracic team into the infradiaphragmatic IVC.

treating tumors extending into the IVC.[40] Urologists at the Cleveland Clinic successfully removed a right atrial tumor thrombus in a calf model using combined laparoscopy and thoracoscopy with deep hypothermic circulatory arrest.[41] Such approaches are sure to surface with the continuing rapid advances in minimally invasive surgical techniques.

NEPHRON-SPARING SURGERY AND TUMOR THROMBUS

The unfortunate patient who has a solitary kidney and RCC with associated tumor thrombus and decent performance status may be a candidate for nephron-sparing surgery. Sengupta and colleagues[42–44] have reported their experience as well as additional case reports. These studies showed limited oncologic success and a relatively high rate of eventual completion radical nephrectomy. The authors recommend that urologists attempting these procedures be skilled in extracorporeal bench surgery, renal autotransplantation, and vena caval reconstruction with the caveat that achieving negative margins is more important than avoiding the need for renal replacement therapy.

INTERRUPTION OF THE INFERIOR VENA CAVA

Using MRI with gadolinium, Blute and colleagues[45] have devised an approach for treating bland tumor thrombus in the setting of RCC to prevent unwanted pulmonary embolism. The authors reviewed 160 patients who had thrombus extending 2 cm and more above the renal vein and identified 40 patients who had total or partial venous occlusion and the presence or absence of associated bland thrombus. (It should be noted that any attempt to resect or ligate the IVC should be preceded by efforts to preserve the integrity of the lumbar drainage system.) Blute and colleagues recommend ligating no more than two lumbar veins. Patients who have a patent cava and no associated distal or bland tumor thrombus can be managed with cavatomy closure only. A partially occluded vena cava with distal pelvic bland thrombus can be managed with an interruption caval filter. Patients who have a totally occluded vena cava with associated bland thrombus are treated by IVC staple ligation. In the latter group, distal margins should be sent to pathology for frozen-section analysis. The outcomes for these groups fail to demonstrate any significant morbidity and thus support the use of these techniques in the management of retrograde bland tumor thrombus in this complex surgical population.

CAVAL RESECTION AND REPAIR

Tumor thrombus may invade the wall of the IVC directly in up to 23% of patients, usually at the ostium of the renal vein.[46] At the Lahey Clinic, the authors have had success using polytetrafluoroethylene substitution grafts. In cases requiring median sternotomy and entry into the heart, the authors also have used a portion of pericardium to repair defects in the vena cava. An additional option includes autologous saphenous vein grafts. Perhaps larger tumor thrombus burden, as suggested by Zini and colleagues, should be treated with cavectomy and interposition grafts where appropriate. Previous publications, however, suggest that these grafts are associated with increased morbidity and mortality, and their use is not recommended at this time.

COMPLICATIONS

The incidence of complications often depends on the level of tumor thrombus and the surgical approach taken. Boorjian and colleagues[47] reviewed their experience with more than 650 patients undergoing nephrectomy and tumor thrombectomy and noted that the incidence of early (<30 days) and late complications correlated with thrombus level. Operative time and blood loss followed the same trend. The present authors have reported their experience with minimal-access

Table 1
Operative and perioperative comparison of traditional (TMS) versus minimal-access (MA) cardiopulmonary bypass[26]

	TMS Median (n = 22)	MA Median (n = 28)	P-value
Operation	600 (295–995)	450 (270–761)	<.001
Cardiopulmonary bypass time	135 (50–217)	148 (86–265)	.527
Circulatory arrest	33 (12–90)	34 (17–62)	.880
Days ventilated	7 (1–110)	4 (1–46)	.032
Length of stay	26 (2–114)	12 (5–45)	.007
Transfusions	11 (4–50)	5 (2–15)	.002
Overall complications	17	21	1.000
Pulmonary	12	7	.264
Cardiac	12	13	.741
Renal	6	4	.311
Infection	10	7	.210
Hepatic	7	5	.331

Data from Wotkowicz C, Libertino J, Sorcini A, et al. Management of renal cell carcinoma with vena cava and atrial thrombus: minimal access vs median sternotomy with circulatory arrest. BJU Int 2006;98(2):289–97.

versus traditional approaches for circulatory arrest with deep hypothermic circulatory arrest, showing the former to have shorter operative time and length of stay, less need for mechanical ventilatory support, and fewer transfusions **Table 1**.[26]

CYTOREDUCTIVE NEPHRECTOMY AND METASTECTOMY

Patients who have metastatic RCC face a poor prognosis, with a median survival of 8 months and a 2-year survival rate of 10% to 20%. A combined analysis of the two sentinel trials elucidating the benefits of cytoreductive nephrectomy (Southwest Oncology Group-8949 and European Organization for Research and Treatment of Cancer) revealed a survival benefit of 13.6 months for nephrectomy combined with interferon-alpha therapy versus 7.8 months for interferon therapy alone.[48] Retrospective data from the UCLA group suggest a more substantial survival benefit when interferon alpha is replaced with interleukin-2.[49] The underlying mechanisms of improved survival with cytoreductive nephrectomy before systemic therapy are not fully understood. The reduction in growth factors, angiogenesis promoters, and inhibitory immunomodulators by primary tumor resection may enhance the efficacy of systemic immunotherapy compared with immunotherapy without prior cytoreductive nephrectomy.

First described by Barney and Churchill[50] in 1939, the resection of pulmonary metastasis remains an effective treatment for select patients. Studies have attempted to define patient populations that would benefit from metastectomy through subgroup analysis. Favorable prognostic factors in resecting isolated pulmonary metastasis include preoperative performance status, completeness of resection, number of lesions (fewer than six), extent of lymph node involvement, and length of disease-free interval. Patients having synchronous lesions have significantly worse outcomes.[51,52] Properly selected patients may have 5-year survival rates exceeding 50%.[51] At the present time, metastectomy in nonpulmonary sites such as the liver and brain is controversial and should be considered investigational.

CLINICAL OUTCOMES

There has been a modest increase in the number of IVC thrombectomies performed by urological oncologists and in improved survival outcomes. These results can be attributed to improved imaging modalities and surgical planning as well as to technological advances in intraoperative anesthesia and postoperative intensive care management. **Table 2** summarizes recent reports from tertiary centers with significant experience in surgical management of RCC with tumor thrombus. The debate concerning the prognostic significance of tumor thrombus level with regards to the current TNM staging system may be resolved best by a multi-institutional meta-analysis.[53–58]

Table 2
Surgical outcomes for patients who had renal cell carcinoma and tumor thrombus

Author, Year	No. Patients	Tumor Thrombus Stratification	Complications (%)	Operative Mortality (%)	Survival Outcomes: Cancer-Specific Survival (CSS) and Disease-Specific Survival (DSS) (%)
Blute 2007	659	0: renal vein (426) I: ≤ 2 cm above renal vein (73) II: at or above hepatic veins (93) III: above hepatic vein (35) IV: above diaphragm (32)	Early surgical complications Level 0: 12.4 Level I: 17.8 Level II: 20.4 Level III: 25.7 Level IV: 46.9 Late complications Level 0: 24.4 Level I: 28.8 Level II: 33.3 Level III: 34.3 Level IV: 37.5 Complications 1970–1989: 13.4 1990–2006: 8.1	1970–1989: 3.8 1990–2006: 2.0	5-year CSS Level 0: 49.1 Level I: 31.7 Level II: 26.3 Level III: 39.4 Level IV: 7 Level 0 versus I ($P = .002$) Level I–IV ($P = .868$) pN0/pNx, pM0: 59 pN1/pN2,pM1: 6 Histologic features With tumor necrosis: 26 Without tumor necrosis: 61 With sarcomatoid: 3 Without sarcomatoid: 47 Perinephric fat invasion Present: 32 Absent: 56
Fijusawa 2007	55	Level 1–IV I: infrahepatic (22) II: intrahepatic (20) III: suprahepatic (10) IV: into atrium (3)	—	3.6	CSS (all levels) 1 year: 74.5 3 years: 51.4 5 years: 30.3
Kalatte and Belldegrun 2007	321	Renal vein: 166 IVC: 137 Atrium: 18	All complications Renal vein; 12 IVC: 28 Atrium: 11	Renal vein: 2 IVC: 7 Atrium: 11	DSS (2/5/10-year) Renal vein (58/41/24) IVC (48/30/25) Atrium (45/22/0) Thrombus level ($P = .53$) Overall immunotherapy response rate: 19 Metastatic disease Median survival: 16 months

Study	N	Classification	Complications		Survival
Parekh and Smoth 2005	49	Nevus classification Level I: renal vein Level II: infrahepatic IVC Level III: retrohepatic to diaphragm Level IV: supradiaphragmatic	Major complications: 6 Minor complications: 16	8	Overall 3-year survival Negative lymph node: 75 Positive lymph node: 0
Ficarra and Patard 2001	142	Renal vein: 118 Subdiaphragmatic IVC: 24	—	—	DSS (5/10 year) Renal vein (51.5/39) IVC (33.4/0) Thrombus level (0.231. NS)
Staehler and Brkovic 2000	74	Level I: <5 cm above renal vein Level II: >5 cm above renal vein and below hepatic veins Level II:I above hepatic veins and below diaphragm Level IV: above diaphragm	Major complications: 28	8	5-year overall survival (no evidence of metastases) Level I: 38 Level II: 38 Level III: 30 Level IV: 0 With evidence of metastatic disease at presentation, median survival = 13 months
Libertino (unpublished data)	243	Renal vein: 87 IVC: 126 Atrium: 30	—	3	CSS (5/10 years) Renal vein: 50/50 IVC: 35/25 Atrium: 20/15 Thrombus level (P =.04)

Abbreviation: NS, not significant.

SUMMARY

The surgical resection of large renal tumors with associated tumor and bland thrombus within the IVC presents a challenge to the urological surgeon. Given the magnitude of many of these procedures, surgeons who have experience at tertiary centers are most adept in their management. The authors' clinical experience is one of the largest to date, and they hope this article serves as guide to physicians treating this unique population. They also commend their colleagues who have encouraged alternative techniques with equivalent outcomes that adhere to the principles of urologic oncology.

REFERENCES

1. Jemal A, Siegel R, Ward E, et al. Cancer statistics. CA Cancer J Clin 2007;57(1):43–66.
2. Lipworth L, Tarone R, McLaughlin J. The epidemiology of renal cell carcinoma. J Urol 2006;176(6 Pt 1): 2353–8.
3. Chow W, Devesa S, Waren J. Rising incidence of renal cell cancer in the United States. JAMA 1999; 281(17):1628–31.
4. Jayson M, Sanders H. Increased incidence of serendipitously discovered renal cell carcinoma. Urology 1998;51(2):203–5.
5. Marshall F, Dietrick D, Baumgartner W, et al. Surgical management of renal cell carcinoma with intracaval neoplastic extension above the hepatic veins. J Urol 1988;139(6):1166–72.
6. Skinner DG, Pfister RF, Colvin R. Extension of renal cell carcinoma into the vena cava: the rationale for aggressive surgical management. J Urol 1972; 107(5):711–6.
7. Neves R, Zincke H. Surgical treatment of renal cancer with vena cava extension. Br J Urol 1987;59(5): 390–5.
8. Montie J, el Amnar R, Pontes J, et al. Renal cell carcinoma with inferior vena cava tumor thrombi. Surg Gynecol Obstet 1991;173(2):107–15.
9. Swierzewski D, Swierzewski M, Libertino J. Radical nephrectomy in patients with renal cell carcinoma with venous, vena caval, and atrial extension. Am J Surg 1994;168(2):205–9.
10. Emmott R, Hayne L, Katz I, et al. Prognosis of renal cell carcinoma with vena cava and renal vein involvement: an update. Am J Surg 1987;154(1): 49–53.
11. Hatcher P, Anderson E, Paulson D, et al. Surgical management of renal cell carcinoma invading the vena cava. J Urol 1991;145(1):20–3.
12. Zini L, Destrieux-Garnier L, Leroy X, et al. Renal vein ostium wall invasion of renal cell carcinoma with an inferior vena cava tumor thrombus: prediction by renal and vena caval vein diameters and prognostic significance. J Urol 2008;179(2):450–4.
13. Belis J, Pae W, Rohner T, et al. Cardiovascular evaluation before circulatory arrest for removal of vena cava extension of renal carcinoma. J Urol 1989; 141(6):1302–7.
14. Treiger B, Humphrey L, Peterson C, et al. Transesophageal echocardiography in renal cell carcinoma: an accurate diagnostic technique for intracaval neoplastic extension. J Urol 1991;145(6):1138–40.
15. Zielinski H, Szmigielski S, Petrovich Z. Comparison of preoperative embolization followed by radical nephrectomy with radical nephrectomy alone for renal cell carcinoma. Am J Clin Oncol 2000;23(1):6–12.
16. Nakano H, Nihira H, Toge T. Treatment of renal cancer patients by transcatheter embolization and its effects on lymphocyte proliferative responses. J Urol 1983;130(1):24–7.
17. Schwartz M, Smith E, Trost D, et al. Renal artery embolization: clinical indications and experience from over 100 cases. BJU Int 2006;99(4):881–6.
18. Moinzadeh A, Libertino J. Prognostic significance of tumor thrombus level in patients with renal cell carcinoma and venous tumor thrombus extension. Is all T3b the same? J Urol 2004;171(2 Pt 1):598–601.
19. Leibovich B, Cheville J, Lohse C, et al. Cancer specific survival for patients with pT3 renal cell carcinoma—can the 2002 Primary Tumor Classification be improved? J Urol 2005;173(3):716–9.
20. Kim H, Zisman A, Han K, et al. Prognostic significance of venous thrombus in renal cell carcinoma. Are renal vein and inferior vena cava involvement different? J Urol 2004;171(2 Pt 1):588–91.
21. Patard J, Kim H, Lam J, et al. Use of the University of California Los Angeles integrated staging system to predict survival in renal cell carcinoma: an international multicenter study. J Clin Oncol 2004;22(16):3316–22.
22. Kattan M, Reuter V, Motzer R, et al. A postoperative prognostic nomogram for renal cell carcinoma. J Urol 2001;166(1):63–7.
23. Frank I, Blute M, Cheville J, et al. An outcome prediction model for patients with clear cell renal cell carcinoma treated with radical nephrectomy based on tumor stage, size, grade and necrosis: the SSIGN score. J Urol 2002;168(6):2395–400.
24. Canes D, Wotkowicz C, Vanni A, et al. Prognostic significance of tumor thrombus level and perinephric fat invasion: the debate continues for pT3 disease [abstract 713]. Atlanta (GA): AUA; 2006.
25. Robson C, Churchill B, Anderson W. The results of radical nephrectomy for renal cell carcinoma. J Urol 1969;101:297–301.
26. Wotkowicz C, Libertino J, Sorcini A, et al. Management of renal cell carcinoma with vena cava and atrial thrombus: minimal access vs median sternotomy with circulatory arrest. BJU Int 2006;98(2) 289–97.

27. Svensson L, Crawford E, Hess K, et al. Deep hypothermia with circulatory arrest. Determinants of stroke and early mortality in 656 patients. J Thorac Cardiovasc Surg 1993;106(1):19–28.
28. Fitzgerald J, Tripathy U, Svennson L, et al. Radical nephrectomy with vena caval thrombectomy using a minimal access approach for cardiopulmonary bypass. J Urol 1998;159(4):1292–3.
29. Cosgrove D, Sabik J. Minimally invasive approach for aortic valve operations. Ann Thorac Surg 1996; 62(2):596–7.
30. Svensson L, Libertino J, Sorcini A, et al. Minimal access right atrial exposure for tumor extensions into the inferior vena cava. J Thorac Cardiovasc Surg 2001;121(3):589–90.
31. Foster R, Mahomed Y, Bihrle R, et al. Use of caval-atrial shunt for resection of caval tumor thrombus in renal cell carcinoma. J Urol 1988;140(6):1370–1.
32. Burt M. Inferior vena caval involvement by renal cell carcinoma. Use of venovenous bypass as adjunct during resection. Urol Clin North Am 1991;18(3):437–44.
33. Ciancio G, Livingstone A, Soloway M. Surgical management of renal cell carcinoma with tumor thrombus in the renal and inferior vena cava: the University of Miami experience in using liver transplantation techniques. Eur Urol 2007;51(4):988–94.
34. Ciancio G, Vaidya A, Savoie M, et al. Management of renal cell carcinoma with level III thrombus in the inferior vena cava. J Urol 2002;168(4 Pt 1):1374–7.
35. Ciancio G, Soloway M. Renal cell carcinoma with tumor thrombus extending above diaphragm: avoiding cardiopulmonary bypass. Urology 2005;66(2):266–70.
36. D'Ancona CA, Petrucci O Jr, Otsuka R. Renal cell carcinoma with thrombus in the inferior vena cava: extracorporeal circulation and deep hypothermia without open-chest surgery. Int Braz J Urol 2005;31(1):49–50.
37. Chowdury U, Mishra A, Seth A, et al. Novel techniques for tumor thrombectomy for renal cell carcinoma with intraatrial tumor thrombus. Ann Thorac Surg 2007;83(5):1731–6.
38. Zini L, Haulon S, Leroy X, et al. Endoluminal occlusion of the inferior vena cava in renal cell carcinoma with retro- or suprahepatic caval thrombus. BJU Int 2006;97(6):1216–20.
39. Kapoor A, Nguan C, Al-Shaiji T, et al. Laparoscopic management of advanced renal cell carcinoma with level I renal vein thrombus. Urology 2006;68(3):514–7.
40. Varkarakis I, Bhayani S, Allaf M, et al. Laparoscopic-assisted nephrectomy with inferior vena cava tumor thrombectomy: preliminary results. Urology 2004; 64(5):925–9.
41. Meraney A, Gill I, Desai M, et al. Laparoscopic inferior vena cava and right atrial thrombectomy utilizing deep hypothermic circulatory arrest. J Endourol 2003;17(5):275–83.
42. Pruthi R, Angell S, Brooks J, et al. Partial nephrectomy and caval thrombectomy for renal cell carcinoma in a solitary kidney with an accessory renal vein. BJU Int 1999;83(1):142–3.
43. Angermeier K, Novick A, Streem S, et al. Nephron-sparing surgery for renal cell carcinoma with venous involvement. J Urol 1990;144(6):1352–5.
44. Sengupta S, Zincke H, Leibovich B, et al. Surgical treatment of stage pT3b renal cell carcinoma in solitary kidneys: a case series. BJU Int 2005;96(1):54–7.
45. Blute M, Boorjian S, Leibovich B, et al. Results of inferior vena caval interruption by Greenfield filter, ligation or resection during radical nephrectomy and tumor thrombectomy. J Urol 2007;178(2):440–5.
46. Rabbani F, Hakimian P, Reuter V, et al. Renal vein or inferior vena caval extension in patients with renal cortical tumors: impact of tumor histology. J Urol 2004;172(3):1057–61.
47. Boorjian S, Sengupta S, Blute M. Renal cell carcinoma: vena caval involvement. BJU Int 2007;99(5 Pt B):1239–44.
48. Flanigan RC, Mickisch G, Sylvester R, et al. Cytoreductive nephrectomy in patients with metastatic renal cancer: a combined analysis. J Urol 2004; 171(3):1071–6.
49. Pantuck A, Belldegrun A, Figlin R. Nephrectomy and interleukin-2 for metastatic renal cell carcinoma. N Engl J Med 2001;345(23):1711–2.
50. Barney J, Churchill E. Adenocarcinoma of the kidney with metastases to the lung: cured nephrectomy and lobectomy. J Urol 1939;42:269–76.
51. Hofmann HS, Neef H, Krohe K, et al. Prognostic factors and survival after pulmonary resection of metastatic renal cell carcinoma. Eur Urol 2005;48:77–82.
52. Assouad J, Petkova B, Berna P, et al. Renal cell carcinoma lung metastases surgery: pathologic findings and prognostic factors. Ann Thorac Surg 2007;84:1114–20.
53. Blute M, Leibovich B, Lohse C, et al. The Mayo Clinic experience with surgical management, complications and outcome for patients with renal cell carcinoma and venous tumor thrombus. BJU Int 2004;94:33–41.
54. Terakawa T, Miyake H, Takenaka A, et al. Clinical outcome of surgical management for patients with renal cell carcinoma involving the inferior vena cava. Int J Urol 2004;14:781–4.
55. Klatte T, Pnatuck A, Riggs S, et al. Prognostic factors for renal cell carcinoma with tumor thrombus extension. J Urol 2007;178:1189–95.
56. Parekh D, Cookson M, Chapman W, et al. Renal cell carcinoma with renal vein and inferior vena caval involvement: clinicopathological features, surgical techniques and outcomes. J Urol 2005;173:1897–902.
57. Ficarra V, Righetti R, D'Amico, et al. Renal vein and vena cava involvement does not affect prognosis in patients with renal cell carcinoma. Oncology 2001;61:10–5.
58. Staehler G, Brkovic D. The role of radical surgery for renal cell carcinoma with extension into the vena cava. J Urol 2000;163:1671–5.

Lymph Node Dissection in the Management of Renal Cell Carcinoma

Bradley C. Leibovich, MD, Michael L. Blute, MD*

KEYWORDS

- Carcinoma, renal cell • Kidney neoplasms
- Nephrectomy • Lymph node excision

Radical nephrectomy and regional lymphadenectomy have been the cornerstone of therapy for renal cell carcinoma (RCC) for several decades;[1] however, debate regarding the potential advantages of lymph node dissection for RCC continues. Currently, there are no definitive data indicating a survival advantage to lymphadenectomy. Furthermore, systematic complete lymph node dissection adds time to the procedure and requires manipulation of the great vessels, which some surgeons may find challenging. This article examines the rationale for lymphadenectomy in the management of renal cell carcinoma and reviews the limited literature on the subject.

Carcinoma of the kidney and renal pelvis is expected to be newly diagnosed in over 54,000 patients in the United States and will result in over 13,000 deaths, accounting for approximately 3% of all cancer deaths in 2008.[2] About one-third of new patients presenting with RCC have metastatic disease. Another third of patients presenting with localized disease eventually experience recurrence and progression. Approximately 25% of patients with metastatic RCC have clinically evident lymphadenopathy. While metastatic disease is highly resistant to chemotherapy, systemic therapy options now include targeted therapy in addition to immunotherapy.[3] Thankfully, survival for patients with RCC appears to be improving, with decreasing death rates per 100,000 from 6.16 to 5.91 in men and from 2.95 to 2.72 in women between the early 1990s and today.[2] This is reflected in improved 5-year survival rates from 52% between 1974 and 1976 to 63% in 1999.[4] Positive nodes have been clearly shown to have an independent adverse effect on outcome, regardless of other prognostic factors.[5–7] For patients with node-positive disease, 5-year survival rates range between 5% and 35%. Most studies of node-positive renal cell carcinoma report 5-year survival rates of about 15%.[8] **Fig. 1** demonstrates the impact of lymph node status on cancer-specific survival among patients treated surgically for RCC at the Mayo Clinic.

Proponents of lymphadenectomy point to higher survival rates for patients undergoing radical nephrectomy plus extended lymph node dissection, compared with historical studies that did not include routine lymphadenectomy. Opponents point to the high rates of hematogenous metastases and question the value of lymph node dissection in a disease that follows an unpredictable course. To definitively address the potential benefit of lymphadenectomy in RCC, the European Organization for Research and Treatment of Cancer Genitourinary Group launched a head-to-head randomized phase 3 trial at multiple European centers in 1988. The trial, which completed enrollment in 1992, is designed to compare the long-term results of radical nephrectomy with complete lymphadenectomy (n = 383) against radical nephrectomy alone (n = 389) in patients without evidence of metastases. Early results indicate that complete lymph node dissection did not increase morbidity associated with radical nephrectomy. Pathology confirmed lymph node metastases in 3.3% of clinically negative nodes after lymphadenectomy. However, survival in the study so far had been reported to be excellent overall and more follow-up time is needed to compare tumor-free survival and overall survival

Mayo Clinic, 200 First Street, SW, Rochester, MN 55905, USA
* Corresponding author.
E-mail address: blute.michael@mayo.edu (M.L. Blute).

Urol Clin N Am 35 (2008) 673–678
doi:10.1016/j.ucl.2008.07.011

urologic.theclinics.com

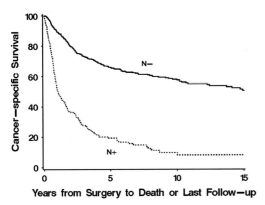

Fig. 1. Cancer–specific survival from time of radical nephrectomy by lymph node status.

between the lymphadenectomy and non-lymphadenectomy groups.[9] While results are pending, debate will continue regarding the need for lymphadenectomy in RCC patients.

Although the role of nephron-sparing surgery for renal masses under 7 cm continues to evolve,[10,11] the appropriate surgical treatment for large renal masses has not changed substantively since Robson and colleagues[1] first reported increased survival in a small cohort of patients who received lymphadenectomy in 1969. Surgical excision of solid tumors was common by the late nineteenth century.[12] After Halsted demonstrated the efficacy of extensive regional lymphadenectomy for breast cancer in 1894, radical excision and regional lymphadenectomy gradually evolved as the standard of care for most carcinomas. During the first half of the twentieth century simple nephrectomy became the standard treatment for localized RCC. The procedure typically involved removal of the kidney from the surrounding Gerota's fascia. Surgeons generally left the perirenal fat, adrenal gland, and regional lymph nodes in situ.

The first radical nephrectomy, removing the kidney, adrenal gland, and the surrounding Gerota's fascia, was reported by Mortensen in 1948.[13] The reported rationale for the extent of surgery was the observation that pathology studies revealed perirenal fat infiltration in 13% of renal tumors; therefore, removal of the fat and the organs contained within was postulated to increase survival. In the 1960s, Robson and colleagues[1,14] added retroperitoneal lymphadenectomy to radical nephrectomy and reported improved 5-year survival rates.

The first systematic survey of lymphatic drainage from the kidneys was published in 1935, when Parker[15] reported on the dissection of cadavers and stillborn infants to detail the renal lymphatic system. For the right kidney, the first-echelon nodes are the precaval, retrocaval, and interaortocaval lymph nodes. The paracaval nodes are not a primary drainage route for the right kidney. For the left kidney, the primary drainage nodes include the para-aortic, preaortic, and retroaortic lymph nodes. By the early 1990s other groups had confirmed Parker's findings by mapping the sites of involved nodes in node-positive patients who underwent extended lymph node dissection.[12] Right kidney metastases were most commonly found in the interaortocaval and retrocaval area. The hilar and paracaval nodes were less frequently involved. Most left kidney metastases were found in the hilar, para-aortic, and retroaortic areas. Isolated metastases were also found in the ipsilateral iliac nodes and in the supraclavicular nodes.

A hilar lymphadenectomy removes only the lymph nodes surrounding the renal vessels, while a regional dissection typically includes the para-aortic region on the left and the paracaval area on the right. Such a procedure may be adequate for tumors of the left kidney, but would miss the most common site for lymphatic metastases from the right kidney, the interaortocaval area. If the urologist wishes to minimize the risk of leaving nodal metastases in situ, the authors advocate an extended lymphadenectomy. On the left side, an extended dissection includes removal of the preaortic, para-aortic, retroaortic, interaortocaval, and precaval lymphatic tissue from the diaphragm to the bifurcation of the aorta. On the right side, extended dissection includes removal of the precaval, paracaval, retrocaval, interaortocaval, and preaortic lymph nodes.

There are only two reasons to perform an extended lymphadenectomy in conjunction with a radical nephrectomy: one is to improve staging accuracy. Although modern imaging techniques, such as computed tomography, magnetic resonance imaging, ultrasound, and positron emission tomography offer excellent diagnostic and staging, none are able to reliably predict nodal involvement. In terms of staging RCC, the overall accuracy of CT scanning, generally accepted as the most sensitive and accurate imaging method for staging, ranges from 61% to 91%. Future advances in imaging, such as the use of lymphotrophic ferromagnetic nanoparticles in conjunction with MRI, may allow detection of lymphatic metastases in patients without overt lymphadenopathy.[16] Perhaps a more debatable rationale for lymphadenectomy is to improve patient outcomes by removing overt or subclinical lymph node metastases. It is possible that lymphadenectomy may be beneficial because of other mechanisms, such as removal of potential immunosuppressive factors in antigen-primed lymph nodes in the absence of metastases.

Terrone and colleagues recently examined the relationship between the accuracy of tumor staging and the number of nodes examined by retrospectively reviewing the number of lymph nodes removed during radical nephrectomy for RCC in 725 patients. Of the 725 cases, 608 (84%) had lymph nodes removed. Of the 608 patients with nodes identified pathologically, 13.6% had lymphatic metastases. Interestingly, the rate of positive lymph nodes was higher if more than 12 nodes were found with 21% positive nodes in patients with greater than or equal to 13 nodes and 10% positive for patients with fewer than 13 nodes in the specimen. The investigators concluded that lymphadenectomy is essential to properly stage a tumor, regardless of the potential therapeutic impact. With the recent introduction of several targeted therapies for RCC, and in the setting of ongoing clinical trials of adjuvant therapy for high risk resected RCC without hematogenous metastases, accurate staging will become increasingly important.[17]

The radiographic finding of enlarged lymph nodes in patients with renal masses has been shown to have poor correlation with pathology. Studer and colleagues[18] reviewed the CT scans of 163 patients with RCC. CT scans were falsely negative in five patients. Furthermore, among 43 patients with retroperitoneal lymphadenopathy by CT criteria (lymph nodes 1 cm–2.2 cm), only 18 (42%) had lymph node metastases. The 58% of patients with lymphadenopathy by CT criteria and no pathologically confirmed lymph node metastases were found to have only inflammatory changes or follicular hyperplasia. Lymphadenopathy on CT because of inflammatory changes or follicular hyperplasia was more common among patients with venous tumor thrombus or tumor necrosis. This study further supports the need for extended lymphadenectomy in patients where accurate staging is important.

Modern evidence for the potential therapeutic benefit of lymphadenectomy in conjunction with radical nephrectomy is mounting. In 1991 Herrlinger and colleagues[19] reported a significant survival advantage in a study of 511 patients who were treated with extended lymphadenectomy with radical nephrectomy, compared with those whose lymph nodes were removed only if clinically abnormal or for staging purposes (the investigators referred to this group as "facultative lymphadenectomy"). In patients with left kidney tumors, extended lymphadenectomy involved the removal of all preaortic, para-aortic, and retroaortic lymph nodes from the diaphragm to the bifurcation of the aorta. For right kidney tumors, all paracaval, precaval, retrocaval, and interaortocaval nodes were removed from the diaphragm to the bifurcation of the vena cava. Operative mortality was 1% in the extended lymphadenectomy group and 3.8% in the facultative lymphadenectomy group.

Herrlinger and colleagues[19] reported substantial differences in the rate of node-positive disease and outcome between the two surgical groups. In the extended lymphadenectomy group, pathologists found 17 or more nodes removed with each radical nephrectomy. In the facultative lymphadenectomy group, more than half of patients had no nodes removed, one to five nodes were removed in 30% of patients, and more than five nodes in 10% of patients. The incidence of positive nodes in the lymphadenectomy group was 17.5% versus 10% for the nonlymphadenectomy group. There was a significant difference in survival between the two treatment groups, with 5- and 10-year survivals of 66% and 56.1%, compared with 58% and 40.9% for the extended lymphadenectomy and facultative lymphadenectomy groups, respectively. The authors reported that the survival advantage was more pronounced for patients with low-stage tumors. In patients with organ-confined RCC, extended lymphadenectomy produced a 5-year survival rate of 91.6% and a 10-year survival rate of 80.2%, compared with 81.3% and 54% for patients who did not receive the extended lymph node dissection. For patients with localized RCC who had extra-renal disease, survival was 76% at 5 years and 58.2% at 10 years, compared with 54.5% and 41.2% without lymphadenectomy. There was no statistically significant difference in survival for more advanced patients. Herrlinger and colleagues concluded that there could be no doubt that extended lymphadenectomy improves survival for patients with low-stage disease. The improvement, they concluded, is a result of the removal of subclinical microscopic metastases in the regional lymph nodes that would otherwise have resulted in dissemination of disease after radical nephrectomy alone. Assuming that patients are reasonable candidates for curative surgery, the group concluded that there is no preoperative or intraoperative staging procedure that could effectively define any group of patients who would not benefit from extended lymphadenectomy.

Phillips and Messing[20] retrospectively reviewed the impact of lymphadenectomy with regard to the subsequent development of local recurrence of RCC following radical nephrectomy in 1993. Patients with nodal metastases who received radical nephrectomy without lymphadenectomy had a local recurrence rate of 86%. None of the patients with node-positive disease who received radical nephrectomy plus lymphadenectomy experienced a local recurrence. There was no increase in morbidity of the surgery as a result of lymphadenectomy.

Schafhauser and colleagues[21] conducted a retrospective review of 1,035 patients with RCC treated between 1974 and 1993. Patients were classified based on the extent of the lymphadenectomy into three groups: group A had a systematic extended lymphadenectomy, group B had only grossly abnormal nodes resected, and group C had no lymph nodes resected. Group A patients had the larger tumors with higher stage and grade RCC relative to groups B and C. Despite the fact that patients in group A had more adverse tumor characteristics, the highest mean survival rate at 5 years (70.1% compared with 61.8% and 65.6%) and 10 years (58.3% compared with 50.4% and 44.5%) was seen in the group A patients. The investigators concluded that radical nephrectomy plus extended lymphadenectomy benefits at least 4% of all patients.

More recently, Pantuck and colleagues[8] retrospectively reviewed 900 patients treated surgically for RCC. The study population was comprised of a high proportion of patients with clinically evident adenopathy and advanced RCC. The investigators found that lymphadenectomy offered no benefit in terms of survival or recurrence of disease in patients with clinically negative lymph nodes. The investigators concluded that the lack of demonstrable benefit in this study was likely a result of the low incidence of positive nodes discovered based on pathology alone. Fewer than 8% of node-positive cases in Pantuck's study were discovered upon pathology after resection. The other 92% of positive nodes had been identified either pre- or intraoperatively. However, among patients with lymph node-positive RCC a distinct advantage in survival was demonstrated for those who underwent lymphadenectomy versus those without lymphadenectomy. Furthermore, patients treated with lymphadenectomy and subsequent interleukin-2 based immunotherapy had a trend toward improved response to systemic therapy. The study concluded that when positive nodes are found, they should be resected when technically feasible.

Recently Minervini and colleagues[22] retrospectively reviewed 167 radical nephrectomy cases and found no difference in survival between 108 patients with radical nephrectomy alone and 59 patients with regional lymphadenectomy. Regional lymphadenectomy was defined as removal of the lymph nodes anterior, posterior, and lateral to the ipsilateral great vessel from the renal pedicle to the level of the inferior mesenteric artery. Among the 59 patients that had a regional lymphadenectomy, 10 had clinically evident lymphadenopathy. Only 1 of 49 patients without lymphadenopathy had pathologically involved lymph nodes. The investigators conclude that in the absence of lymphadenopathy there is no benefit to lymphadenectomy.

Canfield and colleagues[23] recently reviewed the records of 40 patients treated with radical nephrectomy and regional lymphadenectomy (excluding the interaortocaval lymph nodes), all of whom had positive lymph nodes and no evidence of hematogeneous metastases. Median cancer-specific survival was 20 months, and with a median follow-up of 17.7 months 30% of patients remained free of RCC. The investigators suggest that aggressive resection of lymph node metastases may impart a survival advantage based on these findings. The authors have recently reviewed their experience with resection of isolated metachronous recurrence of RCC in the retroperitoneal lymph nodes.[24] Fifteen patients who underwent surgical resection of isolated, metachronous recurrence of RCC in the retroperitoneal lymph nodes following radical nephrectomy were compared with patients who had lymph node-positive RCC at the time of nephrectomy and to patients who underwent complete resection of a solitary metachronous metastasis of RCC at another site. No intra- or postoperative mortality occurred. Six of the 15 patients that underwent resection of metachronous lymph node metastasis subsequently died from RCC at a median of 18 months (range 6–33.6) following resection. The median cause-specific survival was 33.3 months for patients with metachronous lymph node metastases versus 20.8 months and 46.9 months for patients with synchronous lymph node metastases and metachronous nonlymph node metastases, respectively.

It is clear that without prospective studies of standardized lymph node resection, no survival advantage can be proven based on the varied retrospective data to date. The question, then, is how to identify the small (3%–8%) cohort of patients with unidentified positive nodes for whom extended lymphadenectomy is most likely to be useful and which nodes should be removed. The authors have recently analyzed more than 1,600 patients with clear cell RCC from the Mayo Clinic Nephrectomy Registry.[25] The study identified five features that were associated with lymph node metastases: primary tumor stage T3 or T4, nuclear grade 3 or 4, tumor size 10 cm or greater, presence of a sarcomatoid component, and presence of histologic tumor necrosis.

Patients with none of the risk features or any one feature have a low likelihood of regional lymph node involvement (0.6%). But patients exhibiting any two of the five features have a 4.4% risk of regional lymph node involvement and patients with all five features have a greater than 50% risk of lymph node-positive disease. The authors therefore suggest that lymphadenectomy is indicated for patients with any two or more risk features, which can be determined by frozen section analysis intraoperatively.

In summary, there are adequate data to suggest that patients can benefit from resection of clinically evident lymphadenopathy at the time of radical nephrectomy. There are currently insufficient data regarding patients with clinically negative retroperitoneal lymph nodes to mandate lymphadenectomy at the time of radical nephrectomy. The authors' bias is that patients with large tumors, high grade or stage, or other adverse features should have a lymphadenectomy, and that more extensive lymph node resection will be more likely to confer maximum benefits. For right side tumors, lymphadenectomy should include dissection of the vena cava from the diaphragm to the bifurcation of the vessels, including the precaval, paracaval, retrocaval, and interaortocaval nodes. For left side tumors, dissection should include the preaortic, para-aortic, and retroaortic nodes from diaphragm to the bifurcation.

REFERENCES

1. Robson CJ, Churchill BM, Anderson W. The results of radical nephrectomy for renal cell carcinoma. J Urol 1969;101:297–301.

2. Jemal A, Siegel R, Ward E, et al. Cancer statistics, 2008. CA Cancer J Clin 2008;58:71–96.

3. Garcia JA, Rini BI. Recent progress in the management of advanced renal cell carcinoma. CA Cancer J Clin 2007;57:112–25.

4. Pantuck AJ, Zisman A, Dorey F, et al. Renal cell carcinoma with retroperitoneal lymph nodes. Impact on survival and benefits of immunotherapy. Cancer 2003;97:2995–3002.

5. Frank I, Blute ML, Cheville JC, et al. An outcome prediction model for patients with clear cell renal cell carcinoma treated with radical nephrectomy based on tumor stage, size, grade and necrosis: the SSIGN score. J Urol 2002;168:2395–400.

6. Leibovich BC, Blute ML, Cheville JC, et al. Prediction of progression after radical nephrectomy for patients with clear cell renal cell carcinoma: a stratification tool for prospective clinical trials. Cancer 2003;97: 1663–71.

7. Leibovich BC, Cheville JC, Lohse CM, et al. A scoring algorithm to predict survival for patients with metastatic clear cell renal cell carcinoma: a stratification tool for prospective clinical trials. J Urol 2005;174:1759–63 [discussion: 1763].

8. Pantuck AJ, Zisman A, Dorey F, et al. Renal cell carcinoma with retroperitoneal lymph nodes: role of lymph node dissection. J Urol 2003;169:2076–83.

9. Blom JH, van Poppel H, Marechal JM, et al. Radical nephrectomy with and without lymph node dissection: preliminary results of the EORTC randomized phase III protocol 30881. EORTC Genitourinary Group. Eur Urol 1999;36:570–5.

10. Leibovich BC, Blute ML, Cheville JC, et al. Nephron sparing surgery for appropriately selected renal cell carcinoma between 4 and 7 cm results in outcome similar to radical nephrectomy. J Urol 2004;171: 1066–70.

11. Thompson RH, Boorjian SA, Lohse CM, et al. Radical nephrectomy for pT1a renal masses may be associated with decreased overall survival compared with partial nephrectomy. J Urol 2008;179:468–71 [discussion: 472–3].

12. Wood DP Jr. Role of lymphadenectomy in renal cell carcinoma. Urol Clin North Am 1991;18:421–6.

13. Mortensen H. Transthoracic nephrectomy. J Urol 1948;60:855–8.

14. Robson CJ. Radical nephrectomy for renal cell carcinoma. J Urol 1963;89:37–42.

15. Parker A. Studies on the main posterior lymph channels of the abdomen and their connections with the lymphatics of the genito-urinary system. Am J Anat 1935;56:409–43.

16. Saksena MA, Saokar A, Harisinghani MG. Lymphotropic nanoparticle enhanced MR imaging (LNMRI) technique for lymph node imaging. Eur J Radiol 2006;58:367–74.

17. Terrone C, Guercio S, De Luca S, et al. The number of lymph nodes examined and staging accuracy in renal cell carcinoma. BJU Int 2003;91(1):37–40.

18. Studer UE, Scherz S, Scheidegger J, et al. Enlargement of regional lymph nodes in renal cell carcinoma is often not due to metastases. J Urol 1990; 144:243–5.

19. Herrlinger A, Schrott KM, Schott G, et al. What are the benefits of extended dissection of the regional renal lymph nodes in the therapy of renal cell carcinoma. J Urol 1991;146:1224–7.

20. Phillips E, Messing E. Role of lymphadenectomy in the treatment of renal cell carcinoma. Urology 1993;41:9–15.

21. Schafhauser W, Ebert A, Brod J, et al. Lymph node involvement in renal cell carcinoma and survival chance by systematic lymphadenectomy. Anticancer Res 1999;19:1573–8.

22. Minervini A, Lilas L, Morelli G, et al. Regional lymph node dissection in the treatment of renal cell carcinoma: is it useful in patients with no suspected adenopathy before or during surgery? BJU Int 2001; 88:169–72.

23. Canfield SE, Kamat AM, Sanchez-Ortiz RF, et al. Renal cell carcinoma with nodal metastases in the absence of distant metastatic disease (clinical stage TxN1-2M0): the impact of aggressive surgical resection on patient outcome. J Urol 2006;175:864–9.

24. Boorjian SA, Crispen PL, Lohse CM, et al. Surgical resection of isolated retroperitoneal lymph node recurrence of renal cell carcinoma following nephrectomy. J Urol 2008;180(1):99–103.

25. Blute ML, Leibovich BC, Cheville JC, et al. A protocol for performing extended lymph node dissection using primary tumor pathological features for patients treated with radical nephrectomy for clear cell renal cell carcinoma. J Urol 2004;172:465–9.

Surgical Intervention in Patients with Metastatic Renal Cancer: Metastasectomy and Cytoreductive Nephrectomy

Paul Russo, MD, FACS[a],*, Matthew Francis O'Brien, MD[b]

KEYWORDS

- Renal cancer • Cytoreductive
- Kidney cancer • Metastasectomy

There will be an estimated 54,390 new renal tumors and 13,010 deaths from renal cancer in the United States in 2008.[1] Approximately 30% to 40% of patients with malignant renal cortical tumors will either present with or later develop metastatic disease. In metastatic renal cancer, surgical intervention may be performed alone or in combination with systemic therapy. Although the evolution of metastatic disease usually occurs within 2 years after the radical or partial nephrectomy, disease-free intervals of up to 30 years and metastases to unusual sites (eg, endocrine glands, digits) can cause diagnostic dilemmas. Unlike patients with renal cortical tumors detected incidentally during abdominal imaging obtained for other reasons, the vast majority of patients with metastatic renal tumors have large, locally advanced tumors often with regional nodal and or renal vein or inferior venal extension. Approximately 90% of the metastatic renal tumors are of the conventional clear cell histologic subtype. Unfortunately for metastatic renal cancer patients, systemic chemotherapy, cytokine therapy, and hormonal manipulations alone or in combination have low overall response rates (10%–15%) and are rarely associated with a complete remission. Median patient survival for metastatic renal cancer patients is in the range of 10 to 12 months.[2] Rare spontaneous remissions of metastatic disease sites occur in less than 1% of cases and have been reported in both surgical series and the control arms of clinical trials with or without previous surgical intervention. New systemic chemotherapy agents, including multitargeted tyrosine kinase inhibitors (TKIs) (sunitinib, sorafenib) and mammalian target of rapamycin kinase inhibitors (temsirolimus, RAD001) are proving highly effective in clinical trials[3,4] and are now actively being investigated in neoadjuvant and adjuvant surgical trials in patients with poor prognostic renal tumors.

Surgical intervention in any patient with metastatic renal cancer has one of two aims: (1) through metastasectomy, to render a patient clinically free of all sites of metastases, or (2), through cytoreductive nephrectomy to resect the primary tumor in the face of unresectable metastatic disease before the initiation of systemic therapy. The occasionally unpredictable natural history of renal cancer and varying patient selection criteria can make the interpretation of results from different centers difficult. Operative intervention in the

[a] Department of Surgery, Urology Service, Weill Cornell College of Medicine, Memorial Sloan Kettering Cancer Center, 1275 York Avenue, New York, N Y 10021, USA
[b] Urological Oncology, Memorial Sloan Kettering Cancer Center, 1275 York Avenue, New York, N Y 10021, USA
* Corresponding author.
E-mail address: russop@mskcc.org (P. Russo).

Urol Clin N Am 35 (2008) 679–686
doi:10.1016/j.ucl.2008.07.009

face of metastatic renal cancer is controversial and is the subject of this review.

METASTASECTOMY

In 1939 Barney and Churchill[5] first reported a patient who underwent nephrectomy and a resection of an isolated pulmonary metastasis for a renal cancer only to die 23 years later of coronary artery disease. Over the last 60 years, the surgical resection of limited metastatic disease (metastasectomy) was offered to patients and selectively performed in the absence of effective systemic therapies. The reported selection criteria for this aggressive surgical approach varied from study to study and reported significant prognostic factors included the site and number of metastatic deposits, completeness of resection, patient performance status, and the disease-free interval from treatment of the primary tumor to the diagnosis of metastatic disease. Complete resection of isolated metastases was associated with 5-year survival rates of between 35% and 60%. Despite successful resection of metastatic disease and associated patient survival, these studies lacked definitive proof that the surgical intervention itself, as opposed to patient selection factors and the natural history of renal cancer, led to the observed outcomes.[6–9] Pogrebniak and colleagues[10] reported 23 patients who underwent resection of pulmonary metastases from renal cell carcinoma (RCC), 15 of whom had previously been treated with IL-2–based immunotherapy. Patients with resectable lesions had a longer survival (mean 49 months) than those patients with unresectable lesions (mean 16 months). Furthermore, in this study, survival was not dependent upon the number of nodules removed. The investigators concluded that patients with metastatic RCC should be offered an operation if the likelihood that complete resection of all sites of disease were high. Favorable subgroups include those patients with a solitary site of metastases and disease-free interval to the development of metastases of greater than 1 year. It should be noted that occasionally sites of disease presumed to be metastatic RCC are instead secondary tumors (eg, pancreatic islet cell tumor) of either benign or malignant histology. This diagnostic dilemma may be addressed in the future with the further development of conventional clear cell specific immuno–positron emission tomographic scanning with 124-I cG250 scanning.[11]

In a report from Memorial Sloan Kettering Cancer Center (MSKCC), prognostic factors associated with enhanced survival in 278 patients who underwent surgical metastasectomy included a disease-free interval of greater than 12 months (55% versus 9% 5-year overall survival), solitary versus multiple sites of metastases (54% versus 29% 5-year overall survival), and age younger than 60 years (49% versus 35% 5-year survival). Patient survival was longer when the solitary site of resection was lung (54% 5-year survival) compared with brain (18% 5-year survival). Twenty-nine percent of patients with completely resected multiple sites of metastases within a given organ survived 5 years, again suggesting that complete resection of all metastatic deposits was more important than the number metastatic deposits within a given site.[12] Although the curative impact of metastasectomy is uncertain, operative intervention can also provide effective palliation for symptomatic metastatic disease to such sites as bone, brain, and adrenal gland.[13,14] MSKCC investigators recently reported their experience with 61 patients who underwent nephrectomy followed by complete metastasectomy from 1989 to 2003. Of these patients, 59% had a Karnofsky performance status (KPS) greater than 90, 90% had conventional clear cell histology, and 62% had renal tumors that were greater than stage T2. Median survival was 30 months (**Fig. 1**).[15] A prospective and randomized clinical trial comparing metastasectomy to best standard systemic therapy could define the exact role of this approach.

CYTOREDUCTIVE NEPHRECTOMY

The role of radical nephrectomy in patients with extensive metastatic renal cancer, when complete metastasectomy is not possible, has long been debated. Given the lack of effective systemic therapies and the unpredictable natural history of metastatic RCC, many oncologists referred patients to surgeons for resection of the primary tumor before cytokine-based therapy. In theory, cytoreductive radical nephrectomy is performed to remove a large, potentially immunosuppressive, tumor burden; to obtain accurate tumor histologic subtyping; and to prevent complications related to the primary tumor during systemic therapy. On rare occasions, a highly symptomatic tumor is removed for symptom palliation after the failure of conservative palliation measures (eg, unremitting gross hematuria or flank pain not relieved by conservative care or angioinfarction). Radical nephrectomy should not be done to induce spontaneous remission, a phenomena observed only in 4 of 474 patients (0.8%) treated with radical nephrectomy alone in a study from the Cleveland Clinic.[16] Surgical mortality has been reported from 2% to 11% for patients with large primary

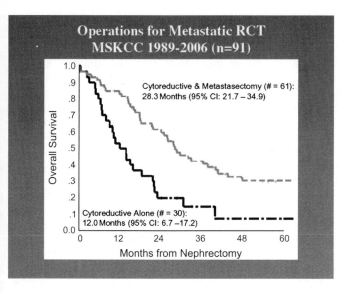

Fig. 1. Overall survival distribution of 91 patients undergoing operation in the face of metastatic RCC at MSKCC from 1989 to 2006. This includes 61 patients undergoing cytoreductive nephrectomy/ metastasectomy (median survival 28.3 months) and 30 patients undergoing cytoreductive nephrectomy alone (median survival 12.0 months).

renal tumors and metastatic disease. The possibility that the patient may not recover sufficiently to receive systemic immunotherapy after preparatory radical nephrectomy is of concern to surgeons and medical oncologists alike. In a study of 195 patients with metastatic RCC treated at the National Cancer Institute, 121 patients (62%) were eligible for high-dose IL-2 following cytoreductive nephrectomy, leading to a response rate of 18%. Yet, 38% of the patients in this series who underwent nephrectomy never received any immunotherapy either because of complications of nephrectomy or because of rapid clinical deterioration from disease progression.[17] Some oncology groups recommend adjuvant radical nephrectomy only if initial systemic therapy was effective in initiating clinical regression of metastatic sites. This avoids the surgical morbidity.[18,19]

Two randomized and prospective clinical trials have attempted to further define the role of cytoreductive nephrectomy in the treatment of metastatic renal cancer—one in the United States organized by the Southwest Oncology Group (SWOG), and the other in Europe organized by the European Organization Research and Treatment of Cancer (EORTC). Both used similar entry criteria comparing treatment for metastatic renal cancer with cytoreductive nephrectomy plus interferon alpha-2b versus interferon alpha-2b alone.

In the SWOG trial, between 1991 and 1998, 246 patients with metastatic renal cancer and with the tumor-bearing kidney in place from 80 participating institutions were randomly assigned to the two groups of 123 patients each. Eligible patients had a histologically confirmed diagnosis of metastatic RCC in tissue obtained by needle biopsy or aspiration of a least one measurable metastatic

site or the primary tumor with metastases beyond the regional lymphatics involving a tumor of any size or any nodal status. Renal tumors with inferior vena caval extension below the hepatic veins were included. Patients were excluded if they received any prior systemic chemotherapy, hormonal therapy, cytokine therapy, biological response modifier therapy, or radiation therapy either to the primary tumor or any metastatic site. They were also excluded if the serum bilirubin was threefold higher than normal, if the serum creatinine was greater than 3.0 mg/dL, or if there was a history of significant cardiac arrhythmias or concomitant cancers less than 5 years before. Patients needed an Eastern Cooperative Oncology Group performance status of 0 or 1. Five patients were found to be ineligible because the pathologic diagnosis was incorrect (3 in the surgery arm and 2 in the interferon-alone arm). Of the 120 eligible patients analyzed in the nephrectomy-plus-interferon arm, 17 patients did not undergo the operation (7 refused, 5 were deemed medically unfit, 3 were unresectable, and 2 died before the operation). In the 98 patients evaluated for surgical complications, 1 patient died after operation for unresectable tumor with wound dehiscence and abdominal abscess with peritonitis, 2 patients had cardiac ischemia or infarction, 2 had postoperative infections, and 1 had hypotension. Sixteen patients had mild to moderate complications. In 76 of 98 patients (78%), no complications were reported. The mean hospitalization time was 8.2 days[3–22] and the mean time to receive interferon alfa-2b was 19.9 days. Two eligible patients, 1 in each group, refused interferon therapy. One patient in the interferon group died of a treatment-related myocardial infarction and 23 patients

(10 in surgical arm, 13 in interferon-only arm) had severe complications due to interferon. The therapeutic effect of interferon in both arms of the study was minimal for patients with measurable lesions at the time of treatment initiation with 3 partial responses in the surgery arm and 3 responses, 1 complete and 2 partial, in the interferon-alone arm. The extremely low rate of interferon responses in this study as opposed to other studies may be attributable to more stringent criteria for response used in the SWOG trial. At the time of the final analysis before publication, only 20 of the 241 (8%) eligible patients were alive. The patients who underwent cytoreductive nephrectomy and interferon alfa-2b had a significantly improved median survival of 11.1 months compared with 8.1 months for the interferon alfa-2b–alone group.[20]

The EORTC study accrued 85 patients with metastatic renal cancer between 1995 and 1998 and, using a similar study design to the above-described SWOG protocol, randomly assigned patients to receive interferon alfa-2b alone or cytoreductive radical nephrectomy plus interferon alfa-2b. Two patients, 1 from each group, were ineligible and 4 patients in the cytoreductive surgery arm did not undergo operation. Forty of the 75 patients received at least 16 weeks of interferon alfa-2b therapy. Time to disease progression (5 versus 3 months) and median duration of survival (17 versus 7 months) significantly favored the patients in the cytoreductive nephrectomy–plus–interferon alfa-2b arm of the study. In this study, there were 5 complete remissions registered (1 in the interferon-alone arm and 4 in the cytoreductive nephrectomy arm). There were 6 postoperative complications, which included wound infection, pneumothorax, pneumonia, fever of unknown origin, cardiac arrhythmia, and cerebellar syndrome.[21] Investigators from SWOG and EORTC later combined their data to analyze a total of 331 patients stratified at prerandomization by performance status (0 or 1), sites of metastases (lung or other), and disease measurability. The combined analysis of these two trials yielded a median survival of 13.6 months for the cytoreductive nephrectomy–plus–interferon alpha-2b arm versus 7.8 months for interferon alpha-2b alone. There was no difference in treatment effects according to prerandomization stratification factors. Unlike historical series, operative mortality in the combined experience was 1.5% (2 patients) and only 5.6% of patients did not proceed to interferon therapy. These improved surgical outcomes are likely a result of modern surgical techniques and contemporary perioperative care.[22] In a recent update of 30 patients undergoing cytoreductive radical nephrectomy at MSKCC, median survival was 12 months, which is considerably less than the 30 months observed in the nephrectomy/metastasectomy patients (see **Fig. 1**).[15]

While these trials show an apparent survival benefit of cytoreductive nephrectomy, such benefits may in part be attributed to referral patterns, surgical judgment, and patient selection, according to Bromwich and colleagues[23] from Glasgow, United Kingdom. In their study of 94 patients with metastatic renal cancer evaluated from 1998 to 2001 for possible cytoreductive nephrectomy, 38 patients (40%) were considered inoperable and 36 patients (38%) were felt to have an Eastern Cooperative Oncology Group performance status of greater than 1. Cytoreductive radical nephrectomy was offered to 20 patients (22%) with a performance status of 0 or 1 and performed in 19. Of the 19, 13 patients began a course of immunotherapy (interferon) postoperatively. Seven patients had treatment-related toxicity necessitating withdrawal from the study and 4 patients had progressive cancer despite the interferon. Four patients were alive after cytoreductive nephrectomy (mean 8 months, range 3–16 months) and 15 have died of disease (mean time to death 9.5 months, range 3–28 months).[23] The general impact of cytoreductive surgery and systemic therapy in this group of patients was minimal.[23]

IMPORTANT PROGNOSTIC VARIABLES

Results of contemporary cytokine-based clinical trials differ based on the clinical characteristics of the patients such that some studies show a modest benefit and others do not.[24] Insight into this inconsistency came from a study of 670 patients with metastatic RCC treated at MSKCC. Risk factors associated with a shorter survival included low KPS (<80%), high lactate dehydogenase (LDH) (>1.5 × upper limit of normal), low hemoglobin, high corrected serum calcium (>10 mg/dL), and the absence of nephrectomy. Median survival ranged from 4 to 13 months with the increasing presence of the above risk factors strongly associated with decreased survival.[25] Only 12 patients (1.8%) in this data set, all assigned to good or intermediate pretreatment risk groups (KPS >80, prior nephrectomy), were long-term survivors (>5 years), 6 following cytokine treatment (interferon alfa-2b, IL-2 alone, or in combination) chemotherapeutic agents (flutamide, topotecan, N-methyl-formadmide) and 6 following metastasectomy. These same risk factors also predicted survival in 251 patients previously treated on clinical trials and then entered into second-line clinical trials. For patients without any of the risk factors (favorable group), the median time to death was 22.1 months; for patients with one of the risk factors (intermediate group), the median time to death was 12 months; and for patients with two or three risk factors (poor risk), median time to death was 5 months.[26] The presence or absence of systemic symptoms at the time of operation also strongly predicted for a poor survival in surgical series.[27,28]

These risk stratification studies are likely a reflection of the complex interactions between host defenses and the variable malignant potential of renal tumors that directly effect patient survival. Investigators at MSKCC applied these same prognostic variables to 118 initially nonmetastatic nephrectomy patients and also found that survival was segregated by risk factors. At the time of the diagnosis of metastatic disease, a risk score based upon time from nephrectomy (1 point if <12 months), serum corrected calcium (1 point if >10mg/dL), hemoglobin (1 point if below normal), serum LDH (1 point if >1.5 times upper limit of normal), and KPS (1 point if <80%) was applied to develop three risk groups. Patients were categorized into low (score of 0), intermediate (score of 1 or 2), and high-risk subgroups (score of 3–5) (**Fig. 2**). The median survival from the time of metastatic recurrence was 21 months and overall survival was strongly associated with risk groups. Median survival for low risk, intermediate risk, and high risk was 76, 25, and 6 months respectively.[29] In subsequent analysis of 44 patients undergoing metastasectomy involving 10 different organs, patients designated as low risk (51%) were more likely to undergo resection than intermediate risk (28%) or high risk (21%), confirming that surgeons were selecting a healthier group of metastatic patients to operate upon. In this subset of patients, metastasectomy in low-risk patients was significantly associated with improved survival compared with those low-risk patients who did not have metastasectomy (hazards ratio 2.9,

P = .03, median survival not reached versus 56 months).[30]

NEOADJUVANT AND ADJUVANT THERAPY CLINICAL TRIALS

For poor prognostic renal cancer patients with massive tumors that are not resectable and for patients with massive renal tumors with regional adenopathy or other poor prognostic features that are resected completely, numerous neoadjuvant and adjuvant clinical trials have been initiated in an attempt to improve survival. A variety of agents are in now in clinical trials including cytokines (IL-2, IL-12, interferon alpha), monoclonal antibodies (cG250), heat shock protein (heat shock protein-peptide complex–96 [HSPPC-96]), and vaccines (autologous human tumor–derived vaccine, cd-40 ligand vaccine).

An enhanced understanding of the molecular biology of the conventional clear cell histologic subtype, which accounts for 90% of the tumors that metastasize, has led to the development of promising new Food and Drug Administration–approved systemic chemotherapy agents for metastatic disease. These include the TKIs sunitinib and sorafenib, and the mammalian target of rapamycin inhibitor temsorilimus. These agents function in the clear cell carcinoma pathway, which begins with a mutation in the Von Hippel-Lindau gene (*VHL*), causing a loss of function of its gene product,[3,4] which normally targets hypoxia inducible factor (HIF) genes for ubiquination and degradation, leading to up-regulation of HIF-responsive genes responsible for angiogenesis, including the platelet-derived growth factor gene (*PDGF*), the vascular endothelial growth factor gene (*VEGF*), and the carbonic anhydrase 9 gene (*CalX*). This up-regulation is thought to induce the renal tumor–associated neovascularity observed with many primary and metastatic

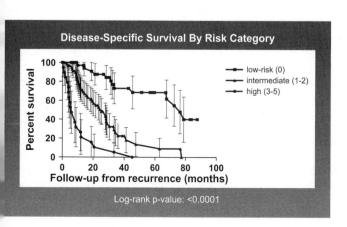

Fig. 2. Disease-specific survival based on risk category in 118 previously resected surgical patients who developed interval metastases (log-rank *P* < .0001).

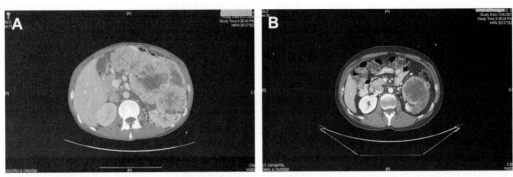

Fig. 3. (*A*) Massive 21.2-cm left RCC in 43-year-old male with numerous pulmonary metastases started on sunitinib, 50 mg/d. (*B*) Ten-months later, near complete resolution in pulmonary metastases and marked reduction in left kidney primary to 15 cm. Radical nephrectomy revealed viable poorly differentiated clear cell carcinoma with areas of necrosis.

conventional clear cell cancers.[31,32] For the papillary and chromophobe carcinomas of the kidney, patterns and sites of metastases are similar to those for the conventional clear cell carcinoma, but the molecular mechanisms are likely different.[33] For unknown reasons, metastatic papillary and chromophobe carcinomas are virtually unresponsive to systemic cytokine and TKI therapy.[34] A complete description of these clinical trials is available at ClinicalTrials.gov.

Medical oncologists and surgeons alike have noticed remarkable regression of both the metastatic sites and primary tumor following TKI (sunitinib and sorafenib) administration and, in some cases, resolution of distant metastases followed by marked regression of the primary tumor, allowing for radical nephrectomy to be integrated into the patient management of patients felt to be previously unresectable (**Fig. 3**). However, during the break from TKI administration during the period of postnephrectomy recovery, rapidly recurrent distant metastatic disease has been noticed. Reinitiation of the TKI has lead to secondary response in the same metastatic sites, suggesting that in these patients chronic administration of TKI is required. In a recent report from MD Anderson Cancer Center, 44 patients treated with multitargeted therapies before cytoreductive nephrectomy and resections of locally recurrent RCC were compared with 58 matched patients treated with cytoreductive nephrectomy or resection alone. In this study, 27.5% of the nephrectomies were done using laparoscopic techniques. Complications occurred in 39% of patients treated with preoperative TKI versus 28% treated with operation alone ($P = .287$). The investigators concluded that the preoperative treatment of patients before cytoreductive nephrectomy and resection does not significantly increase operative morbidity, which was substantial in both groups, and, although the

ultimate value of this approach remains to be determined, it appears to be a comparable to cytoreductive nephrectomy and resection alone.[35]

SUMMARY

RCC represents a family of neoplasms possessing unique molecular and cytogenetic defects with 90% of the metastases emanating from the conventional clear cell carcinoma subtype. For patients with metastatic renal cancer, prognostic factors defined in systemic therapy clinical trials stratify patients into good, intermediate, and poor risk groups with median survival varying from 4 to 13 months. These same factors also stratify patients whose renal cancers were initially resected completely and who then developed subsequent metastatic disease. Metastasectomy performed in low-risk patients was significantly associated with enhanced survival when compared with low-risk patients not undergoing metastasectomy. Careful case selection by surgeons of relatively healthy patients with disease-free intervals of greater than 1 year, which is associated with subsequent survival, makes it difficult to distinguish between the natural history of metastatic renal cancer and direct therapeutic effect. Two randomized, prospective clinical trials from the EORTC and SWOG, analyzed both separately and then together, demonstrated a modest survival advantage of approximately 6 months for patients undergoing cytoreductive nephrectomy followed by interferon alfa-2b. The mechanism by which the cytoreductive nephrectomy benefits the patient is not known but may relate to removing an immunosuppressive tumor burden. It is our opinion that, once effective systemic agents are developed, both metastasectomy and cytoreductive nephrectomy will play greater roles in consolidating clinical responses. Numerous adjuvant and neoadjuvant clinical trials are underway using a variety of agents in an attempt to improve overall survival in surgical patients with locally advanced and metastatic renal cancer. Preliminary reports indicate that cytoreductive operations following TKI administration does not increase perioperative morbidity.

REFERENCES

1. Jemal A, Siegel R, Ward E, et al. Cancer statistics, 2008. CA Cancer J Clin 2008;58:71–96.

2. Motzer RJ, Russo P. Systemic therapy for renal cell carcinoma. J Urol 2000;163:408–17.

3. Bukowski RM, Wood LS. Renal cell carcinoma: state of the art diagnosis and treatment. Clin Oncol 2008; 11:9–21.

4. O'Brien F, Motzer R, Russo P. Sunitinib therapy in renal cell carcinoma. BJU Int 2008;101:1339–42.

5. Barney JD, Churchill EJ. Adenocarcinoma of the kidney with metastasis to the lung: cured by nephrectomy and lobectomy. J Urol 1939;42:269–76.

6. Giuliani L, Giberti C, Martorana G, et al. Radical extensive surgery for renal cell carcinoma: long-term results and prognostic factors. J Urol 1990;143:468–73.

7. Golimbu M, Joshi P, Sperber A, et al. Renal cell carcinoma: survival and prognostic factors. Urology 1986;27:291–301.

8. Maldazys JD, deKernion JB. Prognostic factors in metastatic renal carcinoma. J Urol 1986;136:376–9.

9. Neves RJ, Zincke H, Taylor WF. Metastatic renal cell cancer and radical nephrectomy: identification of prognostic factors and patient survival. J Urol 1988;139:1173–6.

10. Pogrebniak HW, Haas G, Linehan WM, et al. Renal cell carcinoma: resection of solitary and multiple metastases. Ann Thorac Surg 1992;54:33–8.

11. Divgi CR, Pandit-Taskar N, Jungbluth AA, et al. Preoperative characterization of clear-cell carcinoma using iodine-124-labelled antibody chimeric G250 (^{124}I-cG250) and PET in patients with renal masses: a phase I trial. Lancet Oncol 2007;8:304–10.

12. Kavolius JP, Mastorakos DP, Pavolvich C, et al. Resection of metastatic renal cell carcinoma. J Clin Oncol 1998;16:2261–6.

13. Wronski M, Russo P, Galicich J, et al. Surgical resection of brain metastases from renal cell carcinoma. Urology 1996;47:187–93.

14. Kim SH, Brennan MF, Russo P. The role of surgery in the treatment of adrenal metastasis. Cancer 1998; 82:389–94.

15. Russo P, Snyder M, Vickers A, et al. Cytoreductive nephrectomy and nephrectomy/complete metastasectomy for metastatic renal cancer. The Scientific World Urology 2007;2:42–52.

16. Montie JE, Stewart BH, Straffon RA, et al. The role of adjuvant nephrectomy in patients with metastatic renal cell carcinoma. J Urol 1977;117:272–5.

17. Walther MM, Yang JC, Pass HI, et al. Cytoreductive surgery before high dose interleukin-2 based therapy in patients with metastatic renal cell carcinoma. J Urol 1997;158:1675–8.

18. Rackley R, Novick A, Klein E, et al. The impact of adjuvant nephrectomy on multimodality treatment of metastatic renal cell carcinoma. J Urol 1994; 152:1399–403.

19. Sella A, Swanson DA, Ro JY, et al. Surgery following response to interferon-alpha-based therapy for residual renal cell carcinoma. J Urol 1993;149:19–21.

20. Flanigan RC, Salmon SE, Blumenstein BA, et al. Nephrectomy followed by interferon alfa 2-b compared with interferon alfa-2b alone for metastatic renal cell carcinoma. N Engl J Med 2001;345:1655–9.

21. Mickisch GH, von Poppel H, de Prijck L, et al. Radical nephrectomy plus interferon–alfa based immunotherapy compared with interferon alfa alone in metastatic renal-cell carcinoma: a randomized trial. Lancet 2001;358:966–70.

22. Flanigan RC, Mickisch G, Sylvester R, et al. Cytoreductive npherectomy in patients with metastatic renal cancer: a combined analysis. J Urol 2004;171: 1071–6.

23. Bromwich E, Hendry D, Aitchison M. Cytoreductive nephrectomy: Is it a realistic option in patients with renal cancer. BJU Int 2002;89:523–5.

24. Fossa SD. Interferon in metastatic renal cell carcinoma. Semin Oncol 2000;27:187–93.

25. Motzer RJ, Mazumdar M, Bacik J, et al. Survival and prognostic stratification of 670 patients with advanced renal cell carcinoma. J Clin Oncol 1999; 17:2859–67.

26. Motzer RJ, Bacik J, Schwartz LH, et al. Prognostic factors for survival in previously treated patients with metastatic renal cell carcinoma. J Clin Oncol 2004;22:454–63.

27. Kattan MW, Reuter VE, Motzer RJ, et al. A postoperative prognostic nomogram for renal cell carcinoma. J Urol 2001;166:63–7.

28. Lee CT, Katz J, Fearn PA, et al. Mode of presentation of renal cell carcinoma provides prognostic information. Urol Oncol 2002;7:135–40.

29. Eggener SE, Yossepowitch O, Pettus JA, et al. Renal cell carcinoma recurrence after nephrectomy for localized disease. Predicting survival from time of recurrence. J Clin Oncol 2006;24:3101–31.

30. Eggener SE, Yossepowitch O, Kudhu S, et al. Objective (risk stratification) and subjective (metastasectomy) factors impact prognosis in patients with recurrent renal cell carcinoma following nephrectomy. J Urol 2008;180(3):873–8.

31. Iliopoulous O, Levy AP, Jiang C, et al. Negative regulation of hypoxia-inducible genes by the von

Hippel-Lindau protein. Proc Natl Acad Sci U S A 1996;93:10595–9.

32. Wykoff CC, Beasley NJ, Watson PH, et al. Hypoxia-inducible expression of tumor-associated carbonic anhydrases. Cancer Res 2000;60: 7075–83.

33. Beck SD, Patel MI, Snyder ME, et al. Renal cortical tumors: variable metastatic potential. Ann Surg Oncol 2004;11:71–7.

34. Motzer RJ, Bacik J, Mariani T, et al. Treatment outcome and survival associated with metastatic renal cell carcinoma of non–clear cell histology. J Clin Oncol 2002;20:2376–81.

35. Margulis V, Matin SF, Tannir N, et al. Surgical morbidity associated with administration of targeted molecular therapies before cytoreductive nephrectomy or resection of locally recurrent renal cell carcinoma. J Urol 2008;180:94–8.

Systemic Therapy for Metastatic Renal Cell Carcinoma

Glenn S. Kroog, MD*, Robert J. Motzer, MD

KEYWORDS

- Renal cell cancer • Kidney cancer • Sunitinib
- Sorafenib • Temsirolimus • Targeted therapy

Kidney and renal pelvis tumors represented approximately 3.5% of cancers and 2.3% of the deaths due to cancer in 2007 in the United States,[1] where renal cell cancer (RCC) accounts for an estimated 85% of all kidney tumors. Therefore, in 2008, approximately 44,000 cases of RCC will be diagnosed with more than 11,000 RCC-related deaths in the United States. RCC can be categorized as conventional (clear cell, 70%–85% of cases), papillary (chromophil, 10%–15%), chromophobe (5%), collecting duct (<1%), and unclassified (3%–5%).[2,3] There are also the recently described Xp11 translocation RCCs, all of which bear gene fusions involving the TFE3 transcription factor gene. They account for at least one third of pediatric tumors and are a rare cause of aggressive RCC in adults.[4] Each subtype may have a sarcomatoid component. Since there is no evidence that sarcomatoid RCC develops de novo, it is not viewed as a subtype on its own. Instead it is a high-grade variant of the type from which it arose. When no antecedent subtype can be identified, sarcomatoid RCCs are categorized as unclassified RCCs.

At presentation, up to 30% of patients with RCC have metastatic disease and recurrence develops in approximately 40% of patients treated for localized disease.[5] Hence a large proportion of RCC patients require systemic therapy. However, renal cell carcinoma is in general resistant to traditional cytotoxic chemotherapeutic agents and investigators have sought novel approaches to treatment. These approaches have until recently focused upon immune modulation. Cytokine therapy with either interferon or interleukin-2 (IL-2) was the standard of care for patients with metastatic RCC and allogeneic stem cell transplantation showed promise.

Improved understanding of the biology of RCC led to the study of so-called "targeted therapies." As a result, over the last few years, therapeutic options have improved dramatically as broad-spectrum receptor tyrosine kinase inhibitors, vascular endothelial growth factor (VEGF) antibodies, and mammalian target of rapamycin (mTOR) inhibitors have shown impressive antitumor activity or prolonged survival relative to cytokines. Since 2005, two multitargeted tyrosine kinase inhibitors (TKIs) and one mTOR inhibitor have been approved by the US Food and Drug Administration (FDA) for the treatment of advanced RCC: sorafenib (FDA approved in December 2005), sunitinib (FDA approved in January 2006), and temsirolimus (FDA approved in May 2007). Since each histologic subtype of RCC is associated with distinct genetic and molecular alterations, the use of these signal transduction inhibitors in metastatic RCC highlights the fact that the unique biology associated with specific histologic subtypes of RCC therapy will likely be associated with different response rates with current and future agents. Therapy will probably eventually be tailored to the biology of the tumor, as is currently being done for other malignancies, such as breast cancer. This review summarizes the current state of systemic therapy for metastatic RCC.

Genitourinary Oncology Service, Division of Solid Tumor Oncology, Department of Medicine, Memorial Sloan-Kettering Cancer Center, 1275 York Avenue, New York, NY 10065, USA
* Corresponding author.
E-mail address: kroogg@mskcc.org (G.S. Kroog).

Urol Clin N Am 35 (2008) 687–701
doi:10.1016/j.ucl.2008.07.007

TUMORIGENESIS OF RENAL CELL CANCER

The improved survival and quality of life for patients with metastatic RCC over the last several years are direct results of advances in understanding the development of RCC. The genetics of RCC tumorigenesis has been reviewed elsewhere[6–8] and is briefly summarized here with attention to the consequences for systemic therapy for RCC.

The von Hippel-Lindau (VHL) syndrome is an autosomal dominant disease characterized by the development of tumors in the cerebellum, spine, retina, inner ear, pancreas, adrenal glands, and kidneys. The kidney cancer in VHL syndrome is uniformly clear cell RCC, and affected individuals have hundreds of clear cell RCCs per kidney. The VHL tumor suppressor gene was identified in 1993. Both sporadic and inherited forms of clear cell RCC are strongly associated with mutations, deletions, or hypermethylations in the VHL gene (*VHL*), which inactivate the gene. The *VHL* protein functions as part of a multiprotein complex involved in targeting proteins for degradation by marking them with ubiquitin. Major targets that the *VHL* complex ubiquitinates are the transcription factors hypoxia-inducible factor 1α (HIF-1α) and hypoxia-inducible factor 2α (HIF-2α). Under normal oxygen conditions and with normal *VHL* function, HIFs are degraded. When hypoxia develops or if *VHL* is inactivated, HIF levels increase and HIF-dependent genes are transcribed (**Fig. 1**). This leads to changes in expression of various proteins and constitutes the cellular response to hypoxia. HIF levels can also be regulated by growth factor and cell adhesion pathways, leading to activation of the Ras-Raf–mitogen-activated protein kinase pathway and the phosphatidylinositol 3-kinase-AKT-mTOR pathway. The HIF-dependent response is characterized by increased levels of VEGF, epidermal growth factor receptor (EGFR), platelet-derived growth factor (PDGF), glucose transporters (eg, GLUT-1), transforming growth factor-α (TGF-α, ligand for EGFR), and erythropoietin. In the context of a clear cell RCC, this results in stimulation of angiogenesis and tumor cell proliferation. Because VEGF has a central role during pathologic angiogenesis and restricted expression in healthy adults, a variety of therapeutic strategies aimed at blocking VEGF-induced signal transduction have been attempted. See Ferrara and colleagues[9] for an excellent review of VEGF biology. Other RCC histologies are also associated with specific mutations. For example, type 1 papillary RCC is characterized by dysregulation or mutation in the tyrosine kinase domain of the c-Met oncogene.

CYTOTOXIC CHEMOTHERAPY

Multiple reviews have summarized the poor results with traditional cytotoxic chemotherapeutic agents and hormonal therapies in metastatic RCC.[10–14] Response rates were usually much less than 15%. Chemotherapeutic strategies for RCC were reviewed by Milowsky and Nanus[14] 5 years ago in *Urologic Clinics of North America*. The investigators concluded that single-agent chemotherapy trials had been disappointing. They discussed the continued modest enthusiasm for combination chemotherapy, highlighting gemcitabine- and fluoropyrimidine-based regimens. However, two recently published trials of gemcitabine and capecitabine showed response rates of only 11% to 16% with significant toxicity.[15,16] Stadler and colleagues[16] concluded from their trial that the activity seen and degree of toxicity would not support the evaluation of gemcitabine plus capecitabine in a phase III trial. The combination of doxorubicin and gemcitabine has shown some activity in sarcomatoid and rapidly progressing RCC.[17,18] In the study, the investigators collected the experience of two institutions (outside of a formal clinical trial) in treating patients with sarcomatoid and rapidly progressing RCC and found that, of 18 patients, 2 had a complete response and 5 had a partial response. A prospective cooperative group study with this regimen in patients with sarcomatoid features has completed enrollment and is currently being analyzed.

IMMUNOTHERAPY

Relapse of RCC many years after nephrectomy, prolonged disease stabilization without systemic treatment, and occasional spontaneous regressions suggested that host immune mechanisms might control tumor growth. This led to the study of immunotherapy for RCC.[13] Interferon and IL-2 were reported to have antitumor activity in the 1980s and were the only proven therapy for metastatic RCC until recently. Immunotherapy for RCC has been the subject of a recently updated analysis by Coppin and colleagues[19] for the Cochrane Collaboration. Combined data for a variety of immunotherapies gave an overall response rate of 12.4% (8.9% partial response and 3.5% complete response) compared with 2.4% in nonimmunotherapy control arms. High-dose IL-2 is associated with increased vascular permeability and requires inpatient monitoring, often in an intensive care unit. A limited number of centers now offer high-dose IL-2. It has been associated with a 4% incidence of treatment-related death and should be offered only to patients with normal

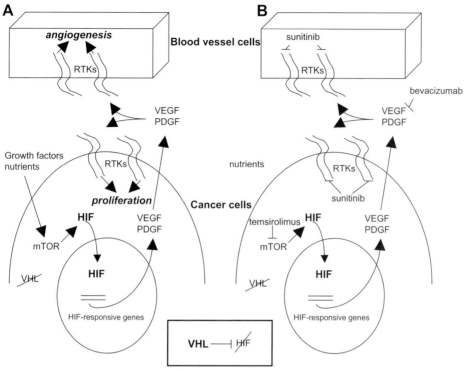

Fig. 1. The *VHL* pathway in clear cell cancer of the kidney and inhibition by targeted therapies. Under normoxic conditions, *VHL* promotes HIF degradation (*box*). When *VHL* mutates (*A*), HIF-dependent genes, including *VEGF* and *PDGF*, are transcribed and angiogenesis is stimulated. Targeted therapies (*B*) block various aspects of these events, leading to antiproliferative and antiangiogenic effects. Sunitinib and temsirolimus are shown as examples of TKIs and mTOR inhibitors respectively. See text for details. RTKs, receptor tyrosine kinases.

cardiac, renal, and pulmonary function. However, response was poorly correlated with survival so that remission rate is not a good surrogate marker for survival for advanced RCC. High-dose IL-2 did not give better overall survival compared with low-dose IL-2 or to subcutaneous cytokine therapy, but may improve survival in the patients with bad prognostic factors based on subset analysis.

High-dose IL-2 was approved as treatment for RCC in the United States on the basis of phase II studies because of durable complete remissions seen in 5% to 7% of patients.[20,21] The results of several studies indicate that interferon alpha (IFN-α) is superior to controls with a hazard ratio for death of 0.74. Doses ranging from 5 to 20 million units (MU) per day have been studied, although the optimal dose and schedule is not known. The addition of a variety of enhancers has failed to improve survival compared with IFN-α alone. Due to the limited availability of high-dose IL-2, its toxicity profile, and the survival associated with interferon, randomized studies of signaling inhibitors used interferon as the control arm. In addition, studies on cytokines have proven that surgery has a role in the treatment of

metastatic RCC. In highly selected patients with metastases at diagnosis and minimal symptoms, cytoreductive nephrectomy before IFN-α therapy improves survival over IFN-α alone.[22,23] Therefore, cytoreductive nephrectomy is a common part of systemic therapy for metastatic RCC. As a result, studies with signaling inhibitors (discussed below) have usually been performed in patients who have had prior nephrectomy.

ALLOGENEIC STEM CELL TRANSPLANTATION

Other approaches to improve immunotherapy have been tried. It was hypothesized that graft-versus-tumor effects analogous to those seen in leukemias might occur in RCC. Childs and colleagues[24] performed nonmyeloablative allogeneic peripheral-blood stem cell transplantation in 19 patients with suitable donors. The preparative regimen consisted of 60 mg/kg cyclophosphamide on day 7 and day 6 before transplantation, followed by 25 mg/m² fludarabine on each of the last 5 days before transplantation. Three patients (16%) had complete response and 7 had a partial response (37%) for an overall response rate of 53%. Two patients (11%) died of transplantation-related toxicity. In addition, consistent with a graft-versus-tumor effect, regression of metastases occurred a median of 129 days after transplantation, and often followed the withdrawal of cyclosporine and the establishment of complete donor–T-cell chimerism. These results were scientifically consistent with the initial hypothesis and were clinically extremely encouraging. A series of trials followed, including an intergroup trial[25] that attempted to confirm these exciting results. Ueno and Childs[26] recently summarized and reviewed the data from all trials. Most trials were small (7–25 patients) and used a variety of conditioning regimens and graft–versus–host disease prophylaxis. Response rates varied from 0% to 57%, and treatment-related mortality ranged from 0% to 40%. In the largest series, reported by Barkholt and colleagues,[27] 124 patients were treated at 21 European centers with a variety of regimens. Transplant-related mortality was seen in 16% of patients. Out of 98 evaluable patients, 4 had complete response, 24 had partial response, and 24 had stable disease. Therefore, although autologous stem cell transplantation has not been optimized in this disease, it is clear that a graft-versus-tumor effect can be evoked against RCC. However, because the development of growth factor signaling inhibitors, the clinical necessity of this high-risk approach has lessened. Therefore, the risk/benefit profile of nonmyeloablative allogeneic peripheral-blood stem cell transplantation in RCC may relegate this approach to patients refractory to growth factor signaling inhibitors. Although allogeneic stem cell transplantation remains investigational in RCC, the improved treatments available may potentially diminish the suitability of patients who receive transplantation and lessen the chance of observing an antitumor effect.

TARGETED THERAPIES

VEGF antibodies, broad spectrum TKIs, and mTOR inhibitors are generally referred to as "targeted therapies." However, most of the clinically useful TKIs would be better described as multitargeted. They are small molecules that bind to the ATP binding pocket of a group of evolutionarily related kinases with varying affinities (**Table 1**). Some, such as sorafenib (which also inhibits raf), have an even broader spectrum of inhibition. The reason or reasons for the varying efficacy in the clinic with these agents is not clear. Therefore, although usually rationally designed, their use is therapy for RCC is somewhat empiric. Targeted therapies have recently been reviewed.[28–30] Because the treatment of RCC is in rapid flux, we focus on targeted therapies in detail. Results of major randomized phase III trials are summarized in **Table 2**.

Sunitinib (SU11248)

Sunitinib was developed as an oral inhibitor of VEGF receptor 2 and PDGF receptor β[31] although its spectrum of activity is broad. Sunitinib is primarily metabolized by cytochrome CYP3A4, resulting in formation of a major, pharmacologically

Table 1
Concentration required for 50% inhibition in vitro (IC$_{50}$) for selected tyrosine kinase inhibitors

Kinase	Sunitinib (nmol/L)[31,90]	Sorafenib (nmol/L)[91]	Pazopanib (nmol/L)[92]	Vatalanib (PTK787/ZK 222,584) (nmol/L)[93]
VEGF receptor 1	—	26	10	77
VEGF receptor 2	9–80	15–90	30	37
VEGF receptor 3	—	20	47	660
PDGF receptor α	—	—	71	—
PDGF receptor β	2–8	57	84	580
EGFR	> 20,000	>10,000	> 20,000	—
Fibroblast growth factor receptor 1	830–2900	580	140	—
Flt-3 and mutants	10–300	33–58	> 20,000	—
Stem cell factor receptor (c-kit)	1–10	68	74	730
Ret	—	47	2800	—
Colony stimulating factor 1 receptor/c-fms	—	—	146	1400

Table 2
Major positive randomized phase III trials of targeted therapies in metastatic renal cell carcinoma

Drug(s)	Number of Patients	Overall Response Rate (%)[a]	Dz Control Rate (%)[b]	Median Progression-Free Survival (mo)	Overall Survival (mo)	MSKCC Prognostic Groups	Setting
Sorafenib vs placebo[38]	903	2 vs 0	80 vs 55	5.5 vs 2.8	—	Good/intermediate	2nd line
Sunitinib vs Interferon[5]	750	31 vs 6	79 vs 55	11 vs 5	—	Good/intermediate	1st line
Temsirolimus vs temsirolimus + interferon vs interferon[55]	626	8.6 vs 8.1 vs 4.8	32.1 vs 28.1 vs 15.5	5.5 vs 4.7 vs 3.1	10.9 vs 8.4 vs 7.3	Intermediate/poor	1st line
Bevacizumab + interferon vs interferon[45]	649	31 vs 13	77 vs 63	10.2 vs 5.4	—	Good/intermediate	1st line

Abbreviation: MSKCC, Memorial Sloan-Kettering Cancer Center.
[a] Complete response plus partial response.
[b] Overall response rate plus stable disease.

active N-desethyl metabolite, SU012662. This metabolite was shown to be equipotent to the parent compound in biochemical tyrosine kinase and cellular proliferation assays, acting toward VEGF receptors, PDGF receptors, and stem cell factor receptors. Due to concerns about potential bone marrow and adrenal toxicity observed in animal models, a 4-week-on, 2-week-off schedule (rather than continuous administration) was selected for phase I at the request of the health authorities to allow patients to recover. During the course of the phase I study, pharmacokinetic analysis revealed that variability in exposure was not reduced by normalizing for body surface area, so flat dosing was used.[32] There was wide interpatient variation in plasma sunitinib and SU012662 levels. Two consecutive open-label, phase II studies were conducted with sunitinib starting at 50 mg per day in patients with metastatic RCC and progressive disease while patients were receiving cytokine-based immunotherapy. In the first trial,[33] 25 of 63 patients (40%) achieved partial responses with sunitinib, and 17 of 63 (27%) had stable disease lasting at least 3 months. Although open to all histologic subtypes of RCC, most patients (87%) had clear cell RCC. Out of the remaining patients, 1 patient with papillary RCC achieved partial response. Median time to tumor progression was 8.7 months. A second, 106-patient single-arm trial was conducted solely in metastatic clear cell RCC to confirm the antitumor activity and safety observed in the first phase II trial.[34] Of 105 assessable patients, the independently assessed response rate was 34%, stable disease rate 29%, and median progression-free survival 8.3 months. The most common adverse events experienced by patients in both studies were fatigue and diarrhea. Additional grade 3 toxicities included nausea, stomatitis, and hypertension. Grade 4 neutropenia was rare.

A randomized phase III trial compared sunitinib with interferon alpha-2a (IFNα-2a) in first-line treatment of metastatic clear cell RCC.[5] Seven hundred fifty patients were randomly assigned to sunitinib (n = 375) or IFNα-2a (n = 375). The primary end point was progression-free survival. In a planned preliminary analysis, median progression-free survival, as assessed by third-party independent review, was 11 months for sunitinib versus 5 months for IFNα-2a ($P < .001$). The response rate by third-party independent review was 31% for sunitinib versus 6% for IFNα-2a ($P < .001$). The toxicity profile was similar to that reported in second-line studies. Patients in the sunitinib group reported a significantly better quality of life than did patients in the IFNα-2a group ($P < .001$). The results demonstrate a significant improvement in progression-free survival and objective response rate for sunitinib over interferon in first-line treatment of metastatic RCC. Based on the results of this interim analysis, the FDA approved sunitinib, which has become standard therapy for first-line treatment for metastatic RCC.

An alternative dosing schedule of sunitinib is currently being studied. In a study of 107 patients treated with a continuous daily sunitinib with a starting dose of 37.5 mg per day, patients received either AM or PM doses of sunitinib and could be dose-escalated or -decreased, depending upon toxicity. Partial response was seen in 20% and stable disease in 52% (>3 months in 40%). Median progression-free survival was 36 weeks. Few differences were seen between AM and PM dosing in tolerability or response. Sunitinib administered by continuous dosing was relatively well tolerated, with only a few patients requiring treatment breaks or dose reduction. A current trial is comparing this schedule to the standard 4-week-on, 2-week-off schedule (NCT00267748).

Sorafenib (BAY 43-9006)

Sorafenib was designed as an inhibitor of the Raf-1 protein. Subsequently, sorafenib was found to inhibit VEGF receptors and PDGF receptors.[35] Strumberg and colleagues[36] performed a phase I study of daily sorafenib. Disease stabilization was observed in a patient with metastatic RCC. No dose-limiting toxicity was observed at 400 mg by mouth twice daily. However, dose-limiting toxicity was seen at 800 mg twice daily (grade 3 diarrhea in 2 of 6 patients) and 600 mg twice daily (dose-limiting skin toxicity in 4 of 14 patients). In addition, there was great interpatient variability in serum sorafenib levels and there seemed to be no difference in mean steady-state serum levels between these three dose levels. Therefore, the dose level recommended for phase II trials was 400 mg twice daily.

Because of the expectation for disease stabilization, a large phase II study was designed as a "randomized discontinuation trial," intended to evaluate tumor growth inhibition rather than tumor shrinkage.[37] All patients enrolled onto the study initially received 400 mg twice daily sorafenib for 12 weeks. Disease evaluation was conducted, and patients who had 25% or more tumor shrinkage continued with open-label drug. Patients with less than 25% decrease or less than 25% increase in tumor size were randomly assigned to either continue sorafenib for 12 weeks or receive placebo. Patients who progressed with an increase of tumor size of 25% or more were considered as having progressive disease and removed from study. More than 500 patients with various solid tumors were treated in this study. Due to activity detected in patients with RCC, the investigators amended the trial to focus on RCC and a total of 202 patients with metastatic RCC were treated. Of the 202 RCC patients, 73 had tumor shrinkage of more than 25% during the initial 12 weeks of therapy. Partial response rate by modified World Health Organization criteria was only 11%. Another 65 patients with stable disease during this run-in period were randomly assigned at week 12 to therapy with either placebo or continuation of sorafenib. The median progression-free survival from random assignment was significantly longer with sorafenib (24 weeks) compared with placebo (6 weeks). Adverse effects included skin rash, hand-foot skin reaction, and fatigue. The study demonstrated significant disease-stabilizing activity in metastatic RCC and tolerability with chronic daily therapy.

Based on these results, the Treatment Approaches in Renal Cancer Global Evaluation Trial (TARGET), a randomized phase III trial comparing sorafenib (n = 451) with placebo (n = 452) was performed in patients with treatment-refractory metastatic clear cell RCC.[38] Even though treatment-refractory, the patient population had a relatively favorable prognosis with approximately 50% good prognosis and 50% intermediate prognosis, as determined by the Memorial Sloan-Kettering Cancer Center (MSKCC) prognosis score.[39] A planned interim analysis after 353 events demonstrated that the median duration of progression-free survival was 5.5 months in sorafenib patients compared with 2.8 months in the placebo group ($P < .001$). Independent review of the response data at a January 2005 cutoff demonstrated that 80% of patients were progression-free in the sorafenib arm (2% partial response and 78% stable disease) compared with 55% in the placebo arm (0% partial response and 55% stable disease). At a May 2005 cutoff, investigator review showed 11% overall response rate (1% complete response, 10% partial response) and 74% stable disease in the sorafenib group compared with 2% overall response rate (2% partial response) and 53% stable disease in the placebo group. The most common adverse effects significantly associated with sorafenib included skin rash (40%), hand-foot skin reaction (30%), diarrhea (43%), alopecia (27%), pruritus (19%), and hypertension (17%). These data demonstrated the efficacy of sorafenib in metastatic RCC, and led to FDA approval for advanced RCC.

As first-line therapy, sorafenib (400 mg twice daily) was compared with interferon (9 MU three times weekly) in a randomized phase II study in patients with metastatic clear cell RCC.[40] A unique feature of the design was a second phase of the trial in which patients who progressed on sorafenib then received 600 mg twice weekly and patients who progressed on interferon received sorafenib 400 mg twice weekly. Although some tumor shrinkage occurred more frequently in the sorafenib arm (68% vs. 39%), and patients on sorafenib went longer before a deterioration in health status, progression-free survival was disappointing in the first part of the study. Progression-free survival was similar in both arms (5.7 months for sorafenib vs. 5.6 months for IFN) and more patients in the interferon arm continued on therapy at 1 year. Consistent with other trials,[33] plasma VEGF increased and soluble VEGF receptor 2 decreased in the sorafenib group while soluble VEGF receptor 2 increased in the interferon group. A larger decrease in soluble VEGF receptor 2 on sorafenib correlated with longer progression-free survival. In the second phase, 60% of the patients who progressed on 400 mg twice daily sorafenib dose-escalated to 600 mg twice daily. Dose escalation was well tolerated, progression-free survival was 4.1 months, and 46% of patients experienced stable disease. For patients who crossed over from interferon to sorafenib, results were comparable to the TARGET data: 22% responded (2% complete response, 20% partial response) and 54% had stable disease. These data suggest that sorafenib can be sequentially escalated to 600 mg twice daily and that more patients may have clinical benefit.

Consistent with the data in the second phase of the first-line sorafenib study, Amato and colleagues[41] presented data from a dose-escalation phase II trial of sorafenib. In this study, 44 patients with a component of clear cell RCC, some of whom had progressed on cytokine therapy, were treated with 400 mg twice daily for 28 days, then 600 mg twice daily for 28 days, then 800 mg twice daily continuously. Dose modification was made for grade 3/4 toxicity. Forty-one of 44 patients tolerated dose escalation to 600 mg twice daily, and 25 of 41 were able to maintain a dose of 800 mg twice daily. Results were extremely encouraging with 7 of 44 (16%) having complete response, 17 of 44 (39%) having partial response, and 9 of 44 (20%) stable disease. Median time to progression has not yet been reached and is greater than 8.4 months. If confirmed in subsequent trials, this would lead to a reevaluation of sorafenib dosing and its role in metastatic RCC.

Bevacizumab

Bevacizumab is a humanized monoclonal antibody agent that binds and neutralizes all the major isoforms of VEGF-A.[42] Bevacizumab was initially investigated in a randomized, double-blind, placebo-controlled phase 2 trial in patients with clear cell carcinoma of the kidney.[43] Bevacizumab at doses of 3 and 10 mg per kilogram of body weight or placebo was given every 2 weeks and crossover from placebo to antibody treatment was allowed. All patients had either received previous therapy with IL-2 or had a contraindication to use of IL-2 and almost all had prior nephrectomy. The primary end points were time to disease progression and response rate. A total of 116 patients were randomly assigned to the three treatment groups. At the time of a planned interim analysis, the median time to progression was significantly increased to 4.8 months in the patients receiving the 10-mg/kg dose of bevacizumab, compared with 2.5 months for placebo. Four partial responses occurred, all in the group treated with bevacizumab at 10 mg/kg, for a partial response rate of 10%. Based on the significant increase in time to progression, accrual to the trial was stopped. The lack of an effect on survival was attributed to the crossover design. Most patients had VEGF levels below the lower limit of detection and there was no significant association between response and VEGF level. However, the low sensitivity did not rule out a correlation between VEGF and clinical benefit.

Two randomized phase III studies examined combinations of bevacizumab with interferon in patients with predominantly clear cell histology. A study comparing interferon alpha-2b (IFN-α-2b) with or without bevacizumab coordinated through the Cancer and Leukemia Group B (CALGB-90,206; NCT00072046) has closed to accrual.[44] Results of this study are not currently available. The results of the Avoren trial was recently published and compared bevacizumab (10 mg/kg every 2 weeks) plus IFN-α-2a (9 MU subcutaneously three times weekly; n = 327) to placebo plus IFN-α-2a (control group, n = 322) in patients with previously untreated metastatic RCC who had prior nephrectomy.[45] The study did not include a bevacizumab monotherapy arm because, at the time of trial design, this was considered unethical. The planned primary end point was overall survival. Secondary end points included progression-free survival and safety. An interim analysis of overall survival was prespecified after 250 deaths. However, while the trial was in progress, new therapies became available that could have confounded analyses of overall survival data, so the investigators agreed with regulatory agencies that the preplanned final analysis of progression-free survival would be acceptable for regulatory submission. The protocol was amended to allow the study to be unblinded at this point. At the time of unblinding, progression had occurred in 230 patients in the bevacizumab-plus-interferon group and 275 in the control group with 114 deaths in the bevacizumab-plus-interferon group and 137 in the control group. Median duration of progression-free survival was significantly longer in the bevacizumab–plus–interferon alpha group than it was in the control group (10.2 months vs. 5.4 months; $P = .0001$). Overall response rates were 31% for bevacizumab plus interferon versus 11% for placebo plus interferon. However, there was no independent radiologic assessment included in the study design. MSKCC prognostic group distribution was similar to that for the patients studied by Motzer and colleagues,[5] and progression-free survival and overall response rate were similar to sunitinib as a single agent. Combination therapy was generally well tolerated. In both groups the most commonly reported grade 3 or worse adverse events were established interferon-related toxicities (eg, fatigue, asthenia, and neutropenia). Grade 3 and 4 adverse events in patients who received bevacizumab included gastrointestinal perforations (1%) and thromboembolic events (3%). Patients receiving bevacizumab also discontinued treatment due to hypertension (2%) and proteinuria (5%). Although 33% of patients on bevacizumab suffered bleeding of any grade, only 2 patients (<1%) died from bleeding complications.

Since a bevacizumab monotherapy arm was not included in these studies, they do not justify the use of bevacizumab alone in first-line therapy. Whether combination with interferon will be the preferred regimen long term, is an issue to be addressed. The Avoren trial cannot be directly compared with the study by Yang and colleagues[43] because in the placebo-controlled bevacizumab study almost all of the patients had progressed on prior IL-2 therapy whereas the Avoren trial required patients to have not had prior systemic therapy for metastatic RCC.

Other bevacizumab-containing combinations have also been tried recently. Based on encouraging preclinical and phase I and II data implicating EGFR signaling in the pathogenesis of RCC,[46] a randomized phase II trial of bevacizumab with and without the EGFR TKI erlotinib has been completed in patients with a nephrectomy who had not received prior systemic therapy.[47] However, there was no additional clinical benefit to the addition of erlotinib to bevacizumab. Response rates of about 14%, stable disease rates of 68%, and progression-free survival of 9 to 10 months were seen in both arms.

Mammalian Target of Rapamycin Inhibitors: Temsirolimus (CCI-779) and Everolimus (RAD001)

The mTOR is an enzyme involved in regulating cellular responses to nutrients and growth factors and is one of the main regulators of cell growth and proliferation.[48–50] The signaling pathways that activate mTOR are altered in many human cancers. mTOR is a large multidomain protein that complexes with other proteins and belongs to a group of kinases that includes phosphatidylinositol 3-kinases (PI3Ks). The complexes in which mTOR participates are termed mTOR complex 1 (mTORC1) and mTOR complex 2 (mTORC2). Rapamycin forms a complex with the 12-kDa FK506 binding protein (FKBP12), and this complex then binds to and inhibits mTORC1. Therefore, rapamycin and its analogs exert their effects by inhibiting TORC1 signaling. The best-understood roles of mTOR in mammalian cells are related to the control of mRNA translation. However, HIF-1α expression and function can be regulated by mTOR, and loss of *VHL* sensitizes cells to temsirolimus via regulation of HIF-1α.[51,52]

Temsirolimus (CCI-779) has been the most thoroughly studied mTOR inhibitor. In a phase II trial, 111 patients with advanced (primarily MSKCC intermediate and poor risk), heavily pretreated, refractory RCC were randomized to 25, 75, or 250 mg of temsirolimus.[53] Only 7% of patients achieved an objective response. There were no significant differences in outcome noted between dose levels. The median time to progression was 5.8 months, with a median survival for the entire population of 15.0 months.

Temsirolimus was combined with IFNα-2b in a phase I/II clinical trial of 71 metastatic RCC patients. The trial had many patients with intermediate or poor prognosis (21% favorable, 55% intermediate, and 24% poor prognosis) and 39 (55%) of patients had received prior systemic therapy, 36 (51%) of whom had received IL-2.

Partial responses were observed in 11% of all patients, with a median time to progression of 9.1 months.[54] In view of the patient population, the median progression-free survival in this trial was encouraging, and led to the inclusion of combination therapy as an arm in a randomized phase III trial in patients with poor-risk features. Hudes and colleagues[55] compared temsirolimus (25 mg) alone versus temsirolimus (15 mg) plus IFNα-2a versus IFNα-2a alone as first-line treatment. Poor-risk eligibility for the trial was based on modified MSKCC criteria (approximately three fourths of the patients in each arm met standard MSKCC poor-risk criteria). Six hundred twenty-six patients were randomly assigned. Although objective response rates were low (8.6% vs. 8.1% vs. 4.8%) and differences among the three arms were not statistically significant, the median survival for temsirolimus was 10.9 months compared with 8.4 months with temsirolimus plus interferon and 7.3 months with interferon. There was a significant improvement in survival for temsirolimus compared with interferon (P = .0069; hazard ratio of 0.73 in favor of temsirolimus). Although the combination of temsirolimus and IFNα-2a provided no additional benefit, temsirolimus, compared with IFNα-2a, significantly increases the survival and quality-adjusted survival[56] of first-line, poor-risk advanced RCC patients. Temsirolimus was FDA approved based on the results of this study. Patients with all histologies of RCC were included in the trial and non–clear cell histologies had particularly good outcomes relative to interferon. However, of the 18% of patients without clear cell histology in the study, approximately 12% had "indeterminate" histology and only 6% had defined non–clear cell histology.[57] Therefore, the utility of temsirolimus in non–clear cell histologies is not known for certain.

Further studies are also needed to define the role of temsirolimus in first-line therapy for patients with a more favorable prognosis (intermediate and poor risk) and as second line after sunitinib therapy. The low response rates seen currently make it a less appealing choice as a single agent for patients who can tolerate sunitinib or who have symptoms that need palliation. As for temsirolimus as second-line therapy, a study currently enrolling patients (NCT00474786) is randomizing patients who progressed on sunitinib to sorafenib or temsirolimus. In addition, several studies have begun to look at temsirolimus in combination with other targeted therapies (see section on combination therapy below).

Everolimus (RAD001) is an orally active mTOR inhibitor with a similar mechanism of action to temsirolimus. It has been studied alone and in combination with TKIs. A phase II trial of RAD001 as a single agent has been presented at the American Society of Clinical Oncology.[58] Out of 37 evaluable patients, 12 (32%) had partial responses and 19 (51%) were stable for 3 or more months. Treatment-related adverse events included mucositis, skin rash, pneumonitis, hypophosphatemia, hyperglycemia, hypertriglyceridemia, hypercholesterolemia, thrombocytopenia, anemia, and elevated liver function tests. A multicenter phase III double-blind randomized placebo-controlled trial comparing RAD001 plus best supportive care to best supportive care alone has completed enrollment (NCT00410124). Phase I and II doublet combination studies with bevacizumab, sunitinib, or vatalanib[59] are in progress.

COMBINATION THERAPY

The available targeted and multitargeted therapies represent a significant advance in the treatment of RCC. However, none are associated with significant rates of long-term disease-free survival. Intensive research has begun over the last several years to determine if combinations of targeted therapies or targeted therapies plus immunomodulatory therapies are superior to sequential therapy with these agents.

Attempts to combine sunitinib with other agents have been met with significant toxicity. A trial of temsirolimus plus sunitinib was stopped due to dose-limiting toxicity observed in two of three patients in the first cohort of a dose-finding study using temsirolimus 15 mg weekly and sunitinib 25 mg daily.[60] A phase I trial of sunitinib plus bevacizumab has been performed. Hypertension was reported to be the most common adverse event and grade 4 hemorrhage was observed in 2 out of 20 patients.[61] Finally, a dose-finding study has been completed combining sunitinib with interferon.[62] The study enrolled 25 patients. Sunitinib 37.5 mg per day (4 weeks on, 2 weeks off) and interferon 3 MU three times weekly was tolerated, although all patients on the study experienced grade 3 adverse events. Of the 6 patients at sunitinib 37.5 mg per day and interferon 3 MU three times weekly, grade 3 adverse events included neutropenia, dyspnea, hypertension, swelling face, and syncope. One patient at this dose level experienced a serious adverse event. For the entire group, 12% had partial response and 80% stable disease. The investigators concluded that the toxicity of this regimen does not justify continued study.

Sorafenib-based combinations have recently been reviewed.[63] Two phase II trials of sorafenib plus interferon were published in 2007. Both used sorafenib 400 mg twice daily plus IFN-α-2b 10 MU subcutaneously three times weekly and studied patients with similar prognosis to those treated by Motzer and colleagues in the randomized study of sunitinib versus interferon. Ryan and colleagues[64] examined patients who had not received prior systemic therapy and found responses in 12 of 62 patients (19%) and stable disease in 31 of 62 patients (50%). Median progression-free survival was 7 months. Toxicity was more severe than with either agent alone. Fatigue (29%) and diarrhea (16%) were the most common grade 3 toxicities. In a smaller trial, Gollob and colleagues[65] found a 33% overall response rate (5% complete response and 28% partial response) and 45% stable disease. Median progression-free survival was 10 months. Grade 3/4 toxicities included hypophosphatemia (37%), neutropenia (25%), fatigue (13%), and rash (13%). In both trials, toxicity and response rates were higher than what has been seen with either agent alone.

Two phase I studies of sorafenib plus bevacizumab have been completed.[66–68] A dose of sorafenib 200 mg twice daily and bevacizumab 5 mg/kg every other week appeared tolerable in a study open to multiple tumor types.[66,67] The other study was limited to patients with metastatic RCC.[68] Sorafenib 200 mg every day and bevacizumab 5 mg/kg every other week appeared tolerable. The investigators found a very impressive response rate with 21 of 46 evaluable patients (46%) having a partial response as defined by the Response Evaluation Criteria in Solid Tumors. In addition, 23 patients had stable disease. Forty-one of 46 (89%) patients experienced some tumor shrinkage ranging from 5% to 80% from baseline.

A phase I study of sorafenib plus temsirolimus[69] determined that the combination of sorafenib 200 mg twice daily and temsirolimus 25 mg intravenous once per week appears tolerable. Combination therapy was limited by mucocutaneous and hematologic toxicity.

A phase I study of temsirolimus and bevacizumab[70] determined that the recommended phase II doses are temsirolimus 25 mg/wk and bevacizumab 10 mg every other week. A very high response rate was seen with 8 partial responses, 3 with stable disease, and only 1 progressive disease out of 12 evaluable patients. Therapy was generally well tolerated with grade 3 anorexia, nausea, mucositis, and hemorrhage being seen in 2 patients each.

Based on some of the phase I and II data described above, the BeST trial (NCT00378703) has begun. It is a phase II trial of randomizing a total of 360 patients to one of four arms: bevacizumab 10 mg/kg every 2 weeks; bevacizumab 10 mg/kg plus temsirolimus 25 mg weekly; bevacizumab 5 mg/kg plus sorafenib 200 mg twice a day on days 1 through 5, 8 through 12, 15 through 19, and 22 through 26; or temsirolimus 25 mg per week plus sorafenib 200 mg twice a day. It opened in the fall of 2007. The trial includes a bevacizumab-alone arm and several promising combinations. However, it does not include an arm with sunitinib alone.

SEQUENCING OF AGENTS
Sunitinib/Sorafenib Sequencing

In two small series examining sequencing of sunitinib and sorafenib, some patients who progressed on sorafenib had partial response from sunitinib and vice versa.[71,72] In addition, some patients for whom their best response was progressive disease had a partial response or stable disease when sunitinib followed sorafenib. Therefore, the molecular targets and therapeutic efficacy of these agents are different enough that patients are not necessarily cross-resistant.

Bevacizumab → Sorafenib or Sunitinib

In an expanded access program for sorafenib, the subset of patients who had received prior bevacizumab was compared with the entire population.[73] Partial response rate (3%), stable disease rate (78%), and toxicity were similar to those for the entire population. Therefore prior bevacizumab treatment does not make patients less likely to have stable disease in response to sorafenib. In addition, responses are seen to sunitinib after progression on bevacizumab. A phase II trial of 61 patients reported 23% partial response and 57% stable disease in patients treated with sunitinib who had prior bevacizumab.[74]

Sorafenib → Bevacizumab or Tyrosine Kinase Inhibitor

Similarly, small series suggest that prior sorafenib does not preclude partial response or stable disease in patients subsequently treated with bevacizumab, sunitinib, or axitinib.[75,76]

ADDITIONAL AND NOVEL AGENTS

Several studies have recently been presented or published evaluating additional or novel agents in metastatic RCC. Many of these drugs target HIF-dependent aberrant signaling in the same way that currently approved agents do. Several are small-molecule, multitargeted TKIs, with unique spectra of kinase inhibition compared with sunitinib and sorafenib. Like sunitinib and sorafenib, pazopanib (GW786034) has high affinity for a variety of receptor tyrosine kinases (see **Table 1**). A 225-patient randomized discontinuation study of pazopanib has been presented in abstract form and shows response and stable disease rates similar to those for sunitinib (27% partial response and 46% stable disease by independent review).[77] Treatment was generally well tolerated. Less than 30% of patients required dose reduction or interruption. Six percent of patients experiencing grade 4 toxicity and 1% grade 5. The spectrum of toxicity was similar to that for sunitinib with diarrhea, hypertension, nausea, and fatigue being most common.[77] A phase III placebo-controlled study (NCT00334282) has completed enrollment and results are pending.

Axitinib (AG-013,736) is an oral potent inhibitor of VEGF receptors 1, 2, and 3 and PDGF receptors. It was studied in a recently published phase II study of 52 patients with cytokine-refractory RCC.[78] All patients except one had clear cell RCC. The overall response rate was 44% and stable disease was seen in an additional 44% of patients. The median time to progression was 15.7 months and the group overall had a similar percentage with MSKCC good risk features as in the randomized phase III trial of sunitinib versus interferon with a similar disease-control rate. Further studies are continuing.

Preclinical data has implicated TGFα/EGFR signaling in the pathogenesis of RCC.[79] However, in contrast to the results using inhibitors of VEGF and PDGF signaling, there is no published evidence that targeting EGFR signaling alone or in combination with other agents is therapeutic in RCC. Two studies found no evidence of single-agent activity with gefitinib in RCC[80,81] and erlotinib did not add to the effect of bevacizumab[47] or sunitinib.[82]

Several antibodies targeting cell surface proteins selectively expressed in RCC are in various stages of development. The G250 antigen (carbonic anhydrase IX [CAIX]) is expressed with fairly high specificity on clear cell RCC. Expression is dependent upon hypoxia-related molecules, including HIFα. After no success with radiolabeled mouse monoclonal G250 in the late 1990s,[83] several phase I and II studies of cG250, a chimeric (humanized) CAIX antibody have been performed with or without low-dose IL-2 (to improve the immune response). Although the antibody targeted very well to tumor masses in all patients when examined, and occasional patients had a complete response in early studies,[84,85] cG250 had little or no activity in a phase II study as a single agent or in combination with low-dose IL-2.[84,86,87] It appears that tumor targeting alone is not sufficient for significant antitumor activity of this humanized clear cell RCC antibody. Other antibodies are in development. For example, volociximab, an α5β1 integrin antibody, showed stable disease in 80% of patients (including one partial response) in a phase II trial.[88]

NON–CLEAR CELL HISTOLOGIES

Much less is known about the optimal treatment of non–clear cell RCC. Trials of specific agents (such as c-Met inhibitors) targeting the unique molecular profile of non–clear cell histologies are beginning. As noted above, due to the distribution of patients and the trial design, most trials evaluating currently approved targeted therapies have been limited to or heavily biased toward clear cell RCC. Even the phase III study of temsirolimus included very few patients with documented non–clear cell histology. Experience is just being obtained in non–clear cell histologies. For example, a recently published data set[89] reported patients with papillary or chromophobe RCC treated with sunitinib or sorafenib as part of extended access programs at five cancer centers. Out of 41 patients with papillary RCC, 13 received sunitinib and 28 sorafenib. Two partial responses were seen, both in the sunitinib group, and progression-free survival was 11.9 months in sunitinib-treated patients versus 5.1 months in sorafenib-treated patients ($P < .001$). Out of 12 chromophobe RCC patients, 7 were treated with sunitinib, and 5 with sorafenib. Two patients treated with sorafenib and 1 patient treated with sunitinib achieved a partial response, and stable disease was achieved in the other patients. Sorafenib-treated patients tended to have a prolonged median progression-free survival time (27.5 months). These data are preliminary and suggest subtype-specific responses to different agents. However, they are limited by small numbers of patients and the absence of randomization. Further studies are ongoing.

SUMMARY

Until recently, only interferon and IL-2 were of proven efficacy in the treatment of metastatic RCC. Improved understanding of the biology of RCC led to the development, study, and approval by the FDA of sunitinib, sorafenib, and temsirolimus for treatment of metastatic RCC. Both sunitinib and temsirolimus are proven to be superior to interferon. In addition, the combination of bevacizumab and interferon has also shown superiority to interferon alone. However, none of the available targeted therapies are associated with significant rates of long-term disease-free survival. Clinical research is ongoing to answer many questions including:

What is the optimal sequence of available agents?

Do combinations of targeted therapies provide additional clinical benefit over sequential treatment with single agents?

What new small molecules and antibodies are effective against kidney cancer?

What treatments are best for non–clear cell histologies?

REFERENCES

1. Jemal A, Siegel R, Ward E, et al. Cancer statistics, 2007. CA Cancer J Clin 2007;57(1):43–66.
2. Störkel S, Eble JN, Adlakha K, et al. Classification of renal cell carcinoma: workgroup No. 1. Union Internationale Contre le Cancer (UICC) and the American Joint Committee on Cancer (AJCC). Cancer 1997; 80(5):987–9.
3. Zisman A, Chao DH, Pantuck AJ, et al. Unclassified renal cell carcinoma: clinical features and prognostic impact of a new histological subtype. J Urol 2002;168(3):950–5.
4. Argani P, Olgac S, Tickoo SK, et al. Xp11 translocation renal cell carcinoma in adults: expanded clinical, pathologic, and genetic spectrum. Am J Surg Pathol 2007;31(8):1149–60.
5. Motzer RJ, Hutson TE, Tomczak P, et al. Sunitinib versus interferon alfa in metastatic renal-cell carcinoma. N Engl J Med 2007;356(2):115–24.
6. Linehan WM, Vasselli J, Srinivasan R, et al. Genetic basis of cancer of the kidney: disease-specific approaches to therapy. Clin Cancer Res 2004;10(18): 6282S–9S.
7. Patel PH, Chaganti RS, Motzer RJ. Targeted therapy for metastatic renal cell carcinoma. Br J Cancer 2006;94(5):614–9.
8. Linehan WM, Pinto PA, Srinivasan R, et al. Identification of the genes for kidney cancer: opportunity for disease-specific targeted therapeutics. Clin Cancer Res 2007;13(2 Pt 2):671s–9s.
9. Ferrara N, Gerber HP, LeCouter J. The biology of VEGF and its receptors. Nat Med 2003;9(6):669–76.
10. Yagoda A, Abi-Rached B, Petrylak D. Chemotherapy for advanced renal-cell carcinoma: 1983–1993. Semin Oncol 1995;22(1):42–60.
11. Yagoda A, Petrylak D, Thompson S. Cytotoxic chemotherapy for advanced renal cell carcinoma. Urol Clin North Am 1993;20(2):303–21.
12. Hartmann JT, Bokemeyer C. Chemotherapy for renal cell carcinoma. Anticancer Res 1999;19(2C):1541–3.
13. Motzer RJ, Bander NH, Nanus DM. Renal-cell carcinoma. N Engl J Med 1996;335(12):865–75.
14. Milowsky MI, Nanus DM. Chemotherapeutic strategies for renal cell carcinoma. Urol Clin North Am 2003;30(3):601–9, x.
15. Waters JS, Moss C, Pyle L, et al. Phase II clinical trial of capecitabine and gemcitabine chemotherapy in patients with metastatic renal carcinoma. Br J Cancer 2004;91(10):1763–8.
16. Stadler WM, Halabi S, Rini B, et al. A phase II study of gemcitabine and capecitabine in metastatic renal cancer: a report of Cancer and Leukemia Group B protocol 90008. Cancer 2006;107(6):1273–9.
17. Nanus DM, Garino A, Milowsky MI, et al. Active chemotherapy for sarcomatoid and rapidly progressing renal cell carcinoma. Cancer 2004;101(7):1545–51.
18. Milowsky MI, Rosmarin A, Tickoo SK, et al. Active chemotherapy for collecting duct carcinoma of the kidney: a case report and review of the literature. Cancer 2002;94(1):111–6.
19. Coppin C, Porzsolt F, Awa A, et al. Immunotherapy for advanced renal cell cancer. Cochrane Database Syst Rev 2005;1:CD001425.
20. McDermott DF, Regan MM, Clark JI, et al. Randomized phase III trial of high-dose interleukin-2 versus subcutaneous interleukin-2 and interferon in patients with metastatic renal cell carcinoma. J Clin Oncol 2005;23(1):133–41.
21. Yang JC, Sherry RM, Steinberg SM, et al. Randomized study of high-dose and low-dose interleukin-2 in patients with metastatic renal cancer. J Clin Oncol 2003;21(16):3127–32.
22. Flanigan RC, Salmon SE, Blumenstein BA, et al. Nephrectomy followed by interferon alfa-2b compared with interferon alfa-2b alone for metastatic renal-cell cancer. N Engl J Med 2001;345(23):1655–9.
23. Mickisch GH, Garin A, van Poppel H, et al. Radical nephrectomy plus interferon-alfa–based immunotherapy compared with interferon alfa alone in metastatic renal-cell carcinoma: a randomised trial. Lancet 2001;358(9286):966–70.
24. Childs R, Chernoff A, Contentin N, et al. Regression of metastatic renal-cell carcinoma after nonmyeloablative allogeneic peripheral-blood stem-cell transplantation. N Engl J Med 2000;343(11):750–8.
25. Rini BI, Halabi S, Barrier R, et al. Adoptive immunotherapy by allogeneic stem cell transplantation for metastatic renal cell carcinoma: a CALGB intergroup phase II study. Biol Blood Marrow Transplant 2006;12(7):778–85.
26. Ueno NT, Childs RW. What's past is prologue: lessons learned and the need for further development of allogeneic hematopoietic stem cell transplantation for renal cell carcinoma. Biol Blood Marrow Transplant 2007;13(1):31–3.
27. Barkholt L, Bregni M, Remberger M, et al. Allogeneic haematopoietic stem cell transplantation for metastatic renal carcinoma in Europe. Ann Oncol 2006; 17(7):1134–40.
28. Motzer RJ, Bukowski RM. Targeted therapy for metastatic renal cell carcinoma. J Clin Oncol 2006; 24(35):5601–8.
29. Mancuso A, Sternberg CN. New treatment approaches in metastatic renal cell carcinoma. Curr Opin Urol 2006;16(5):337–41.
30. Vogelzang NJ, Sternberg CN. Signal-transduction inhibitors in renal cell carcinoma. BJU Int 2007; 99(5 Pt B):1289–95.
31. Sun L, Liang C, Shirazian S, et al. Discovery of 5-[5-fluoro-2-oxo-1,2-   dihydroindol-(3Z)-ylidenemethyl]-2,4- dimethyl-1H-pyrrole-3-carboxylic acid (2-diethylaminoethyl)amide, a novel tyrosine kinase inhibitor targeting vascular endothelial and

platelet-derived growth factor receptor tyrosine kinase. J Med Chem 2003;46(7):1116–9.

32. Faivre S, Delbaldo C, Vera K, et al. Safety, pharmacokinetic, and antitumor activity of SU11248, a novel oral multitarget tyrosine kinase inhibitor, in patients with cancer. J Clin Oncol 2006;24(1):25–35.

33. Motzer RJ, Michaelson MD, Redman BG, et al. Activity of SU11248, a multitargeted inhibitor of vascular endothelial growth factor receptor and platelet-derived growth factor receptor, in patients with metastatic renal cell carcinoma. J Clin Oncol 2006;24(1):16–24.

34. Motzer RJ, Rini BI, Bukowski RM, et al. Sunitinib in patients with metastatic renal cell carcinoma. JAMA 2006;295(21):2516–24.

35. Flaherty KT. Sorafenib in renal cell carcinoma. Clin Cancer Res 2007;13(2):747s–52s.

36. Strumberg D, Richly H, Hilger RA, et al. Phase I clinical and pharmacokinetic study of the novel raf kinase and vascular endothelial growth factor receptor inhibitor BAY 43-9006 in patients with advanced refractory solid tumors. J Clin Oncol 2005;23(5):965–72.

37. Ratain MJ, Eisen T, Stadler WM, et al. Phase II placebo-controlled randomized discontinuation trial of sorafenib in patients with metastatic renal cell carcinoma. J Clin Oncol 2006;24(16):2505–12.

38. Escudier B, Eisen T, Stadler WM, et al. Sorafenib in advanced clear-cell renal-cell carcinoma. N Engl J Med 2007;356(2):125–34.

39. Motzer RJ, Mazumdar M, Bacik J, et al. Survival and prognostic stratification of 670 patients with advanced renal cell carcinoma. J Clin Oncol 1999;17(8):2530–40.

40. Szczylik C, Demkow T, Staehler M, et al. Randomized phase II trial of first-line treatment with sorafenib versus interferon in patients with advanced renal cell carcinoma: final results. J Clin Oncol (Meeting Abstracts) 2007;25(18 Suppl):5025.

41. Amato RJ, Harris P, Dalton M, et al. A phase II trial of intra-patient dose-escalated sorafenib in patients (pts) with metastatic renal cell cancer (MRCC). J Clin Oncol (Meeting Abstracts) 2007;25(18 Suppl):5026.

42. Presta LG, Chen H, O'Connor SJ, et al. Humanization of an anti-vascular endothelial growth factor monoclonal antibody for the therapy of solid tumors and other disorders. Cancer Res 1997;57(20):4593–9.

43. Yang JC, Haworth LL, Sherry RM, et al. A randomized trial of bevacizumab, an anti-vascular endothelial growth factor antibody, for metastatic renal cancer. N Engl J Med 2003;349(5):427–34.

44. Rini BI, Halabi S, Taylor J, et al. Cancer and Leukemia Group B 90206: a randomized phase III trial of interferon-alpha or interferon-alpha plus anti-vascular endothelial growth factor antibody (bevacizumab) in metastatic renal cell carcinoma. Clin Cancer Res 2004;10(8):2584–6.

45. Escudier B, Pluzanska A, Koralewski P, et al. Bevacizumab plus interferon alfa-2a for treatment of metastatic renal cell carcinoma: a randomised, double-blind phase III trial. Lancet 2007;370(9605):2103–11.

46. Hainsworth JD, Sosman JA, Spigel DR, et al. Treatment of metastatic renal cell carcinoma with a combination of bevacizumab and erlotinib. J Clin Oncol 2005;23(31):7889–96.

47. Bukowski RM, Kabbinavar FF, Figlin RA, et al. Randomized phase II study of erlotinib combined with bevacizumab compared with bevacizumab alone in metastatic renal cell cancer. J Clin Oncol 2007;25(29):4536–41.

48. Averous J, Proud CG. When translation meets transformation: the mTOR story. Oncogene 2006;25(48):6423–35.

49. Easton JB, Houghton PJ. mTOR and cancer therapy. Oncogene 2006;25(48):6436–46.

50. Wullschleger S, Loewith R, Hall MN. TOR signaling in growth and metabolism. Cell 2006;124(3):471–84.

51. Hudson C, Liu M, Chiang G, et al. Regulation of hypoxia-inducible factor 1alpha expression and function by the mammalian target of rapamycin. Mol Cell Biol 2002;22(20):7004–14.

52. Thomas GV, Tran C, Mellinghoff IK, et al. Hypoxia-inducible factor determines sensitivity to inhibitors of mTOR in kidney cancer. Nat Med 2006;12(1):122–7.

53. Atkins MB, Hidalgo M, Stadler WM, et al. Randomized phase II study of multiple dose levels of CCI-779, a novel mammalian target of rapamycin kinase inhibitor, in patients with advanced refractory renal cell carcinoma. J Clin Oncol 2004;22(5):909–18.

54. Motzer RJ, Hudes GR, Curti BD, et al. Phase I/II trial of temsirolimus combined with interferon alfa for advanced renal cell carcinoma. J Clin Oncol 2007;25(25):3958–64.

55. Hudes G, Carducci M, Tomczak P, et al. Temsirolimus, interferon alfa, or both for advanced renal-cell carcinoma. N Engl J Med 2007;356(22):2271–81.

56. Parasuraman S, Hudes G, Levy D, et al. Comparison of quality-adjusted survival in patients with advanced renal cell carcinoma receiving first-line treatment with temsirolimus (TEMSR) or interferon-α (IFN) or the combination of IFN+TEMSR. J Clin Oncol (Meeting Abstracts) 2007;25(18S) [abstract #5049].

57. Dutcher JP, Szczylik C, Tannir N, et al. Correlation of survival with tumor histology, age, and prognostic risk group for previously untreated patients with advanced renal cell carcinoma (adv RCC) receiving temsirolimus (TEMSR) or interferon-alpha (IFN). J Clin Oncol (Meeting Abstracts) 2007;25(18S) [abstract #5033].

58. Jac J, Giessinger S, Khan M, et al. A phase II trial of RAD001 in patients (Pts) with metastatic renal cell carcinoma (MRCC). J Clin Oncol (Meeting Abstracts) 2007;25(18S) [abstract #5107].

59. Speca JC, Mears AL, Creel PA, et al. Phase I study of PTK787/ZK222584 (PTK/ZK) and RAD001 for patients with advanced solid tumors and dose expansion in renal cell carcinoma patients. J Clin Oncol (Meeting Abstracts) 2007;25(18S) [abstract # 5039].

60. Torisel prescribing information, Wyeth Pharmaceuticals, Inc. Philadelphia, PA.

61. Feldman DR, Kondagunta GV, Ronnen EA, et al. Phase I trial of bevacizumab plus sunitinib in patients (pts) with metastatic renal cell carcinoma (mRCC). J Clin Oncol (Meeting Abstracts) 2007; 25(18 Suppl):5099.

62. Kondagunta GV, Hudes GR, Figlin R, et al. Sunitinib malate (SU) plus interferon (IFN) in first line metastatic renal cell cancer (mRCC): results of a dose-finding study. J Clin Oncol (Meeting Abstracts) 2007;25(18S) [abstract #5101].

63. Takimoto CH, Awada A. Safety and anti-tumor activity of sorafenib (Nexavar((R))) in combination with other anti-cancer agents: a review of clinical trials. Cancer Chemother Pharmacol 2008;61(4):535–48.

64. Ryan CW, Goldman BH, Lara PN Jr, et al. Sorafenib with interferon alfa-2b as first-line treatment of advanced renal carcinoma: a phase II study of the Southwest Oncology Group. J Clin Oncol 2007; 25(22):3296–301.

65. Gollob JA, Rathmell WK, Richmond TM, et al. Phase II trial of sorafenib plus interferon alfa-2b as first-or second-line therapy in patients with metastatic renal cell cancer. J Clin Oncol 2007;25(22):3288–95.

66. Azad NS, Posadas EM, Kwitkowski VE, et al. Increased efficacy and toxicity with combination anti-VEGF therapy using sorafenib and bevacizumab. J Clin Oncol (Meeting Abstracts) 2006;25(18S (June 20 Supplement)):3004.

67. Posadas E, Ksitkowski V, Liel M. Clinical synergism from combinatorial VEGF signal transduction inhibition in patients with advanced solid tumors: early results from a phase I study of sorafenib (BAY 43-9006) and bevacizumab. Eur J Cancer Suppl 2005;3(2):419 [abstract #1450]

68. Puzanov I, Flaherty K, Atkins M. Final results of a phase I trial of sorafenib and bevacizumab in patients with metastatic renal cell cancer (mRCC). American Association for Cancer Research: molecular targets and cancer therapeutics 2007; October 2–26, 2007. San Francisco (CA) 2007 [meeting abstract: A–19].

69. Patnaik A, Ricart A, Cooper J, et al. A phase I, pharmacokinetic and pharmacodynamic study of sorafenib (S), a multi-targeted kinase inhibitor in combination with temsirolimus (T), an mTOR inhibitor in patients with advanced solid malignancies. J Clin Oncol (Meeting Abstracts) 2007;25(18S) [abstract #3512].

70. Merchan JR, Liu G, Fitch T, et al. Phase I/II trial of CCI-779 and bevacizumab in stage IV renal cell carcinoma: phase I safety and activity results. J Clin Oncol (Meeting Abstracts) 2007;25(18 Suppl):5034.

71. Dham A, Dudek AZ. Sequential therapy with sorafenib and sunitinib in renal cell carcinoma. J Clin Oncol (Meeting Abstracts) 2007;25(18S) [abstract #5106].

72. Sablin M, Bouaita L, Balleyguier C, et al. Sequential use of sorafenib and sunitinib in renal cancer: retrospective analysis in 90 patients. J Clin Oncol (Meeting Abstracts) 2007;25(18S) [abstract #5038].

73. Drabkin HA, Figlin RA, Stadler WM, et al. The Advanced Renal Cell Carcinoma Sorafenib (ARCCS) expanded access trial: safety and efficacy in patients (pts) with prior bevacizumab (BEV) treatment. J Clin Oncol (Meeting Abstracts) 2007; 25(18S) [abstract #5041].

74. George DJ, Michaelson MD, Rosenberg JE, et al. Phase II trial of sunitinib in bevacizumab-refractory metastatic renal cell carcinoma (mRCC): updated results and analysis of circulating biomarkers. J Clin Oncol (Meeting Abstracts) 2007;25(18 Suppl):5035.

75. Hajdenberg J, Oberoi S, Cohen N, et al. Evaluation of VEGF targeted therapy efficacy in mRCC after sorafenib failure or intolerance. J Clin Oncol (Meeting Abstracts) 2007;25(18S) [abstract # 15517].

76. Rini BI, Wilding GT, Hudes G, et al. Axitinib (AG-013736; AG) in patients (pts) with metastatic renal cell cancer (RCC) refractory to sorafenib. J Clin Oncol (Meeting Abstracts) 2007;25(18S (June 20 Supplement)):5032.

77. Hutson TE, Davis ID, Machiels JP, et al. Pazopanib (GW786034) is active in metastatic renal cell carcinoma (RCC): interim results of a phase II randomized discontinuation trial (RDT). J Clin Oncol (Meeting Abstracts) 2007;25(18 Suppl):5031.

78. Rixe O, Bukowski RM, Michaelson MD, et al. Axitinib treatment in patients with cytokine-refractory metastatic renal-cell cancer: a phase II study. Lancet Oncol 2007;8(11):975–84.

79. de Paulsen N, Brychzy A, Fournier MC, et al. Role of transforming growth factor-alpha in von Hippel-Lindau (VHL)-/- clear cell renal carcinoma cell proliferation: a possible mechanism coupling VHL tumor suppressor inactivation and tumorigenesis. Proceedings of the National Academy of Sciences 2001;98(4):1387–92.

80. Drucker B, Bacik J, Ginsberg M, et al. Phase II trial of ZD1839 (IRESSA) in patients with advanced renal cell carcinoma. Invest New Drugs 2003;21(3):341–5.

81. Dawson NA, Guo C, Zak R, et al. A phase II trial of gefitinib (Iressa, ZD1839) in stage IV and recurrent

renal cell carcinoma. Clin Cancer Res 2004;10(23): 7812–9.

82. Patel PH, Kondagunta GV, Redman BG, et al. Phase I/II study of sunitinib malate in combination with gefitinib in patients (pts) with metastatic renal cell carcinoma (mRCC). J Clin Oncol (Meeting Abstracts) 2007;25(18 Suppl):5097.

83. Divgi CR, Bander NH, Scott AM, et al. Phase I/II radioimmunotherapy trial with iodine-131–labeled monoclonal antibody G250 in metastatic renal cell carcinoma. Clin Cancer Res 1998;4(11):2729–39.

84. Davis I, Wiseman G, Lee F, et al. A phase I multiple dose, dose escalation study of cG250 monoclonal antibody in patients with advanced renal cell carcinoma. Cancer Immun 2007;7:13.

85. Varga Z, de Mulder P, Kruit W, et al. A prospective open-label single-arm phase II study of chimeric monoclonal antibody cG250 in advanced renal cell carcinoma patients. Folia Biol 2003;49(2):74–7.

86. Davis I, Liu Z, Saunders W, et al. A pilot study of monoclonal antibody cG250 and low dose subcutaneous IL-2 in patients with advanced renal cell carcinoma. Cancer Immun 2007;7:14.

87. Bleumer I, Oosterwijk E, Oosterwijk-Wakka JC, et al. A clinical trial with chimeric monoclonal antibody WX-G250 and low dose interleukin-2 pulsing scheme for advanced renal cell carcinoma. J Urol 2006;175(1):57–62.

88. Yazji S, Bukowski R, Kondagunta V, et al. Final results from phase II study of volociximab, an {alpha}5{beta}1 anti-integrin antibody, in refractory or relapsed metastatic clear cell renal cell carcinoma (mCCRCC). J Clin Oncol (Meeting Abstracts) 2007; 25(18 Suppl):5094.

89. Choueiri TK, Plantade A, Elson P, et al. Efficacy of sunitinib and sorafenib in metastatic papillary and chromophobe renal cell carcinoma. J Clin Oncol 2008;26(1):127–31.

90. Mendel DB, Laird AD, Xin X, et al. In vivo antitumor activity of SU11248, a novel tyrosine kinase inhibitor targeting vascular endothelial growth factor and platelet-derived growth factor receptors: determination of a pharmacokinetic/pharmacodynamic relationship. Clin Cancer Res 2003;9(1):327–37.

91. Wilhelm S, Carter C, Lynch M, et al. Discovery and development of sorafenib: a multikinase inhibitor for treating cancer. Nat Rev Drug Discov 2006; 5(10):835–44.

92. Kumar R, Knick VB, Rudolph SK, et al. Pharmacokinetic-pharmacodynamic correlation from mouse to human with pazopanib, a multikinase angiogenesis inhibitor with potent antitumor and antiangiogenic activity. Mol Cancer Ther 2007;6(7): 2012–21.

93. Wood JM, Bold G, Buchdunger E, et al. PTK787/ZK 222584, a novel and potent inhibitor of vascular endothelial growth factor receptor tyrosine kinases, impairs vascular endothelial growth factor–induced responses and tumor growth after oral administration. Cancer research 2000;60(8):2178–89.

Index

Note: Page numbers of article titles are in **boldface** type.

A

Ablation, thermal, for localized renal masses, 649–650

Acetate metabolism, and positron emission tomography of renal cell carcinoma, 606–607

Acquired cystic disease, of kidney-associated renal cell carcinoma, pathologic features of, 556

Active surveillance. See Surveillance.

Adjuvant therapy, for metastatic renal cell carcinoma, clinical trials of, 683–684

Algorithms, and prognostic models in renal cell carcinoma, **613–625**
  histologic subtypes, 615
  molecular marker-driven therapies, 620–621
  other pathologic factors, 615–620
    molecular factors, 619–620
    postoperative prognostic algorithms for localized, 617–619
    preoperative nomograms for suspected renal malignancy, 615–617
  prognostic algorithms for metastatic, 621
  prognostic factors, 614–615
  TNM staging system, 614

Allogeneic stem cell transplantation, for metastatic renal cell carcinoma, 689–690

Angioinfarction, renal, 658

Antibody positron emission tomography (PET), of renal cell carcinoma, 607

Antigens, tumor-associated, in positron emission tomography of renal cell carcinoma, 607

Axitinib, for metastatic renal cell carcinoma, 697

B

Bevacizumab, for metastatic renal cell carcinoma, 693–694, 696

Bilateral renal tumors, surgical approach to, 650

Biopsy, of renal masses, 630–631

Birt-Hogg-Dubé syndrome, 566–567

C

Cardiopulmonary bypass, minimally invasive, for renal tumors invading the vena cava, 662–663

Cardiovascular disease, chronic kidney disease and risk of, 638–639

Caval thrombus, endoluminal occlusion and, with renal tumors invading the vena cava, 665

cG250, iodine-labeled, in molecular imaging of renal cell carcinoma, 607–609

novel agent for metastatic renal cell carcinoma, 697

Chemotherapy, cytotoxic, for metastatic renal cell carcinoma, 688

Chromophobe renal cell carcinoma, pathologic features of, 554

Chronic kidney disease, and risk of cardiovascular disease, 638–639

Clear cell (conventional) renal cell carcinoma. See also Renal cell carcinoma., pathologic features of, 552–553

Collecting duct carcinoma, pathologic features of, 555

Combination therapy, targeted, for metastatic renal cell carcinoma, 695–696
  sequencing of agents, 696
    bevacizumab/sorafenib or sunitinib, 696
    sorafenib/bevcizumab or tyrosine kinase inhibitor, 696
    sunitinib/sorafenib, 696

Computed tomography (CT) scan, detection of renal cortical tumors with, 594–596
  staging of renal cortical tumors with, 600

Cortical tumors, renal. See Renal cancer.

Cystic disease, acquired, of kidney-associated renal cell carcinoma, pathologic features of, 556

D

Demographics, of renal cell carcinoma, changes in, 582

E

Elective partial nephrectomy. See Nephrectomy.

Endoluminal occlusion, and caval thrombus, with renal tumors invading the vena cava, 665

Epidemiology, of renal cell carcinoma, **581–592**

Everolimus (RAD001), for metastatic renal cell carcinoma, 694–695

F

Familial renal cancer syndromes. See Hereditary renal cancer syndromes.

Function, renal, preservation of with partial nephrectomy, 639–640

G

Genetics, familial and hereditary renal cancer syndromes, **563–572**

Urol Clin N Am 35 (2008) 703–709
doi:10.1016/S0094-0143(08)00111-0

Moving?

Make sure your subscription moves with you!

To notify us of your new address, find your **Clinics Account Number** (located on your mailing label above your name), and contact customer service at:

E-mail: elspcs@elsevier.com

800-654-2452 (subscribers in the U.S. & Canada)
314-453-7041 (subscribers outside of the U.S. & Canada)

Fax number: 314-523-5170

Elsevier Periodicals Customer Service
11830 Westline Industrial Drive
St. Louis, MO 63146

*To ensure uninterrupted delivery of your subscription, please notify us at least 4 weeks in advance of move.

United States Postal Service

Statement of Ownership, Management, and Circulation
(All Periodicals Publications Except Requestor Publications)

1. Publication Title
Urologic Clinics of North America

2. Publication Number
0 0 0 - 7 1 1 1

3. Filing Date
9/15/08

4. Issue Frequency
Feb, May, Aug, Nov

5. Number of Issues Published Annually
4

6. Annual Subscription Price
$249.00

7. Complete Mailing Address of Known Office of Publication *(Not printer) (Street, city, county, state, and ZIP+4)*

Elsevier Inc.
360 Park Avenue South
New York, NY 10010-1710

Contact Person
Stephen Bushing

Telephone *(Include area code)*
215-239-3688

8. Complete Mailing Address of Headquarters or General Business Office of Publisher *(Not printer)*

Elsevier Inc., 360 Park Avenue South, New York, NY 10010-1710

9. Full Names and Complete Mailing Addresses of Publisher, Editor, and Managing Editor *(Do not leave blank)*

Publisher *(Name and complete mailing address)*

John Schrefer, Elsevier, Inc., 1600 John F. Kennedy Blvd. Suite 1800, Philadelphia, PA 19103-2899

Editor *(Name and complete mailing address)*

Kerry Holland, Elsevier, Inc., 1600 John F. Kennedy Blvd. Suite 1800, Philadelphia, PA 19103-2899

Managing Editor *(Name and complete mailing address)*

Catherine Bewick, Elsevier, Inc., 1600 John F. Kennedy Blvd. Suite 1800, Philadelphia, PA 19103-2899

10. Owner *(Do not leave blank. If the publication is owned by a corporation, give the name and address of the corporation immediately followed by the names and addresses of all stockholders owning or holding 1 percent or more of the total amount of stock. If not owned by a corporation, give the names and addresses of the individual owners. If owned by a partnership or other unincorporated firm, give its name and address as well as those of each individual owner. If the publication is published by a nonprofit organization, give its name and address.)*

Full Name	Complete Mailing Address
Wholly owned subsidiary of	4520 East-West Highway
Reed/Elsevier, US holdings	Bethesda, MD 20814

11. Known Bondholders, Mortgagees, and Other Security Holders Owning or Holding 1 Percent or More of Total Amount of Bonds, Mortgages, or Other Securities. If none, check box ☐ None

Full Name	Complete Mailing Address
N/A	

12. Tax Status *(For completion by nonprofit organizations authorized to mail at nonprofit rates) (Check one)*
The purpose, function, and nonprofit status of this organization and the exempt status for federal income tax purposes:
☐ Has Not Changed During Preceding 12 Months
☐ Has Changed During Preceding 12 Months *(Publisher must submit explanation of change with this statement)*

13. Publication Title
Urologic Clinics of North America

14. Issue Date for Circulation Data Below
August 2008

15. Extent and Nature of Circulation		Average No. Copies Each Issue During Preceding 12 Months	No. Copies of Single Issue Published Nearest to Filing Date
a. Total Number of Copies *(Net press run)*		3875	3800
b. Paid Circulation (By Mail and Outside the Mail)	(1) Mailed Outside-County Paid Subscriptions Stated on PS Form 3541. *(Include paid distribution above nominal rate, advertiser's proof copies, and exchange copies)*	1516	1447
	(2) Mailed In-County Paid Subscriptions Stated on PS Form 3541 *(Include paid distribution above nominal rate, advertiser's proof copies, and exchange copies)*		
	(3) Paid Distribution Outside the Mails Including Sales Through Dealers and Carriers, Street Vendors, Counter Sales, and Other Paid Distribution Outside USPS®	1331	1308
	(4) Paid Distribution by Other Classes Mailed Through the USPS (e.g. First-Class Mail®)		
c. Total Paid Distribution *(Sum of 15b (1), (2), (3), and (4))*	▲	2847	2755
d. Free or Nominal Rate Distribution (By Mail and Outside the Mail)	(1) Free or Nominal Rate Outside-County Copies Included on PS Form 3541	75	87
	(2) Free or Nominal Rate In-County Copies Included on PS Form 3541		
	(3) Free or Nominal Rate Copies Mailed at Other Classes Mailed Through the USPS (e.g. First-Class Mail)		
	(4) Free or Nominal Rate Distribution Outside the Mail (Carriers or other means)		
e. Total Free or Nominal Rate Distribution (Sum of 15d (1), (2), (3) and (4))	▲	75	87
f. Total Distribution (Sum of 15c and 15e)	▲	2922	2842
g. Copies not Distributed (See instructions to publishers #4 (page #3))	▲	953	958
h. Total (Sum of 15f and g)	▲	3875	3800
i. Percent Paid (15c divided by 15f times 100)		97.43%	96.94%

16. Publication of Statement of Ownership
If the publication is a general publication, publication of this statement is required. Will be printed in the **November 2008** issue of this publication.   Publication not required ☐

17. Signature and Title of Editor, Publisher, Business Manager, or Owner

[signature] — Executive Director of Subscription Services   Date September 15, 2008

I certify that all information furnished on this form is true and complete. I understand that anyone who furnishes false or misleading information on this form or who omits material or information requested on the form may be subject to criminal sanctions (including fines and imprisonment) and/or civil sanctions (including civil penalties).

PS Form 3526, September 2006 (Page 2 of 3)

PS Form 3526, September 2006 (Page 1 of 3) (Instructions Page 3)   PSN 7530-01-000-9931 PRIVACY NOTICE: See our Privacy policy in www.usps.com